Natural Compounds Applications in Drug Discovery and Development

Natural Compounds Applications in Drug Discovery and Development

Guest Editors

Alina Bora
Luminita Crisan

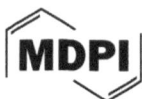

Basel • Beijing • Wuhan • Barcelona • Belgrade • Novi Sad • Cluj • Manchester

Guest Editors

Alina Bora
"Coriolan Dragulescu"
Institute of Chemistry,
Romanian Academy
Timisoara
Romania

Luminita Crisan
"Coriolan Dragulescu"
Institute of Chemistry,
Romanian Academy
Timisoara
Romania

Editorial Office
MDPI AG
Grosspeteranlage 5
4052 Basel, Switzerland

This is a reprint of the Special Issue, published open access by the journal *Processes* (ISSN 2227-9717), freely accessible at: https://www.mdpi.com/journal/processes/special_issues/9T0L5065FV.

For citation purposes, cite each article independently as indicated on the article page online and as indicated below:

Lastname, A.A.; Lastname, B.B. Article Title. *Journal Name* **Year**, *Volume Number*, Page Range.

ISBN 978-3-7258-2279-9 (Hbk)
ISBN 978-3-7258-2280-5 (PDF)
https://doi.org/10.3390/books978-3-7258-2280-5

© 2024 by the authors. Articles in this book are Open Access and distributed under the Creative Commons Attribution (CC BY) license. The book as a whole is distributed by MDPI under the terms and conditions of the Creative Commons Attribution-NonCommercial-NoDerivs (CC BY-NC-ND) license (https://creativecommons.org/licenses/by-nc-nd/4.0/).

Contents

About the Editors vii

Preface ix

Alina Bora and Luminita Crisan
Editorial on the Special Issue "Natural Compounds Applications in Drug Discovery and Development"
Reprinted from: *Processes* **2024**, *12*, 1152, https://doi.org/10.3390/pr12061152 1

Octavia Gligor, Simona Clichici, Remus Moldovan, Dana Muntean, Ana-Maria Vlase, George Cosmin Nadăș, et al.
Red Clover and the Importance of Extraction Processes—Ways in Which Extraction Techniques and Parameters Affect *Trifolium pratense* L. Extracts' Phytochemical Profile and Biological Activities
Reprinted from: *Processes* **2022**, *10*, 2581, https://doi.org/10.3390/pr10122581 4

Gabriela Nistor, Alexandra Mioc, Marius Mioc, Mihaela Balan-Porcarasu, Roxana Ghiulai, Roxana Racoviceanu, et al.
Novel Semisynthetic Betulinic Acid–Triazole Hybrids with In Vitro Antiproliferative Potential
Reprinted from: *Processes* **2023**, *11*, 101, https://doi.org/10.3390/pr11010101 21

Abdur Rauf, Umer Rashid, Zafar Ali Shah, Gauhar Rehman, Kashif Bashir, Johar Jamil, et al.
Anti- Inflammatory and Anti-Diabetic Activity of Ferruginan, a Natural Compound from *Olea ferruginea*
Reprinted from: *Processes* **2023**, *11*, 545, https://doi.org/10.3390/pr11020545 39

Talib Hussain, Muteb Alanazi, Jowaher Alanazi, Tareq Nafea Alharby, Aziz Unnisa, Amir Mahgoub Awadelkareem, et al.
Computational and *In Vitro* Assessment of a Natural Triterpenoid Compound Gedunin against Breast Cancer via Caspase 3 and Janus Kinase/STAT Modulation
Reprinted from: *Processes* **2023**, *11*, 1452, https://doi.org/10.3390/pr11051452 50

Narayanaswamy Radhakrishnan, Vasantha-Srinivasan Prabhakaran, Mohammad Ahmad Wadaan, Almohannad Baabbad, Ramachandran Vinayagam and Sang Gu Kang
STITCH, Physicochemical, ADMET, and In Silico Analysis of Selected *Mikania* Constituents as Anti-Inflammatory Agents
Reprinted from: *Processes* **2023**, *11*, 1722, https://doi.org/10.3390/pr11061722 70

Aneta Baj, Lucie Rárová, Artur Ratkiewicz, Miroslav Strnad and Stanislaw Witkowski
Synthesis and Biological Evaluation of α-Tocopherol Derivatives as Potential Anticancer Agents
Reprinted from: *Processes* **2023**, *11*, 1860, https://doi.org/10.3390/pr11061860 87

Turki Al Hagbani, Afrasim Moin, Talib Hussain, N. Vishal Gupta, Farhan Alshammari, Syed Mohd Danish Rizvi and Sheshagiri Dixit
Anticancer Activity of Anti-Tubercular Compound(s) Designed on Pyrrolyl Benzohydrazine Scaffolds: A Repurposing Study
Reprinted from: *Processes* **2023**, *11*, 1889, https://doi.org/10.3390/ pr11071889 102

Daniela Istrate and Luminita Crisan
Dipeptidyl Peptidase 4 Inhibitors in Type 2 Diabetes Mellitus Management: Pharmacophore Virtual Screening, Molecular Docking, Pharmacokinetic Evaluations, and Conceptual DFT Analysis
Reprinted from: *Processes* **2023**, *11*, 3100, https://doi.org/10.3390/pr11113100 120

**Alexandra Prodea, Andreea Milan, Marius Mioc, Alexandra Mioc, Camelia Oprean,
Roxana Racoviceanu, et al.**
Novel Betulin-1,2,4-Triazole Derivatives Promote In Vitro Dose-Dependent Anticancer Cytotoxicity
Reprinted from: *Processes* **2024**, *12*, 24, https://doi.org/10.3390/pr12010024 . . . . **142**

**Andreea Milan, Marius Mioc, Alexandra Mioc, Narcisa Marangoci, Roxana Racoviceanu,
Gabriel Mardale, et al.**
Exploring the Antimelanoma Potential of Betulinic Acid Esters and Their
Liposomal Nanoformulations
Reprinted from: *Processes* **2024**, *12*, 416, https://doi.org/10.3390/pr12020416 . . . . **166**

About the Editors

Alina Bora

Alina Bora, PhD, Scientific Secretary since 2022 and Senior Researcher at the "Coriolan Dragulescu" Institute of Chemistry, has considerable experience in research centered on the use of computational techniques and chemoinformatics in life sciences to generate translational impact on health and the environment. She contributed to the development of large-scale databases such as WOMBAT, WOMBAT-PK, ChemProt, and DrugCentral, cheminformatic investigation, and identification of new potential HIV protease, MAO-B, and GSK-3 selective inhibitors from natural sources to treat infectious, neurodegenerative, and psychiatric disorders, design new environmentally friendly pesticides. and prioritize novel chemical scaffolds in large chemical libraries. She has served as the PI of one national grant and as a co-investigator in eight other national and international projects, and she has co-authored more than 50 ISI papers, 1 book, and 7 book chapters that have been published with prestigious publishers (e.g., Wiley, Springer) and has served as a reviewer for over 70 international papers. Based on the acquired expertise and knowledge, her current research interests are channeled on the drug discovery process by applying the state-of-the-art computational techniques to develop new safer and more effective candidates.

Luminita Crisan

Luminita Crisan, PhD, is a senior researcher at the "Coriolan Dragulescu" Institute of Chemistry. Her research experience covers a broad range of activities focused on applying computational chemistry techniques that have found general applicability in silico drug design. Throughout her career, she has significantly contributed to developing innovative methods connecting theoretical chemistry with experimental approaches, particularly the rational design of bioactive molecules targeting diabetes, neurodegenerative diseases, and inflammation. Her current research interests focus on the integration of in silico and machine learning techniques to improve the drug discovery process. Her work has yielded over 50 ISI-indexed publications, reflecting her impact and recognition in the scientific community. Furthermore, she played a pivotal role as a reviewer for more than 100 international scientific papers, demonstrating her commitment to maintaining high standards in research. Beyond journal articles, Dr. Crisan has co-authored two book chapters published by prestigious publishers such as John Wiley & Sons, Inc., and Humana NY–Springer Protocols, further showcasing her expertise . Her contributions to scientific conferences, both in Romania and internationally, highlight her active engagement with the global research community.

Preface

As science and modern medicine rapidly advance, natural compounds continue to inspire drug discovery and design, reinforced by complex technologies such as high-throughput screening, computational modeling, and synthetic biology. These innovations lead to new therapeutic developments that hold the promise of addressing previously unmet medical needs and improving the lives of patients. High-throughput screening allows for the rapid evaluation of thousands of potential drug candidates, while computational modeling provides insights into the interactions between drugs and their targets at a molecular level. Synthetic biology enables the creation of novel compounds and pathways, broadening the scope of potential therapeutic agents.

The co-guest editors extend their sincere gratitude to the authors for sharing their latest research, knowledge, and expertise in this field. Their contributions are invaluable in advancing our understanding of how natural compounds can be harnessed for new drug discoveries. This collaborative effort helps pave the way for future breakthroughs and reinforces the critical role of interdisciplinary approaches in tackling complex health challenges.

Alina Bora and Luminita Crisan
Guest Editors

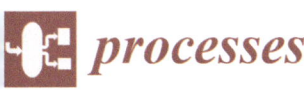

Editorial

Editorial on the Special Issue "Natural Compounds Applications in Drug Discovery and Development"

Alina Bora * and Luminita Crisan *

"Coriolan Dragulescu" Institute of Chemistry, 24 M. Viteazu Avenue, 300223 Timisoara, Romania
* Correspondence: alina_bora@acad-icht.tm.edu.ro (A.B.); lumi_crisan@acad-icht.tm.edu.ro (L.C.)

Nature is an amazing source of natural bioactive compounds derived from numerous species of plants, marine bacteria, and fungi [1]. Today, advanced scientific and technological strategies allow researchers to systematically explore and manipulate the therapeutic potential of these natural resources. The high structural diversity of natural compounds offers important advantages in drug discovery through the wide variety of chemical scaffolds [2,3].

In contrast to synthetic compounds, which often rely on limited chemical libraries, natural products provide a wide range of molecular structures refined by evolution for specific biological activities [4]. This structural complexity and their inherent affinity for biological targets (enzymes, receptors, and signaling pathways implicated in various diseases), make natural compounds valuable starting points for drug development efforts [5]. Besides their pharmacological properties, natural compounds often possess favorable pharmacokinetic and safety profiles, crucial features in drug development. Past research has led to compounds that have improved bioavailability and are well tolerated in the human body, thus minimizing the risk of adverse effects. In addition, the biodegradability and sustainability of natural products aligns with the increasing focus on green drug discovery processes [6].

The applications of natural compounds in drug discovery are vast, encompassing various therapeutic areas such as fungal and bacterial infections, cancer, neurogenerative diseases, and many metabolic disorders [7]. Looking ahead, natural compounds continue to inspire drug discovery design, sustained by technological advances such as high-throughput screening, computational modeling, and synthetic biology. By exploring the richness of biodiversity, researchers can open new therapeutic opportunities and address today's challenging medical needs [4].

In drug discovery and development, searching for effective and safe treatments often leads scientists to explore the wonders of nature. It has always been known that natural compounds have played a key role in medicine, generating a multitude of bioactive molecules with diverse therapeutic potential [8].

Considering the enormous potential of natural products reflected in the design, discovery, and development of new drugs, we introduce a Special Issue in the Processes journal entitled "Natural Compounds Applications in Drug Discovery and Development". This Special Issue comprises 10 original research articles out of 18 submitted for consideration under the rigorous peer review process of the Processes journal (acceptance rate of 55.55%). Open-access ensures high visibility and accessibility of the submitted articles, allowing researchers worldwide to access the latest research in the natural compounds field, regardless of their institutional affiliations or financial resources. It also promotes transparency and reproducibility, leading to broader dissemination of research findings and enhancing articles' impact and citation rates (Figure 1).

Citation: Bora, A.; Crisan, L. Editorial on the Special Issue "Natural Compounds Applications in Drug Discovery and Development". *Processes* **2024**, *12*, 1152. https://doi.org/10.3390/pr12061152

Received: 28 May 2024
Accepted: 30 May 2024
Published: 3 June 2024

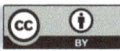

Copyright: © 2024 by the authors. Licensee MDPI, Basel, Switzerland. This article is an open access article distributed under the terms and conditions of the Creative Commons Attribution (CC BY) license (https:// creativecommons.org/licenses/by/ 4.0/).

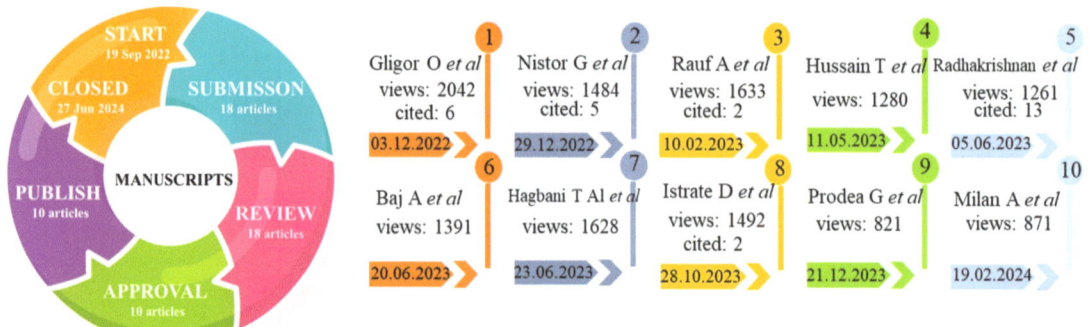

Figure 1. The 10 articles of the Special Issue: authors, views, citations and article publication dates (*citations and views checked on 28 May 2024; for 1 to 10 articles, please see https://www.mdpi.com/journal/processes/special_issues/9T0L5065FV*).

The 10 articles of the Special Issue (Figure 1) cover a wide range of topics that provide new insights into exploring the vast array of natural products and highlight the latest advances and applications in the field. Starting from the extraction, synthesis, and computational exploration of various natural compounds, continuing with the testing of their biological activity, the elucidation of the mechanisms of action and repositioning, and reaching the evaluation of drug-like properties, the influence of extraction methods, synthesis, and characterization, this collection contributes to the ongoing efforts to utilize the therapeutic potential of plants in the fight against challenging diseases. The comprehensive review of these articles showcases the efforts of researchers in the fight against various cancers, inflammation, and diabetes by proposing new candidates with enhanced pharmacological and safety profiles, while highlighting the interdisciplinary nature of modern pharmaceutical research (Figure 2).

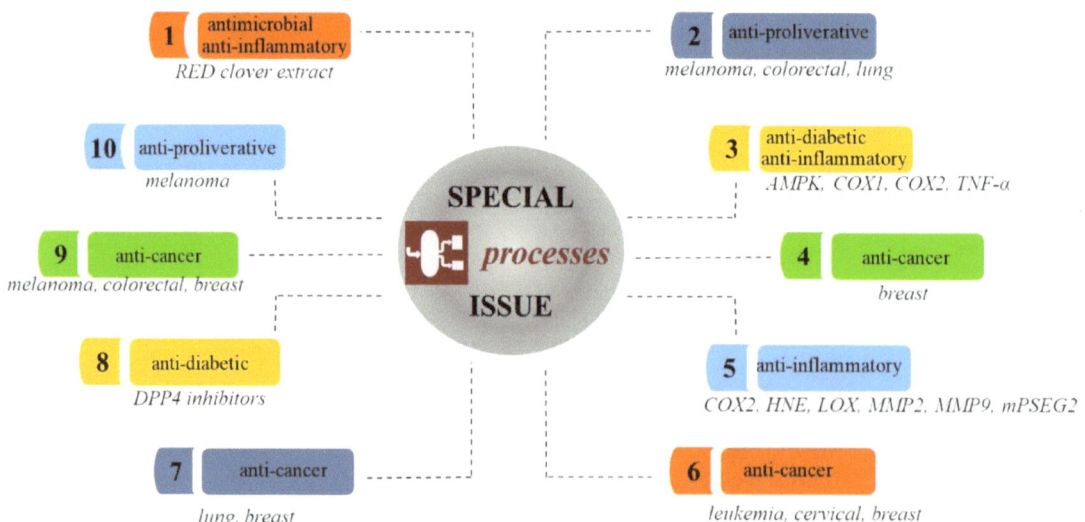

Figure 2. Pharmacological potential of natural products, diseases and targets assessed by Special Issues articles.

In conclusion, the research articles of this Special Issue offer a new perspective on the exploration of natural compounds, representing an infinite quest at the intersection of science, medicine, and nature. By applying innovative approaches and technologies, natural resources remain the best alternative to design new safe and sustainable candidates [9–11]. Leveraging natural resources as active components in medicine offers advantages since numerous bioactive compounds derived from plants are already part of our everyday diets. Even as technologies and methods for drug design and development have evolved, remember to consider the extensive potential of the natural world to deliver new and innovative treatments.

Author Contributions: Conceptualization, A.B. and L.C.; writing—original draft preparation, A.B. and L.C.; writing—review and editing, A.B. and L.C. All authors have read and agreed to the published version of the manuscript.

Acknowledgments: The co-guest editors thank the authors for sharing their latest research, knowledge, and experience. This work was supported by Project No. 1.1 from the "Coriolan Dragulescu" Institute of Chemistry, Timisoara, Romania.

Conflicts of Interest: The authors declare no conflicts of interest.

Abbreviations

DPP-4 (dipeptidyl peptidase-4); AMPK (AMP-activated protein kinase), COX1 (cyclooxygenase 1), COX2 (cyclooxygenase 2), TNF-alfa (tumor necrosis factor), HNE (human neutrophil elastase), LOX (lipoxygenase), MMP2 (matrix metalloproteinase-2), MMP9 (matrix metalloproteinase-9), mPSEG2 (microsomal prostaglandin E synthase 2).

References

1. Pham, J.V.; Yilma, M.A.; Feliz, A.; Majid, M.T.; Maffetone, N.; Walker, J.R.; Yoon, Y.J. A Review of the Microbial Production of Bioactive Natural Products and Biologics. *Front. Microbiol.* **2019**, *10*, 1404. [CrossRef]
2. Dzobo, K. The Role of Natural Products as Sources of Therapeutic Agents for Innovative Drug Discovery. *Compr. Pharmacology* **2022**, 408–422. [CrossRef]
3. Harvey, A.L. Natural products as a screening resource. *Curr. Opin. Chem. Biol.* **2007**, *11*, 480–844. [CrossRef]
4. Atanasov, A.G.; Zotchev, S.B.; Dirsch, V.M.; Supuran, C.T. Natural products in drug discovery: Advances and opportunities. *Nat. Rev. Drug Discov.* **2021**, *20*, 200–216. [CrossRef]
5. Grigalunas, M.; Brakmann, S.; Waldmann, H. Chemical Evolution of Natural Product Structure. *J. Am. Chem. Soc.* **2022**, *144*, 3314–3329. [CrossRef]
6. Castiello, C.; Junghanns, P.; Mergel, A.; Jacob, C.; Ducho, C.; Valente, S.; Mai, A. GreenMedChem—The challenge in the next decade toward eco-friendly compounds and processes in drug design. *Green. Chem.* **2023**, *25*, 2109–2169. [CrossRef]
7. Ulrich-Merzenich, G.; Panek, D.; Zeitler, H.; Vetter, H.; Wagner, H. Drug development from natural products: Exploiting synergistic effects. *Indian. J. Exp. Biol.* **2010**, *48*, 208–219.
8. Choudhury, A. Potential Role of Bioactive Phytochemicals in Combination Therapies against Antimicrobial Activity. *J. Pharmacopunct.* **2022**, *30*, 25, 79–87. [CrossRef] [PubMed]
9. Istrate, D.; Crisan, L. Natural Compounds as DPP-4 Inhibitors: 3D-Similarity Search, ADME Toxicity, and Molecular Docking Approaches. *Symmetry* **2022**, *14*, 1842. [CrossRef]
10. Katz, L.; Baltz, R.H. Natural product discovery: Past, present, and future. *J. Ind. Microbiol. Biotechnol.* **2016**, *43*, 155–176. [CrossRef] [PubMed]
11. Crisan, L.; Bora, A. Small Molecules of Natural Origin as Potential Anti-HIV Agents: A Computational Approach. *Life* **2021**, *11*, 722. [CrossRef] [PubMed]

Disclaimer/Publisher's Note: The statements, opinions and data contained in all publications are solely those of the individual author(s) and contributor(s) and not of MDPI and/or the editor(s). MDPI and/or the editor(s) disclaim responsibility for any injury to people or property resulting from any ideas, methods, instructions or products referred to in the content.

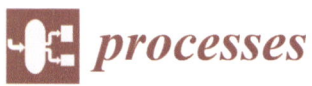

Article

Red Clover and the Importance of Extraction Processes—Ways in Which Extraction Techniques and Parameters Affect *Trifolium pratense* L. Extracts' Phytochemical Profile and Biological Activities

Octavia Gligor [1], Simona Clichici [2], Remus Moldovan [2], Dana Muntean [3], Ana-Maria Vlase [1], George Cosmin Nadăș [4], Cristiana Ștefania Novac [4], Gabriela Adriana Filip [2,*], Laurian Vlase [3,*] and Gianina Crișan [1]

[1] Department of Pharmaceutical Botany, Iuliu Hațieganu University of Medicine and Pharmacy, 8 Victor Babeș Street, 400347 Cluj-Napoca, Romania
[2] Department of Physiology, Iuliu Hațieganu University of Medicine and Pharmacy, 8 Victor Babeș Street, 400347 Cluj-Napoca, Romania
[3] Department of Pharmaceutical Technology and Biopharmaceutics, University of Medicine and Pharmacy, 8 Victor Babeș Street, 400347 Cluj-Napoca, Romania
[4] Department of Microbiology, University of Agricultural Sciences and Veterinary Medicine, 3/5 Mănăștur Street, 400372 Cluj-Napoca, Romania
* Correspondence: gabriela.filip@umfcluj.ro (G.A.F.); laurian.vlase@umfcluj.ro (L.V.)

Citation: Gligor, O.; Clichici, S.; Moldovan, R.; Muntean, D.; Vlase, A.-M.; Nadăș, G.C.; Novac, C.Ș.; Filip, G.A.; Vlase, L.; Crișan, G. Red Clover and the Importance of Extraction Processes—Ways in Which Extraction Techniques and Parameters Affect *Trifolium pratense* L. Extracts' Phytochemical Profile and Biological Activities. *Processes* 2022, *10*, 2581. https://doi.org/10.3390/pr10122581

Academic Editors: Alina Bora and Luminita Crisan

Received: 28 October 2022
Accepted: 28 November 2022
Published: 3 December 2022

Publisher's Note: MDPI stays neutral with regard to jurisdictional claims in published maps and institutional affiliations.

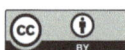

Copyright: © 2022 by the authors. Licensee MDPI, Basel, Switzerland. This article is an open access article distributed under the terms and conditions of the Creative Commons Attribution (CC BY) license (https://creativecommons.org/licenses/by/4.0/).

Abstract: The purpose of this study was to gain an insight into the manner in which several extraction processes (both classical as well as innovative) affected bioactive compound yield, and subsequently to assess several of their biological activities. Red clover extracts were obtained using maceration, Soxhlet extraction, turbo-extraction, ultrasound-assisted extraction, and a combination of the last two. The resulting extracts were analyzed for total phenolic and flavonoid content. The extracts presenting the best results were subjected to a phytochemical assessment by way of HPLC-MS analysis. After a final sorting based on the phytochemical profiles of the extracts, the samples were assessed for their antimicrobial activity, anti-inflammatory activity, and oxidative stress reduction potential, using animal inflammation models. The Soxhlet extraction yielded the most satisfactory results both qualitatively and quantitatively. The ultrasound-assisted extraction offered comparable yields. The extracts showed a high potential against gram-negative bacteria and induced a modest antioxidant effect on the experimental inflammation model in Wistar rats.

Keywords: red clover; extraction methods; biological activity; HPLC; phytochemical profile; antimicrobial activity; oxidative stress reduction; anti-inflammatory activity; ultrasound-assisted extraction; innovative extraction methods

1. Introduction

Having been cultivated no sooner than the third century by European farmers, red clover is still to this day used in agriculture as a cover crop due to its weed suppression capacity, atmospheric nitrogen fixation, soil conservation, and multiple other advantages [1].

The genus *Trifolium* consists of hundreds of annual and perennial species, with short stems, trifoliate compound leaves, and sessile, outwardly spread flowers, as is the case for *Trifolium pratense* L. The corolla ranges in coloring from pink to red or even purple. Flowering periods range from the early months of spring to summer, and even early autumn [2,3].

Apart from its agricultural benefits, numerous applications for red clover have existed in medicine throughout history. The plant is mainly known for its isoflavonic compounds, such as formononetin, biochanin A, ononin, daidzein and genistein, which are considered as phytoestrogens with estrogenic, anti-tumor, anti-inflammatory activity, as well as showing potential effects on cardiovascular risks, neuroprotective effects, and many others [4–10].

Conventional extraction methods have recently been regarded as more disadvantageous due to the necessity of large volumes of solvents, which are often polluting or toxic. These methods also involve many time-consuming steps. Maceration, decoction, infusion, Soxhlet extraction, etc. can be considered major examples of conventional extraction methods. Thus, unconventional extraction methods have come into focus by virtue of their advantages, e.g., decreased solvent volumes, with lower toxicity, reduced extraction time, and so on. Such examples of extraction methods imply the assistance of microwaves, ultrasounds, pressurized fluids, etc. [11,12].

Based on current findings, few reports concerning the influence of extraction methods over the phytochemical profile or biological activity of the species *Trifolium pratense* L. exist [13,14].

The main objective of this study was to evaluate the influence of extraction methods and parameters on the phytochemical profiles and biological activities of *Trifolium pratense* L. extracts. Furthermore, the intention was to offer a comparison between the results of the different extraction methods. The extraction methods that were taken into consideration were maceration, Soxhlet extraction, turbo-extraction, ultrasound-assisted extraction, and finally, a combination of the last two methods. Experimental Wistar rat plantar inflammation models induced by carrageenan administration were employed to elucidate anti-inflammatory and antioxidant effects. Antimicrobial activity was also assessed.

2. Materials and Methods

2.1. Plant Material

Dried aerial parts of *Trifolium pratense* L. were purchased from a local tea company (Hypericum Impex, Baia Sprie, Maramureș, Romania). The plant material was ground to a fine powder with an electric grinder.

2.2. Chemicals, Reagents, and Devices

Folin–Ciocâlteu reagent, sodium carbonate (Na_2CO_3), Aluminum chloride ($AlCl_3$), ABTS (diammonium 2,2′-azino-bis(3-ethylbenzothiazoline-6-sulfonate), DPPH (2,2-Diphenyl-1-(2,4,6-trinitrophenyl)hydrazyl), TPTZ (2,4,6-Tris(2-pyridyl)-s-triazine), indomethacin, carboxymethylcellulose, o-phthalaldehyde, Lambda carrageenan type IV, were purchased from Sigma–Aldrich (Taufkirchen, Germany). 2-thiobarbituric acid and Bradford reagent were acquired from Merck KGaA (Darmstadt, Germany) and ELISA cytokines tests (TNF-α and IL-6, respectively) were purocured from Elabscience (Houston, TX, USA). Bradford total protein assay was purchased from Biorad (Hercules, CA, USA). All analytical grade, HPLC reagents and standards were obtained from Sigma–Aldrich (Taufkirchen, Germany) and Decorias (Valea Lupului, Romania).

The following devices were used: Bosch MKM6003 grinder (Gerlingen, Germany), SER 148 solvent extraction unit (VELP® Scientifica, Usmate Velate, Italy), T 50 ULTRA-TURRAX® disperser (IKA®-Werke GmbH & Co. KG, Staufen, Germany), Sonic-3 ultrasonic bath (Polisonic, Warsaw, Poland), refrigerated high speed centrifuge Sigma 3–30 KS (Sigma Laborzentrifugen GmbH, Osterode am Harz, Germany), Specord 200 Plus spectrophotometer (Analytik Jena, Jena, Germany), Agilent 1100 Series HPLC Value System coupled with an Agilent 1100 mass spectrometer (LC/MSD Ion Trap SL) (Agilent Technologies, Santa Clara, CA, USA), Bioblock Scientific 94,200 rotary evaporator (Heidolph Instruments GmbH & Co. KG, Schwabach, Germany), vacuum controller HS-0245 (Hahnshin Scientific Co., Tongjin-eup, Gimpo-si, Gyeonggi-do, Republic of Korea), Brinkman Polytron homogenizer (Kinematica AG, Littau-Luzern, Switzerland).

2.3. Selected Extraction Methods

The following extraction conditions were maintained constant for all the selected extraction techniques: the solvent was 70% alcohol and the solvent to sample ratio was

10:1 (v/w). This decision was made in order to ensure the correspondence of the results and to permit an accurate comparison between the selected extraction methods. After each completed extraction, separation was further carried out through centrifugation at 12,000 rpm for 10 min.

2.3.1. Maceration

Extraction was carried out according to the specifications of the Romanian Pharmacopoeia. Five grams of plant material were placed in a Falcon flask and 50 mL 70% alcohol were added. The contents of the flask were kept at room temperature for 10 days and mixed periodically. After the extraction was concluded, the sample was separated.

2.3.2. Soxhlet Extraction (SE)

In each extraction cup, 5 g plant material were added, followed by 50 mL 70% alcohol. For this extraction method, the heating plate was set to 210 °C in order to permit the solvent to reach its boiling point of approximately 79 °C. The duration of the extraction process was varied from 20 min to 40 min, and to 60 min, respectively. Separation followed the extraction process.

2.3.3. Turboextraction (TBE)

For each extract, 5 g plant material were added in a beaker, followed by 50 mL 70% alcohol. The parameters selected for study were extraction time and rotation speed. Extraction time was calculated in such a way as to represent 10 min and 20 min, respectively. For this, the extraction time of 10 min was divided into 2 extraction cycles, each of 5 min. In addition, the extraction time of 20 min was divided into 4 cycles, each of 5 min. Dispersion was carried out in the that manner in order to prevent device overheating and evaporation of the solvent. The rotation speed values that were selected for study were as follows: 4.000 rpm, 6.000 rpm, and 8.000 rpm. The extraction process was followed by separation.

2.3.4. Ultrasound-Assisted Extraction (UAE)

Frequency was maintained at a constant of 50 Hz, and power at a constant value of 230 V, respectively. The assessed parameters were time, with values ranging from 10, 20 to 30 min and temperature, with values varying from 30, 40 to 50 °C, respectively. The extracts were then subjected to separation.

2.3.5. Combination of Two Extraction Methods: UAE and TBE (UTE)

The ultrasonic bath was brought to 30 °C. The ULTRA-TURRAX® disperser speed was set to 4.000 rpm. Extraction time was kept to a minimum of one cycle of 5 min. These parameters were selected in order to maintain solvent evaporation to a minimum and to avoid device overheating.

2.4. Determination of Total Phenolic Content (TPC)

The Folin–Ciocâlteu method was selected to determine the total polyphenolic content (TPC). The experiment was carried out according to the specifications of Csepregi et al. with several modifications [15]. Consequently, in a microtube, 270 μL Folin–Ciocâlteu reagent were mixed with 60 μL plant extract, after which 270 μL Na_2CO_3 6% (w/v) were added. Following an incubation period of 30 min, in a dark environment, absorbances of the samples were measured at 765 nm, with the selected standard of gallic acid. The results were expressed as mg gallic acid equivalents per mL extract (GAE mg/mL).

2.5. Determination of Total Flavonoid Content (TFC)

Total flavonoid content was analyzed through a modified version of the method used by Pinacho et al. [16]. 400 μL solution containing $AlCl_3$ 20 mg/mL in 5% acetic acid in ethanol 3:1 (v/v) ratio were added to 200 μL plant extract. Absorbances were determined at

420 nm, with quercetin as standard. Subsequently, results were expressed as mM quercetin equivalents (QE mM).

2.6. Antioxidant Activity Evaluation

2.6.1. DPPH Radical Scavenging Activity

The DPPH assay was carried out according to Martins et al. with slight modifications [17]. 800 µL DPPH radical methanolic solution were added to 200 µL extract. The mixture was incubated for 30 min, in a medium deprived of light, at 40 °C temperature. Absorbances were measured at 517 nm, having Trolox reagent as standard. The results that followed were expressed as mg Trolox equivalents per mL extract (TE mg/mL).

2.6.2. ABTS$^+$ Scavenging Activity

The experiment was performed using a method provided by Erel [18]. 200 µL acetate buffer 0.4 M, pH 5.8 were added to 20 µL ABTS$^+$ in acetate buffer 30 mM, pH 3.6 with 12.5 µL extract added to the previous mixture. The absorbances of the samples were determined at 660 nm, using Trolox as standard. Results were expressed as mM Trolox equivalents (mM TE).

2.6.3. FRAP Assay

The experiment followed the technique used by Csepregi et al. [15], with several alterations. FRAP reagent was obtained by adding 25 mL acetate buffer (300 mM, pH 3.6) to 2.5 mL TPTZ solution (10 mM TPTZ in 40 mM HCl) and 2.5 mL FeCl$_3$ (20 mM in water). The freshly prepared reagent was added to 30 µL plant extract. The mixture was left to incubate for 30 min, then absorbances were measured at 620 nm. Trolox reagent was used as standard. Results were expressed as mM Trolox equivalents (TE mM).

2.7. HPLC-MS Analysis

The apparatus used for phytochemical analysis was an Agilent 1100 HPLC Series system (Agilent Inc., Santa Clara CA, USA) equipped with binary pump, degasser, autosampler, column thermostat, and UV detector. An Agilent 1100 mass spectrometer (LC/MSD Ion Trap SL) was coupled with the HPLC system. For the separation of the phenolic compounds, a reverse-phase analytical column was selected (Zorbax SB-C18, 100 µm × 3.0 µm i.d., 3.5 µm particle size). The working temperature was set at 48 °C. Compounds' detection was performed on both MS mode and UV. The UV detector operated at different wavelengths (330 nm until 17.5 min, followed by 370 nm until the end of analysis). For the MS system, an electrospray ionization source operated in negative mode with a capillary potential of +3000 V, a nebulizer pressure of 60 psi (nitrogen), a flow rate for nitrogen gas of 12 L/min, and a dry gas temperature of 360 °C. The MS operated in monitoring specific ions mode (for polyphenol carboxylic acids) or AUTO Ms (for flavonoids and their aglycones). Separation of the phenolic compounds was carried out with a mobile phase of methanol:acetic acid 0.1% (v/v) and elution was in a binary gradient (at start, elution was with a linear gradient, from 5% to 42% methanol at 35 min, kept at isocratic elution for the following 3 min with 42% methanol, and then rebalance the column with 3% methanol). The flow rate was set at 1 mL/min and the injection volume was of 5 µL [19–21].

Another LC-MS analytical method was used to identify the following polyphenols in the vegetal extracts: epicatechin, catechin, syringic acid, gallic acid, protocatechuic acid, and vanillic acid. Chromatographic separation was carried out on a Zorbax SB-C18 column (100 mm × 3.0 mm i.d., 3.5 µm particle size) under a binary gradient and with a mixture of methanol:acetic acid 0.1% (v/v) as the mobile phase (3% methanol at start, 8% methanol at 3 min, 20% methanol from 8.5 to 10 min, followed by 3% methanol to rebalance the column). The flow rate was set at 1 mL/min, while the injection volume was of 5 µL. The MS mode (SIM-MS) was selected to detect the polyphenolic compounds. The MS system operated under the same conditions as described above [22,23].

Sterolic compounds separation was performed under isocratic elution conditions, with a Zorbax SB-C18 RP analytical column (100 mm × 3.0 mm i.d., 3.5 µm particle size). The mobile phase consisted of methanol:acetonitrile 10:90 (v/v). For MS analyses the positive ion mode was selected and was performed with the apparatus Agilent Ion Trap 1100 SL MS, with an APCI interface. The nitrogen gas temperature was set at 325 °C, with a flow rate of 7 L/min, a nebulizer pressure of 60 psi, and a capillary voltage of −4000 V. For identification of sterolic compounds, the MS spectra and RTs were compared with those obtained under the same conditions for standard compounds. The multiple reactions monitoring analysis mode (MS/MS) was selected to decrease the background interference. Under the described chromatographic conditions, the retention times of the four analyzed sterols were: 2.4 min for ergosterol, 3.7 min for both stigmasterol and campesterol (coelution), and 4.2 min for sitosterol [24,25].

Data Analysis (v5.3) and ChemStation (vA09.03) software from Agilent Inc. (Santa Clara, CA, USA) were used to obtain and analyze the chromatographic data.

2.8. Assessment of Antimicrobial Activity

2.8.1. In Vitro Qualitative Evaluation of Antimicrobial Activity

The antimicrobial potential was assessed by the disk diffusion test, using standard strains of Gram-positive and Gram-negative bacteria as well as yeasts. Four Gram-positive microbial strains were selected: *Staphylococcus aureus* ATCC 6538P, *Listeria monocytogenes* ATCC 13932, *Enterococcus faecalis* ATCC 29212, and *Bacillus cereus* ATCC 11778. Three Gram-negative strains were selected: *Escherichia coli* ATCC 10536, *Salmonella enteritidis* ATCC 13076 and *Pseudomonas aeruginosa* ATCC 27853. The selected yeast strain was *Candida albicans* ATCC 10231. The selected standard antibacterial control was amoxicillin, whereas ketoconazole was selected as a yeast standard control.

Screening was carried out according to EUCAST standards [26]. A suspension was prepared from young microbial colonies (24 h old), grown on Mueller-Hinton (MH) agar for bacteria, and Sabouraud dextrose agar (SDA). It was further adjusted at 0.5 density in saline on McFarland scale using Densichek calibration standard (bioMérieux, Craponne, France). 8.5 cm diameter plastic Petri dishes with MH agar for bacteria and SDA agar for yeast were flooded with the resulted suspension. Once the excess fluid was eliminated, the agar surface was left to dry, and 5 mm diameter filter paper discs were placed in a radial model. 20 µL were added on each filter paper disk and the plates were incubated for 18 h at 35 ± 2 °C for bacteria and 48 h at 28 °C for the fungal strain [26]. The antimicrobial activity was measured by determining the diameter of the growth inhibition area, with results expressed in mm.

2.8.2. In Vitro Quantitative Evaluation of Antimicrobial Activity

The antimicrobial activity was quantitatively measured following the minimum inhibitory concentration (MIC) method for the eight above-mentioned microbial strains. The assessment was accomplished by modified EUCAST protocols [26]. 96-wells titer plates were used. The extracts were added, once diluted in liquid MH medium, and afterwards inoculated with 20 µL microbial suspension. The stock solutions of the extracts were diluted using a two-fold serial dilution system in ten consecutive wells, from the initial concentration (1/1) to the highest (1/512). The total broth volume was adjusted to 200 µL. Positive controls represented by microbial inoculum in MH broth and negative control represented by microbial inoculum in 30% ethanol were also prepared and used to fill wells 11 and 12, respectively. The incubation period of the wells was 24 h at a temperature of 37 °C for bacteria and 48 h at 28 °C for *Candida*, respectively. MIC values were determined as the lowest concentration of the extracts' dilution that inhibited the growth of the microbial cultures (having the same OD as the negative control), compared to the positive control, as established by a decreased value of absorbance at 450 nm (HiPo MPP-96, Biosan, Latvia). MIC50 was also determined, representing the MIC value at which ≥50% of the bacterial/yeast cell growth was inhibited, considered as the well with the OD value similar to the average between the positive and negative control.

2.9. Determination of Biological Activities

Once the phytochemical profile of the extracts was determined, the 60 min SE was selected for further determination of in vivo biological activities. The selection was based on number of identified compounds, and concentration levels of said compounds.

2.9.1. Inflammation Model in Rats Induced by Carrageenan

The in vivo determination was accomplished by way of an inflammation experimental model in male Wistar rats (110–130 g mean weight). The specimens were acclimatized in the ensuing conditions: 12 h light/12 h dark cycles, 35% humidity, free access to water, and a normocaloric standard diet (VRF1), randomization in 4 groups, 8 specimens each. During a period of 4 days, treatment was administered by oral gavage, in a maximum volume of 0.25 mL, such as: group 1—carboxymethylcellulose 2% (positive control group—CMC); group 2—Indomethacin 5 mg/body weight (b.w.) in carboxymethylcellulose 1.5% (Indom); group 3–20 mg TPC/b.w./day (60 min SE).

On the fifth day, inflammation was induced by injecting 100 µL of freshly prepared 1% carrageenan (λ-carrageenan, type IV, Sigma) diluted in normal saline in the right hind footpad (32). An exact saline solution volume was injected at the level of the left hind paw, serving as negative control. Subsequently, at 2 and 24 h after carrageenan administration, soft paw samples were collected under intraperitoneally injected 90 mg/kg ketamine and 10 mg/kg xylazine. The samples were assessed for oxidative stress parameters and cytokine levels, following homogenization in 50 mMTRIS–10 mM EDTA buffer (pH 7.4) [27]. The protein content was evaluated using the Bradford method [28].

The experiments were permitted by the Ethic Committee Board of "Iuliu Hațieganu" University of Medicine and Pharmacy, Cluj-Napoca, Romania (291/23.02.2022) on Animal Welfare according to the Directive 2010/63/EU on the protection of animals used for scientific purposes.

2.9.2. Evaluation of Oxidative Stress

The levels of malondialdehyde (MDA), glutathione reduced and glutathione oxidized levels and GSH/GSSG ratio were determined in the from paw tissue homogenates. Spectrofluorimetry was used to quantify MDA levels, by 2-thiobarbituric acid method [29]. The GSH and GSSG levels were determined by the Hu method [30].

2.9.3. Evaluation of Proinflammatory Cytokines

TNF-α and IL-6 levels from plantar tissue homogenates were evaluated by ELISA assay following the protocol provided by the manufacturer. Results were expressed in pg/mg protein.

2.9.4. Statistical Analysis

One-way analysis of variance (ANOVA) was used to analyze data, followed by the Tukey's multiple comparisons post-test, using GraphPad Prism 8 software. A p value < 0.05 was considered statistically significant. The results were expressed as mean ± standard deviation.

3. Results

A final number of 20 extracts was reached after each extraction process was finished. One extract was performed by maceration (M), three samples were obtained through SE (S), six samples by turboextraction (T), nine samples were prepared through UAE (U) and the last remaining sample was completed by UTE (UT). The initials used to label the samples represent the abbreviation of the extraction method and the parameters that were studied for each item: M for maceration, S for SE, U for ultrasound, and UT for UTE. Table 1 represents the explained nomenclature of the extract samples which were evaluated in this study.

Table 1. Nomenclature of the obtained extract samples of the study.

Extraction Method	Studied Extraction Parameters				Sample Name
Maceration	*				M
Soxhlet extraction (SE)		20			S20
		40			S40
		60			S60
Turboextraction (TBE)	Time (min)	10 min (2 cycles of 5 min)	Rotation speed (rpm)	4.000	T24
				6.000	T26
				8.000	T28
		20 min (4 cycles of 5 min)		4.000	T44
				6.000	T46
				8.000	T48
Ultrasound-assisted extraction (UAE)		10	Temperature (°C)	30	U13
				40	U14
				50	U15
		20		30	U23
				40	U24
				50	U25
		30		30	U33
				40	U34
				50	U35
Combination of two extraction methods: UAE and TBE (UTE)	**				UT

* Parameters remained constant, see Section 2.3.1. Maceration, ** Parameters remained constant, see Section 2.3.5. Combination of two extraction methods: UAE and TBE (UTE).

Finally, the extracts that offered the highest yields were selected for further HPLC analysis. After the phytochemical characterization of the respective extracts, the biological activity of the samples presenting the highest concentration of antitumoral compounds was evaluated.

3.1. Effect of Extraction Parameters on TPC and TFC Values

Table 2 contains the TPC and TFC values of the studied extracts.

Table 2. TPC and TFC of the extracts.

Sample	TPC (GAE mg/mL) *	TFC (QE mM) *
M	0.970 ± 0.022	1.216 ± 0.046
S20	1.146 ± 0.010	1.876 ± 0.019
S40	1.186 ± 0.013	1.331 ± 0.045
S60	1.223 ± 0.017	2.276 ± 0.009
T24	0.818 ± 0.020	1.465 ± 0.039
T26	0.624 ± 0.011	1.320 ± 0.004
T28	0.636 ± 0.014	0.930 ± 0.040
T44	0.708 ± 0.006	1.262 ± 0.024
T46	0.714 ± 0.016	1.070 ± 0.018
T48	0.619 ± 0.017	1.143 ± 0.009
U13	0.522 ± 0.009	0.770 ± 0.041
U14	0.823 ± 0.007	1.303 ± 0.008
U15	0.560 ± 0.017	1.148 ± 0.028
U23	0.728 ± 0.000	0.956 ± 0.028
U24	0.558 ± 0.004	0.970 ± 0.047
U25	0.747 ± 0.015	1.863 ± 0.047
U33	0.673 ± 0.019	1.854 ± 0.034
U34	0.610 ± 0.023	2.161 ± 0.043
U35	0.838 ± 0.030	1.414 ± 0.076
UT	0.687 ± 0.017	0.694 ± 0.038

* concentrations were expressed as mean ± SD.

SE provided the extracts with the highest TPC values. The increase of extraction time was inversely proportional to the polyphenolic content. Thus, in the case of SE, the extraction period of 60 min proved to be the optimal extraction time for this particular plant material and solvent. Maceration followed, having achieved a lower value than SE. Turbo-extraction was comparable to the UAE, although the values resulted from these extraction methods were greatly inferior to the previously mentioned methods. For TBE, increasing extraction time (from two cycles of 5 min to four cycles of 5 min) and speed, particularly from 6.000 rpm to 8.000 rpm, both determined lower yields. The highest TPC value was reached with the parameters of two cycles of 5 min as extraction period and the lowest speed value, 4.000 rpm, respectively. Highest values of TPC for UAE were achieved when the parameter combinations of 10 min extraction time with 40 °C, and 30 min extraction time with 50 °C were used. The combination of UAE and TBE did not reach a comparable value with either SE or maceration.

For TFC, even though SE reached the highest values in this case as well, UAE gave comparable results with SE. Maceration showed a medium value. The lowest value was attained by UTE. Prolonged extraction time, i.e., 60 min for SE enabled the highest yield. This was followed by the UAE extracts, with optimal extraction conditions having been 30 min extraction time and 40 °C. Other UAE conditions comparable with these were the combinations of 20 min with 50 °C and 30 min with 30 °C.

3.2. Effect of Extraction Parameters on Antioxidant Activity

Results are detailed in Table 3.

Table 3. Antioxidant capacity of the extracts.

Sample	DPPH (TE mg/mL) *	FRAP (TE mM) *	ABTS$^+$ (TE mM) *
M	2.721 ± 0.445	5.465 ± 0.196	2.97 ± 1.121
S20	2.541 ± 0.049	8.444 ± 0.165	4.687 ± 0.389
S40	2.718 ± 0.132	8.476 ± 0.365	3.525 ± 0.810
S60	2.822 ± 0.067	8.615 ± 0.326	5.646 ± 0.457
T24	3.740 ± 0.337	8.615 ± 0.217	3.551 ± 0.417
T26	4.430 ± 0.233	9.564 ± 0.405	3.626 ± 0.191
T28	2.270 ± 0.143	8.172 ± 0.027	3.576 ± 0.330
T44	2.894 ± 0.100	8.836 ± 0.270	4.131 ± 0.381
T46	2.549 ± 0.144	9.564 ± 0.377	3.778 ± 0.287
T48	2.801 ± 0.183	9.231 ± 0.190	2.843 ± 0.116
U13	2.271 ± 0.017	3.808 ± 0.027	2.894 ± 0.131
U14	3.452 ± 0.031	9.374 ± 0.142	4.535 ± 0.747
U15	2.241 ± 0.025	1.262 ± 0.047	3.475 ± 0.044
U23	2.231 ± 0.008	6.447 ± 0.123	4.182 ± 0.473
U24	1.648 ± 0.022	5.047 ± 0.179	3.475 ± 0.087
U25	3.345 ± 0.022	10.923 ± 0.152	5.04 ± 0.231
U33	2.802 ± 0.059	7.097 ± 0.207	4.485 ± 0.227
U34	2.434 ± 0.031	5.405 ± 0.072	4.081 ± 0.087
U35	2.444 ± 0.039	7.255 ± 0.198	5.167 ± 0.076
UT	3.253 ± 0.029	6.512 ± 0.152	4.056 ± 0.044

* concentrations were expressed as mean ± SD.

A prime example appeared for the DPPH assay, where the highest value was obtained by TBE, at the shorter extraction time used, i.e., two cycles of 5 min and a medium speed value, i.e., 6.000 rpm. This was followed by a similar combination of parameters, with the exception of the speed value being 4.000 rpm.

FRAP assay results were generally high for multiple methods, i.e., SE and TBE. Medium to low values were achieved for UAE overall. Nevertheless, the highest value of TE was attained by UAE, at 20 min time with 50 °C, respectively.

For the ABTS+ assay however, the highest values were observed for SE, with the longest extraction time of 60 min having been the optimal value in this case. This was followed by UAE, with the parameters most favorable consisting of 20 min extraction time and 50 °C as well as 30 min and 50 °C, respectively.

3.3. HPLC-MS Analysis of the Extracts

Out of the initial 20 extracts, 11 were selected for further HPLC-MS analysis. The selected extracts presented the highest values of the results obtained for the assays carried out as mentioned above, in Section 3.1. and Section 3.2.

3.3.1. Evaluation of Polyphenolic Compounds

Table 4 details the results following the HPLC-MS detection and quantification of polyphenolic compounds in the studied extracts.

Table 4. Polyphenolic compounds in the selected extracts.

Sample	Catechin (µg/mL Extract) *	Syringic Acid (µg/mL Extract) *	Protocatechuic Acid (µg/mL Extract) *	Vanillic Acid (µg/mL Extract) *	Chlorogenic Acid (µg/mL Extract) *	p-Coumaric Acid (µg/mL Extract) *	Caftaric Acid (µg/mL Extract) *
M	ND	0.13 ± 0.004	1.31 ± 0.145	0.45 ± 0.022	3.57 ± 0.393	1.83 ± 0.201	ND
S40	ND	0.16 ± 0.013	0.88 ± 0.124	0.37 ± 0.026	8.78 ± 0.263	1.89 ± 0.283	ND
S60	ND	0.13 ± 0.005	1.11 ± 0.089	0.38 ± 0.042	9.76 ± 0.293	2.49 ± 0.174	ND
T24	ND	0.10 ± 0.011	0.55 ± 0.039	0.23 ± 0.028	5.61 ± 0.393	1.34 ± 0.040	ND
T26	0.05 ± 0.004	0.06 ± 0.004	0.39 ± 0.027	0.17 ± 0.017	5.46 ± 0.164	1.10 ± 0.113	ND
T46	0.08 ± 0.010	0.09 ± 0.003	0.48 ± 0.033	0.27 ± 0.008	6.97 ± 0.836	1.40 ± 0.211	4.51 ± 0.541
U14	0.02 ± 0.003	0.08 ± 0.005	0.56 ± 0.040	0.30 ± 0.024	6.04 ± 0.544	1.65 ± 0.181	ND
U25	ND	0.14 ± 0.012	0.78 ± 0.086	0.31 ± 0.016	5.91 ± 0.296	1.77 ± 0.159	ND
U34	0.05 ± 0.003	0.08 ± 0.009	0.49 ± 0.063	0.19 ± 0.013	4.78 ± 0.478	1.40 ± 0.098	ND
U35	0.11 ± 0.016	0.09 ± 0.013	0.81 ± 0.122	0.32 ± 0.044	7.73 ± 0.618	2.01 ± 0.281	ND
UT	0.04 ± 0.005	0.09 ± 0.014	0.75 ± 0.752	0.39 ± 0.043	8.10 ± 0.810	1.89 ± 0.245	ND

* concentrations were expressed as mean ± SD.

Low levels of catechin were identified. Only TBE, UAE and UTE extracts contained this compound. Seemingly, the increase in extraction time, speed or temperature enabled the extraction of catechin, i.e., four cycles of 5 min and 6.000 rpm for TBE and 30 min and 50 °C for UAE. However, UAE reached the highest yield.

Other polyphenolic compounds such as syringic acid, protocatechuic acid, vanillic acid, chlorogenic acid, and p-coumaric acid were detected in all analyzed samples. The highest levels of syringic acid were found in the SE sample that was subjected to 40 min extraction time, with an increase in temperature showing a decrease in concentration. Other notable extraction methods and conditions that enabled high yield levels for syringic acid were UAE (20 min, 50 °C) and maceration. Protocatechuic acid reached the highest level in the macerate, followed by the SE extract with 60 min extraction time. Vanillic acid was also detected in high concentrations in the macerate, followed by the combination of TBE and UAE, and SE, respectively. The chlorogenic and p-coumaric acids were both detected in high concentrations in the SE extracts that were subjected to a 60 min process time.

Interestingly, the caftaric acid was detected only in one sample, namely the extract obtained through TBE, at four cycles of 5 min and speed of 6.000 rpm, respectively.

3.3.2. Evaluation of Flavonoid Compounds

Results are illustrated in Table 5.

A total of 11 flavonoid compounds were identified in the studied extracts. With eupatilin having been identified in strictly one of the samples. These findings were in accordance with previous reports in scientific literature affirming the wide variety of flavonoid and isoflavonoid compounds in the species pertaining to the genus *Trifolium* [2,3,31,32].

The highest concentrations were reached throughout all extracts for the compounds jaceosidin and hispidulin. These were followed by hyperoside, isoquercitrin and quercitrin, respectively. Generally, SE at 60 min extraction time enabled the highest yields. The exception of rutin, where TBE led to the highest yield, and eupatilin that was identified solely in a UAE extract (30 min extraction time and 40 °C temperature). Overall, low to medium values were detected in samples obtained by maceration, TBE and UAE. However, in the case of rutin, the sample subjected to TBE at four cycles of 5 min and 6.000 rpm enabled a large yield.

Table 5. Flavonoid compounds in the selected extracts.

Sample	Kaempferol (μg/mL Extract) *	Quercetol (μg/mL Extract) *	Isoquercitrin (μg/mL Extract) *	Quercitrin (μg/mL Extract) *	Rutin (μg/mL Extract) *	Hyperoside (μg/mL Extract) *	Luteolin (μg/mL Extract) *	Vitexin (μg/mL Extract) *	Apigenin (μg/mL Extract) *	Eupatilin (ng/mL Extract) *	Jaceosidin (ng/mL Extract) *	Hispidulin (ng/mL Extract) *
M	ND	1.72 ± 0.069	ND	ND	ND	ND	2.27 ± 0.113	1.77 ± 0.247	0.78 ± 0.078	ND	249.29 ± 19.943	371.04 ± 18.552
S40	0.35 ± 0.011	6.95 ± 0.208	2.05 ± 0.061	17.19 ± 1.547	ND	ND	2.27 ± 0.249	2.85 ± 0.285	0.68 ± 0.081	ND	295.57 ± 17.734	343.90 ± 37.829
S60	ND	8.93 ± 0.268	1.58 ± 0.047	7.47 ± 0.672	ND	ND	3.03 ± 0.393	3.26 ± 0.359	1.07 ± 0.128	ND	408.32 ± 48.999	453.76 ± 36.301
T24	ND	4.80 ± 0.144	1.28 ± 0.128	7.66 ± 1.072	ND	ND	1.71 ± 0.086	1.50 ± 0.045	0.68 ± 0.082	ND	199.96 ± 13.997	280.16 ± 16.810
T26	ND	4.80 ± 0.240	0.97 ± 0.087	7.66 ± 0.230	ND	ND	1.51 ± 0.211	1.50 ± 0.209	0.58 ± 0.058	ND	188.79 ± 11.328	260.63 ± 10.425
T46	ND	4.58 ± 0.412	0.66 ± 0.066	4.85 ± 0.146	ND	ND	1.78 ± 0.160	2.58 ± 0.129	0.68 ± 0.088	ND	232.15 ± 20.894	313.70 ± 47.055
U14	0.28 ± 0.014	4.52 ± 0.633	2.35 ± 0.330	10.09 ± 1.513	ND	ND	1.85 ± 0.259	2.17 ± 0.217	0.58 ± 0.081	ND	261.53 ± 28.768	272.18 ± 19.053
U25	0.28 ± 0.020	4.58 ± 0.595	3.59 ± 0.323	12.33 ± 0.740	15.55 ± 1.711	ND	1.99 ± 0.258	2.31 ± 0.277	0.68 ± 0.061	ND	300.05 ± 18.003	300.51 ± 21.036
U34	0.42 ± 0.012	4.03 ± 0.443	3.28 ± 0.492	15.14 ± 0.454	ND	ND	1.51 ± 0.135	1.90 ± 0.133	0.58 ± 0.075	4.00 ± 0.360	224.71 ± 26.966	228.09 ± 6.843
U35	0.55 ± 0.082	5.90 ± 0.413	4.05 ± 0.445	20.56 ± 0.617	ND	ND	2.20 ± 0.066	2.58 ± 0.155	0.78 ± 0.047	ND	301.81 ± 39.235	375.38 ± 15.015
UT	0.42 ± 0.058	5.02 ± 0.452	3.28 ± 0.361	15.14 ± 0.605	ND	1.86 ± 0.167	2.06 ± 0.288	2.45 ± 0.294	0.78 ± 0.023	ND	295.73 ± 17.744	328.26 ± 9.848

* concentrations were expressed as mean ± SD.

3.3.3. Evaluation of Isoflavonoid Compounds

Results of the evaluation of the isoflavonoid compounds are detailed in Table 6.

Table 6. Isoflavonoid compounds in the selected extracts.

Sample	Daidzein (ng/mL Extract) *	Daidzin (ng/mL Extract) *	Genistein (ng/mL Extract) *	Genistin (ng/mL Extract) *	Glycitein (ng/mL Extract) *
M	483.11 ± 53.142	102.14 ± 14.299	388.73 ± 19.437	973.82 ± 48.691	ND
S40	361.67 ± 36.167	161.11 ± 8.055	337.51 ± 50.626	1524.99 ± 76.249	ND
S60	528.48 ± 15.854	235.53 ± 23.553	454.45 ± 59.079	1942.73 ± 58.282	33.11 ± 4.304
T24	367.83 ± 40.461	140.07 ± 9.805	295.98 ± 11.839	944.15 ± 75.532	ND
T26	277.34 ± 8.320	111.00 ± 3.330	240.41 ± 31.253	849.74 ± 101.969	ND
T46	371.48 ± 48.293	147.41 ± 19.164	352.37 ± 31.714	1430.72 ± 174.086	ND
U14	397.66 ± 55.673	223.70 ± 15.659	410.61 ± 49.273	1722.62 ± 241.167	16.24 ± 0.812
U25	431.24 ± 25.874	205.86 ± 10.293	416.65 ± 54.164	1686.72 ± 118.070	35.60 ± 2.136
U34	377.06 ± 37.706	139.86 ± 8.394	341.87 ± 51.280	1374.52 ± 68.726	ND
U35	483.47 ± 72.520	199.96 ± 9.998	443.84 ± 57.699	1714.08 ± 154.267	12.36 ± 1.112
UT	423.72 ± 25.423	177.90 ± 8.895	434.44 ± 26.066	1702.13 ± 85.107	20.84 ± 1.042

* concentrations were expressed as mean ± SD.

Five compounds, daidzein, daidzin, genistein, genistin, and glycitein were detected in the samples, in large concentrations. For these compounds, SE proved to be the most successful extraction method, with the extraction time of 60 min having been the most favorable time parameter, as well. Glycitein was detected only in certain samples, for instance, in the 60 min SE extract, three of the four UAE analyzed extracts and the UTE sample. UAE at 20 min time and 50 °C led to the highest yield in the case of this compound.

3.3.4. Evaluation of Sterolic Compounds

Results discussed in this section are found in Table 7.

Three sterolic compounds were detected in high levels in the samples: stigmasterol, β-sitosterol, and campesterol. For these compounds, UAE proved the most efficient extraction method, with maximum compound levels being extracted at 20 min, 50 °C for campesterol and 30 min, 50 °C for stigmasterol and β-sitosterol.

Table 7. Sterolic compounds in the selected extracts.

Sample	α-Tocopherol (ng/mL Extract)	γ-Tocopherol (ng/mL Extract)	Ergosterol (ng/mL Extract)	Stigmasterol (ng/mL Extract) *	β-Sitosterol (ng/mL Extract) *	Campesterol (ng/mL Extract) *
M	ND	ND	ND	2492.70 ± 99.708	62,032.15 ± 8684.501	1061.37 ± 127.364
S40	ND	ND	ND	1640.04 ± 246.007	34,113.14 ± 3070.183	498.55 ± 24.928
S60	ND	ND	ND	2609.65 ± 339.254	54,007.75 ± 6480.930	1100.60 ± 55.030
T24	ND	ND	ND	2356.91 ± 94.276	50,607.54 ± 5060.754	982.68 ± 29.480
T26	ND	ND	ND	2259.78 ± 293.771	42,076.96 ± 6311.544	710.98 ± 92.427
T46	ND	ND	ND	2370.90 ± 331.926	43,673.45 ± 3493.876	922.40 ± 27.672
U14	ND	ND	ND	3134.05 ± 282.065	56,018.75 ± 2800.938	1006.33 ± 140.887
U25	ND	ND	ND	3202.09 ± 320.210	68,060.97 ± 7486.707	1322.76 ± 52.911
U34	ND	ND	ND	2471.12 ± 197.690	52,752.50 ± 5802.775	1058.24 ± 148.154
U35	ND	ND	ND	3596.66 ± 323.700	83,130.15 ± 10,806.920	1277.69 ± 76.662
UT	ND	ND	ND	2955.13 ± 295.513	63,322.55 ± 5065.804	1014.49 ± 40.579

* concentrations were expressed as mean ± SD.

3.4. Evaluation of Antimicrobial Activity

3.4.1. In Vitro Qualitative Evaluation of Antimicrobial Activity

The potential of microbial growth inhibition of the extracts was screened by the disk diffusion test. The extracts showed high efficiency against Gram-negative bacteria, a moderate level against gram-positive bacteria and *Candida albicans*. Results are shown in Table 8.

Table 8. Results for the risk diffusion test performed for selected samples.

	U35 *	S60 *	Amoxicillin	Ketoconazole
Staphylococcus aureus ATCC 6538P	9.28	9.01	24.38	-
Enterococcus faecalis ATCC 29212	9.51	9.51	16.8	-
Listeria monocytogenes ATCC 13932	9.44	9.44	18.96	-
Bacillus cereus ATCC 11778	8.82	8.82	8.83	-
E. coli ATCC 10536	12.59	12.31	13.72	-
Salmonella enteritidis ATCC 13076	12.73	11.47	18.43	-
Pseudomonas aeruginosa ATCC 27853	11.27	10.3	R	-
Candida albicans 10231	9.11	8.83	-	23.74

* inhibition area diameter in mm; R—resistant.

The diameters of the inhibition areas were: 8.82–9.51 mm in the case of gram-positive strains, 10.3–12.73 mm regarding the gram-negative strains, and 8.83–9.11 mm for Candida albicans. Increased antimicrobial potential was demonstrated against gram-negative bacteria.

3.4.2. In Vitro Quantitative Evaluation of Antimicrobial Activity

Although the antimicrobial screening revealed high potential against gram-negative strains, the MIC method was used to evaluate the quantitative antimicrobial potential of the selected samples against all microbial strains that were used initially, in the qualitative part of the evaluation.

As presented in Table 9, lower MICs could be noted for gram-positive strains in this case, with an overall variation of the antimicrobial potential. A possible reason could be explained by a limited diffusion on the agar surface. A general high inhibitory concentration was observed for the wells with liquid MH medium.

Table 9. Results for the MIC test performed for selected samples.

	U35		S60	
	MIC 100	MIC 50	MIC 100	MIC 50
Staphylococcus aureus ATCC 6538P	1/16	1/32	1/32	1/32
Enterococcus faecalis ATCC 29212	1/64	1/64	1/64	1/64
Listeria monocytogenes ATCC 13932	1/32	1/64	1/32	1/64

Table 9. *Cont.*

	U35		S60	
	MIC 100	MIC 50	MIC 100	MIC 50
Bacillus cereus ATCC 11778	1/32	1/32	1/32	1/64
E. coli ATCC 10536	1/16	1/32	1/16	1/32
Salmonella enteritidis ATCC 13076	1/8	1/16	1/8	1/16
Pseudomonas aeruginosa ATCC 27853	1/16	1/16	1/16	1/32
Candida albicans 10231	1/32	1/32	1/32	1/32

3.5. Evaluation of Oxidative Stress and Inflammation Markers

Oxidative stress was evaluated by determination of lipid peroxidation marker, MDA, and by non-endogenous antioxidants levels such as reduced glutathione (GSH), oxidized glutathione (GSSG), and their respective ratio (GSH/GSSG). The activity of enzymatic antioxidants was also assessed: catalase (CAT) and glutathione peroxidase (GPx). Results are shown in Figure 1.

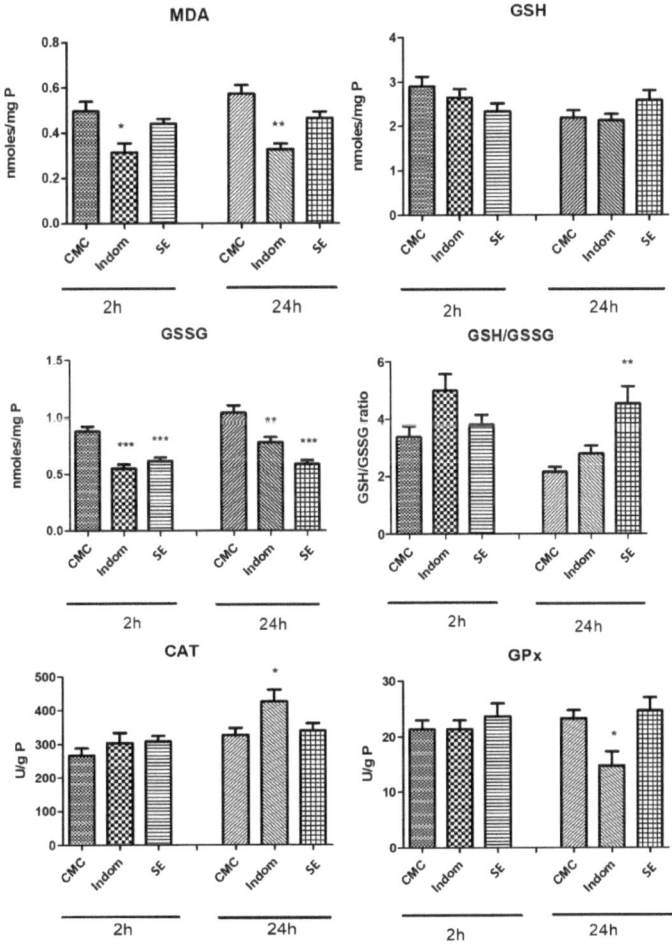

Figure 1. Soft paw tissue levels of MDA, GSG/GSSG ratio and the activity of CAT and GPx at 2, 24 h after carrageenan injection, in rats pretreated with SE extract. Values are means ± SD. Statistical analysis was done by a one-way ANOVA, with Tukey's multiple comparisons post-test (* $p < 0.05$ ** $p < 0.001$ and *** $p < 0.0001$, all treated groups vs. control (CMC) group).

MDA levels decreased significantly only after Indom administration, both at 2 h ($p < 0.05$) and 24 h ($p < 0.01$) while the SE extract did not influence the lipid peroxidation ($p > 0.05$). SE positively influenced the GSSG levels, both at 2 h ($p < 0.001$) and 24 h ($p < 0.001$) after the carrageenan injection, similar to indomethacin and increased the GSH/GSSG ratio at 24 h ($p < 0.01$). CAT activity increased significantly after indomethacin administration at 24 h ($p < 0.05$) while the GPx activity decreased at 24 h in the same group ($p < 0.05$). The TP extract did not influence the antioxidant enzymes activity in paw tissue ($p > 0.05$).

Cytokine levels, such as IL-6 and TNF-α, were assessed in the plantar tissue homogenates compared with indomethacin, at 2 and 24 h after carrageenan injection. Results are illustrated in Figure 2. Compared to Indomethacin, SE administration did not significantly reduce the IL-6 and TNF-α secretions at 2 h and 24 h after induction of inflammation. Only Indomethacin administration decreased the TNF-α levels in the soft tissues at 24 h after carrageenan injection ($p < 0.05$).

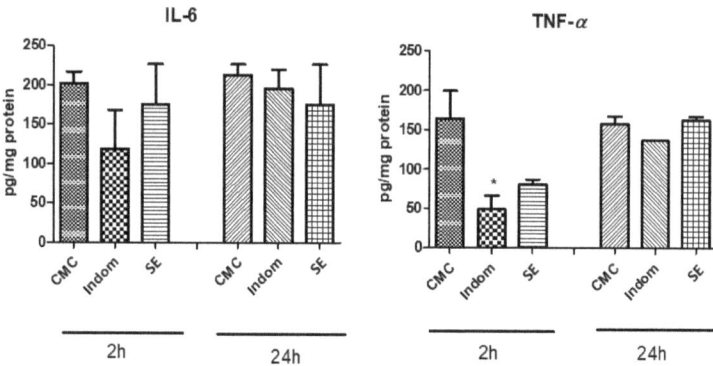

Figure 2. Levels of IL-6 and TNF-α in paw tissue of experimental rats at 2 h and 24 h after injection of carrageenan. Values are means $\pm$ SD. Statistical analysis was performed by a one-way ANOVA, with Tukey's multiple comparisons post-test (* $p < 0.05$ vs. control, CMC, group).

4. Discussion

According to the information available hitherto this study, few scientific reports were recently made concerning the influence of extraction methods or extraction parameters over the phytochemical profile or even biological activity of *Trifolium pratense* L. Two such examples, were focused on compounds belonging to the class of polysaccharides, the first consisting of an optimization of hot water extraction, with the second study following the effect of several extraction methods on these compounds [13,14]. Mikhailov et al. studied the influence of growth site on bioactive compounds, for samples of *T. pratense* L. and *T. repens* L. [33]. Vlaisavljević et al. have also studied the influence of growth phase on phenolic content on *T. pratense* L. extracts, obtained by means of a microwave-assisted extraction [34]. In 2009, two studies using micropreparative techniques, by Zgórka G., attempted to elucidate the effect of extraction methods and the respective parameters over the chemotaxonomy of isoflavonoid compounds from *Trifolium* species [35,36]. Visnevschi-Necrasov et al. have optimized an extraction method based on matrix solid-phase dispersion for isoflavonoid compounds from *T. pratense* L. [37].

Based on the obtained TPC results obtained in this study, it could be presumed that the subjection of the solvent to a higher temperature and prolonged extraction time, enabled greater degradation of cellular walls. This led to a larger release of polyphenolic content. As opposed to the TPC and TFC results, several differences were noticeable, with regards to the antioxidant activity of the extracts. This suggests that this method enabled the extraction of compounds with antioxidant capacity, contrary to the other implemented methods. Other noteworthy differences were represented by the UAE and UTE. In those cases, the parameters that permitted the achievement of higher TE values were 10 min extraction time with the temperature of 40 °C and 20 min extraction time at 50 °C for UAE, and 30 °C with 4.000 rpm and 5 min extraction period for UTE. A possible explanation as to the reason why SE gave medium results might have been the degradation of said antioxidant compounds at high temperature values. Additionally, the low or medium parameters selected for TBE, and UAE showed similar results, in this case, antioxidant compound extraction having been possibly insufficient. The differences between values for each type of assay might reside in the particularity of each of these experiments: type of reagent used, required incubation time, or lack thereof, necessary ambient temperature, and so on.

Supposedly, UTE obtained a somewhat medium value due to the combination of all three parameters (time, temperature, speed) although values for these parameters were kept low due to the possible implications detailed in Section 2.3.5. Akbaribazm et al. have reported similar results, using a liquid chromatography-electrospray ionization mass spectrometry analysis method for hydroalcoholic extracts [32]. These findings were contrary to the results reported by Tundis et al. in which case rutin and quercitrin exhibited the highest values [31].

For isoflavonoid compounds, the findings were in accordance with previous scientific reports not only for the *T. pratense* L. species, but also concerning other members of this genus [32,38,39].

Despite newly developed industrial antibiotics, the resistance of microorganisms to these substances has grown. Generally, bacteria possess the genetical capacity to transmit and gain resistance towards therapeutic compounds. This fact becomes worrisome due to the increase of in-hospital patients which are immunosuppressed, but also due to the new multi-resistant strains. For this reason, new bacterial infections may arise, resulting in the increase of infectious pathologies. Such medical issues, derived from bacterial resistance, have found to be increasing. Thus, the use of antibacterial compounds has become troublesome. In this manner, healthcare specialists face the need of taking measures in order to reduce bacterial multi-resistance, by monitoring antibiotic use. Thus, the improvement of antibiotic treatment is desired. For a long period of time, plants have been a valuable resource of natural compounds used to maintain human health, and to this day, are still considered a possible alternative treatment, by way of natural therapies. For this reason, the pharmaceutical use of plant bioactive compounds has become a frontrunner. Current research suggests the effectiveness of plant bioactive compounds in treating infectious diseases. Therefore, plant-derived products can be considered promising, being used as antimicrobial agents. Plant-derived compounds also lack secondary effects, are easily available, and are low-cost [40].

Regarding the results of the antimicrobial activity of the presently studied extracts, the samples were found to present a high potential against gram-negative strains high potential against gram-negative strains. However, Khan et al. reported that for the extracts of the species *Trifolium alexandrium* L., the studied extracts presented a greater efficiency against gram-positive bacteria, rather than gram-negative bacteria [41].

Inflammation represents a defensive, restoring process, with the major objective of protecting the organism. Causes of the inflammatory process may lie in the initial lesion, e.g., bacteria, fungi, parasites, toxins, etc., or in the consequences resulting from such said lesions, e.g., cellular and tissular necrosis [42]. The most important phenomenon consists in the permanent migration and recruitment of macrophages from within the capillary microcirculation. The regenerative tissular capacity is the result of two categories of factors. The first consists of the capacity of resting cells to reenter the division cycle. The second factor is represented by the efficient differentiation of stem cells from the lesioned tissue. The regeneration capacity of tissues and organs is specific to animal organisms. Many of the regeneration processes in mammals represent compensatory growth processes which imply cell hyperplasia and hypertrophy [43].

The effect of SE on plantar inflammation was modest, probably due to the low dose or the transitory effect of the phenolic compounds administered through the extracts. These findings are similar to previous reports in the literature, which attested the antioxidant and anti-inflammatory activities of several *Trifolium* species determined by both in vitro and in vivo studies, employing various cell lines as well as mice models. These pharmacological properties are attributed to the genus' abundance of phenolic and isoflavonic compounds, as detailed in the previous subchapters of this study. These compounds have been reported to inhibit cyclooxygenase activity in human monocytes as well as macrophages [2,44–46]. In this sense, plant-derived natural compounds have been recognized as safe substances, with moderate effectiveness for the treatment of several inflammatory diseases [47]

5. Conclusions

A major observation was the tendency of extraction yields to increase proportionately along with the values of extraction parameters. However, this progression in yields halted abruptly once compound degradation temperatures were achieved, being also favored by other amplified conditions such as extraction time or speed. This phenomenon was most notable for TBE and UAE. One could conclude that the SE presented biological activity, considering the results of the phytochemical profile of the red clover extracts. Therefore, red clover could also constitute a medicinal herbal species with potential applications in complementary therapies, demonstrating safety and efficacy for antioxidant and antimicrobial activities.

Author Contributions: O.G.: conceptualization, investigation, writing—original draft preparation, data interpretation; S.C.: supervision, review; R.M.: methodology, investigation; D.M. and A.-M.V.: methodology, investigation, formal analysis; resources, interpretation of data; G.C.N. and C.Ș.N.: methodology, formal analysis, data curation; G.A.F.: writing—review and editing, supervision, L.V.: project administration, funding acquisition; supervision, editing; G.C.: supervision, review. All authors have read and agreed to the published version of the manuscript.

Funding: This research was funded by UEFISCDI Romania, project PN-III-P1-1.1-PD-2019-0774, and "Iuliu Hațieganu" University of Medicine and Pharmacy, Cluj-Napoca, Romania, PhD grant PCD No. 1170/3/14.01.2021.

Data Availability Statement: Not applicable.

Acknowledgments: The authors would like to gratefully acknowledge Nicoleta Decea for her aid in the determination of the biological activities of the obtained extracts.

Conflicts of Interest: The authors declare no conflict of interest.

References

1. McKenna, P.; Cannon, N.; Conway, J.; Dooley, J.; Davies, W.P. Red clover (*Trifolium pratense*) in conservation agriculture: A compelling case for increased adoption. *Int. J. Agric. Sustain.* **2018**, *16*, 342–366. [CrossRef]
2. Sabudak, T.; Guler, N. *Trifolium* L.—A review on its phytochemical and pharmacological profile. *Phyther. Res.* **2009**, *23*, 439–446. [CrossRef]
3. Tripathi, N.; Chaudhary, S. A review on chemical and biological activity of *Trifolium pretense*. *PharmaTutor* **2014**, *2*, 93–101. Available online: http://www.pharmatutor.org/magazines/articles/march-2014/review-chemical-biological-activity-trifolium-pratense (accessed on 22 July 2022).
4. Chen, H.-Q.; Wang, X.-J.; Jin, Z.-Y.; Xu, X.-M.; Zhao, J.-W.; Xie, Z.-J. Protective effect of isoflavones from *Trifolium pratense* on dopaminergic neurons. *Neurosci. Res.* **2008**, *62*, 123–130. [CrossRef]
5. Kanadys, W.; Baranska, A.; Jedrych, M.; Religioni, U.; Janiszewska, M. Effects of red clover (*Trifolium pratense*) isoflavones on the lipid profile of perimenopausal and postmenopausal women—A systematic review and meta-analysis. *Maturitas* **2020**, *132*, 7–16. [CrossRef]
6. Atkinson, C.; Oosthuizen, W.; Scollen, S.; Loktionov, A.; Day, N.E.; Bingham, S.A. Modest Protective Effects of Isoflavones from a Red Clover-Derived Dietary Supplement on Cardiovascular Disease Risk Factors in Perimenopausal Women, and Evidence of an Interaction with ApoE Genotype in 49–65 Year-Old Women. *J. Nutr.* **2004**, *134*, 1759–1764. [CrossRef]
7. Chen, X.; Zhang, M.; Ahmed, M.; Surapaneni, K.M.; Veeraraghavan, V.P.; Arulselvan, P. Neuroprotective effects of ononin against the aluminium chloride-induced Alzheimer's disease in rats. *Saudi J. Biol. Sci.* **2021**, *28*, 4232–4239. [CrossRef]
8. Luo, L.; Zhou, J.; Zhao, H.; Fan, M.; Gao, W. The anti-inflammatory effects of formononetin and ononin on lipopolysaccharide-induced zebrafish models based on lipidomics and targeted transcriptomics. *Metabolomics* **2019**, *15*, 153. [CrossRef]
9. Gong, G.; Zheng, Y.; Kong, X.; Wen, Z. Anti-angiogenesis Function of Ononin via Suppressing the MEK/Erk Signaling Pathway. *J. Nat. Prod.* **2021**, *84*, 1755–1762. [CrossRef]

10. Fang, Y.; Ye, J.; Zhao, B.; Sun, J.; Gu, N.; Chen, X.; Ren, L.; Chen, J.; Cai, X.; Zhang, W.; et al. Formononetin ameliorates oxaliplatin-induced peripheral neuropathy via the KEAP1-NRF2-GSTP1 axis. *Redox Biol.* **2020**, *36*, 101677. [CrossRef]
11. Alara, O.R.; Abdurahman, N.H.; Olalere, O.A. Optimization of microwave-assisted extraction of flavonoids and antioxidants from *Vernonia amygdalina* leaf using response surface methodology. *Food Bioprod. Process.* **2018**, *107*, 36–48. [CrossRef]
12. Lefebvre, T.; Destandau, E.; Lesellier, E. Selective extraction of bioactive compounds from plants using recent extraction techniques: A review. *J. Chromatogr. A* **2020**, *1635*, 461770. [CrossRef]
13. Zhang, H.; Zhao, J.; Shang, H.; Guo, Y.; Chen, S. Extraction, purification, hypoglycemic and antioxidant activities of red clover (*Trifolium pratense* L.) polysaccharides. *Int. J. Biol. Macromol.* **2020**, *148*, 750–760. [CrossRef]
14. Shang, H.; Li, R.; Wu, H.; Sun, Z. Polysaccharides from *Trifolium repens* L. extracted by different methods and extraction condition optimization. *Sci. Rep.* **2019**, *9*, 6353. [CrossRef]
15. Csepregi, K.; Neugart, S.; Schreiner, M.; Hideg, É. Comparative evaluation of total antioxidant capacities of plant polyphenols. *Molecules* **2016**, *21*, 208. [CrossRef]
16. Pinacho, R.; Cavero, R.Y.; Astiasarán, I.; Ansorena, D.; Calvo, M.I. Phenolic compounds of blackthorn (*Prunus spinosa* L.) and influence of in vitro digestion on their antioxidant capacity. *J. Funct. Foods* **2015**, *19*, 49–62. [CrossRef]
17. Martins, N.; Barros, L.; Dueñas, M.; Santos-Buelga, C.; Ferreira, I.C.F.R. Characterization of phenolic compounds and antioxidant properties of *Glycyrrhiza glabra* L. rhizomes and roots. *RSC Adv.* **2015**, *5*, 26991–26997. [CrossRef]
18. Erel, O. A novel automated direct measurement method for total antioxidant capacity using a new generation, more stable ABTS radical cation. *Clin. Biochem.* **2004**, *37*, 277–285. [CrossRef]
19. Benedec, D.; Hanganu, D.; Filip, L.; Oniga, I.; Tiperciuc, B.; Olah, N.K.; Gheldiu, A.-M.; Raita, O.; Vlase, L. Chemical, antioxidant and antibacterial studies of Romanian *Heracleum sphondylium*. *Farmacia* **2017**, *65*, 252–256.
20. Toiu, A.; Vlase, L.; Gheldiu, A.M.; Vodnar, D.; Oniga, I. Evaluation of the antioxidant and antibacterial potential of bioactive compounds from *Ajuga reptans* extracts. *Farmacia* **2017**, *65*, 351–355.
21. Toiu, A.; Vlase, L.; Vodnar, D.C.; Gheldiu, A.-M.; Oniga, I. *Solidago graminifolia* L. Salisb. (*Asteraceae*) as a Valuable Source of Bioactive Polyphenols: HPLC Profile, In Vitro Antioxidant and Antimicrobial Potential. *Molecules* **2019**, *24*, 2666. [CrossRef] [PubMed]
22. Rusu, M.E.; Fizesan, I.; Pop, A.; Mocan, A.; Gheldiu, A.-M.; Babota, M.; Vodnar, D.C.; Jurj, A.; Berindan-Neagoe, I.; Vlase, L.; et al. Walnut (*Juglans regia* L.) Septum: Assessment of Bioactive Molecules and In Vitro Biological Effects. *Molecules* **2020**, *25*, 2187. [CrossRef]
23. Pop, A.; Fizeșan, I.; Vlase, L.; Rusu, M.; Cherfan, J.; Babota, M.; Gheldiu, A.-M.; Tomuta, I.; Popa, D.-S. Enhanced Recovery of Phenolic and Tocopherolic Compounds from Walnut (*Juglans Regia* L.) Male Flowers Based on Process Optimization of Ultrasonic Assisted-Extraction: Phytochemical Profile and Biological Activities. *Antioxidants* **2021**, *10*, 607. [CrossRef] [PubMed]
24. Toiu, A.; Mocan, A.; Vlase, L.; Pârvu, A.E.; Vodnar, D.C.; Gheldiu, A.-M.; Moldovan, C.; Oniga, I. Comparative Phytochemical Profile, Antioxidant, Antimicrobial and In Vivo Anti-Inflammatory Activity of Different Extracts of Traditionally Used Romanian *Ajuga genevensis* L. and *A. reptans* L. (Lamiaceae). *Molecules* **2019**, *24*, 1597. [CrossRef] [PubMed]
25. Rusu, M.E.; Fizeșan, I.; Pop, A.; Gheldiu, A.-M.; Mocan, A.; Crișan, G.; Vlase, L.; Loghin, F.; Popa, D.-S.; Tomuta, I. Enhanced Recovery of Antioxidant Compounds from Hazelnut (*Corylus avellana* L.) Involucre Based on Extraction Optimization: Phytochemical Profile and Biological Activities. *Antioxidants* **2019**, *8*, 460. [CrossRef] [PubMed]
26. Matuschek, E.; Brown, D.F.J.; Kahlmeter, G. Development of the EUCAST disk diffusion antimicrobial susceptibility testing method and its implementation in routine microbiology laboratories. *Clin. Microbiol. Infect.* **2014**, *20*, O255–O266. [CrossRef] [PubMed]
27. Moldovan, B.; Filip, A.; Clichici, S.; Suharoschi, R.; Bolfa, P.; David, L. Antioxidant activity of Cornelian cherry (*Cornus mas* L.) fruits extract and the in vivo evaluation of its anti-inflammatory effects. *J. Funct. Foods* **2016**, *26*, 77–87. [CrossRef]
28. Patil, C.R.; Gadekar, A.R.; Patel, P.N.; Rambhade, A.; Surana, S.J.; Gaushal, M.H. Dual effect of *Toxicodendron pubescens* on Carrageenan induced paw edema in rats. *Homeopathy* **2009**, *98*, 88–91. [CrossRef]
29. Conti, M.; Morand, P.C.; Levillain, P.; Lemonnier, A. Improved fluorometric determination of malonaldehyde. *Clin. Chem.* **1991**, *37*, 1273–1275. [CrossRef]
30. Hu, M.-L. Measurement of protein thiol groups and glutathione in plasma. *Methods Enzymol.* **1994**, *233*, 380–385. [CrossRef]
31. Tundis, R.; Marrelli, M.; Conforti, F.; Tenuta, M.C.; Bonesi, M.; Menichini, F.; Loizzo, M.R. *Trifolium pratense* and *T. repens* (Leguminosae): Edible Flower Extracts as Functional Ingredients. *Foods* **2015**, *4*, 338–348. [CrossRef] [PubMed]
32. Akbaribazm, M.; Khazaei, M.R.; Khazaei, M. Phytochemicals and antioxidant activity of alcoholic/hydroalcoholic extract of *Trifolium pratense*. *Chin. Herb. Med.* **2020**, *12*, 326–335. [CrossRef] [PubMed]
33. Mikhailov, A.L.; Timofeeva, O.A.; Ogorodnova, U.A.; Stepanov, N.S. Comparative analysis of biologically active substances in *Trifolium pratense* and *Trifolium repens* depending on the growing conditions. *J. Environ. Treat Technol.* **2019**, *7*, 874–877.
34. Vlaisavljević, S.; Kaurinović, B.; Popović, M.; Vasiljević, S. Profile of phenolic compounds in *Trifolium pratense* L. extracts at different growth stages and their biological activities. *Int. J. Food Prop.* **2017**, *20*, 3090–3101. [CrossRef]
35. Zgórka, G. Ultrasound-assisted solid-phase extraction coupled with photodiode-array and fluorescence detection for chemotaxonomy of isoflavone phytoestrogens in *Trifolium* L. (Clover) species. *J. Sep. Sci.* **2009**, *32*, 965–972. [CrossRef]
36. Zgórka, G. Pressurized liquid extraction versus other extraction techniques in micropreparative isolation of pharmacologically active isoflavones from *Trifolium* L. species. *Talanta* **2009**, *79*, 46–53. [CrossRef]

37. Visnevschi-Necrasov, T.; Cunha, S.C.; Nunes, E.; Oliveira, M.B.P. Optimization of matrix solid-phase dispersion extraction method for the analysis of isoflavones in *Trifolium pratense*. *J. Chromatogr. A* **2009**, *1216*, 3720–3724. [CrossRef]
38. Reis, A.; Scopel, M.; Zuanazzi, J.A.S. *Trifolium pratense*: Friable calli, cell culture protocol and isoflavones content in wild plants, in vitro and cell cultures analyzed by UPLC. *Rev. Bras. Farm.* **2018**, *28*, 542–550. [CrossRef]
39. Hanganu, D.; Vlase, L.; Olah, N. LC/MS analysis of isoflavones from Fabaceae species extracts. *Farmacia* **2010**, *58*, 177–183.
40. Khameneh, B.; Iranshahy, M.; Soheili, V.; Bazzaz, B.S.F. Review on plant antimicrobials: A mechanistic viewpoint. *Antimicrob. Resist. Infect. Control.* **2019**, *8*, 118. [CrossRef]
41. Khan, A.V.; Ahmed, Q.U.; Shukla, I.; Khan, A.A. Antibacterial activity of leaves extracts of *Trifolium alexandrinum* Linn. against pathogenic bacteria causing tropical diseases. *Asian Pac. J. Trop. Biomed.* **2012**, *2*, 189–194. [CrossRef] [PubMed]
42. Kishore, N.; Kumar, P.; Shanker, K.; Verma, A.K. Human disorders associated with inflammation and the evolving role of natural products to overcome. *Eur. J. Med. Chem.* **2019**, *179*, 272–309. [CrossRef]
43. Hwang, J.H.; Ma, J.N.; Park, J.H.; Jung, H.W.; Park, Y. Anti-inflammatory and antioxidant effects of MOK, a polyherbal extract, on lipopolysaccharide-stimulated RAW 264.7 macrophages. *Int. J. Mol. Med.* **2018**, *43*, 26–36. [CrossRef] [PubMed]
44. Kolodziejczyk-Czepas, J. Trifolium species-derived substances and extracts—Biological activity and prospects for medicinal applications. *J. Ethnopharmacol.* **2012**, *143*, 14–23. [CrossRef] [PubMed]
45. Sarfraz, A.; Javeed, M.; Shah, M.A.; Hussain, G.; Shafiq, N.; Sarfraz, I.; Riaz, A.; Sadiqa, A.; Zara, R.; Zafar, S.; et al. Biochanin A: A novel bioactive multifunctional compound from nature. *Sci. Total. Environ.* **2020**, *722*, 137907. [CrossRef]
46. Raheja, S.; Girdhar, A.; Lather, V.; Pandita, D. Biochanin A: A phytoestrogen with therapeutic potential. *Trends Food Sci. Technol.* **2018**, *79*, 55–66. [CrossRef]
47. Kim, Y.; Oh, Y.J.; Han, K.Y.; Kim, G.H.; Ko, J.; Park, J. The complete chloroplast genome sequence of *Hibiscus syriacus* L. 'Mamonde' (*Malvaceae*). *Mitochondrial DNA Part B* **2019**, *4*, 558–559. [CrossRef]

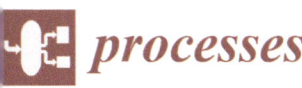

Article

Novel Semisynthetic Betulinic Acid—Triazole Hybrids with In Vitro Antiproliferative Potential

Gabriela Nistor [1,2], Alexandra Mioc [2,3,*], Marius Mioc [1,2], Mihaela Balan-Porcarasu [4], Roxana Ghiulai [2,5], Roxana Racoviceanu [1,2], Ștefana Avram [2,6], Alexandra Prodea [1,2], Alexandra Semenescu [2,7], Andreea Milan [1,2], Cristina Dehelean [2,7] and Codruța Șoica [2,5]

[1] Department of Pharmaceutical Chemistry, Faculty of Pharmacy, "Victor Babeș" University of Medicine and Pharmacy Timisoara, Eftimie Murgu Square, No. 2, 300041 Timisoara, Romania
[2] Research Centre for Pharmaco–Toxicological Evaluation, "Victor Babeș" University of Medicine and Pharmacy, Eftimie Murgu Square, No. 2, 300041 Timisoara, Romania
[3] Department of Anatomy, Physiology, Pathophysiology, Faculty of Pharmacy, Victor Babeș University of Medicine and Pharmacy, Eftimie Murgu Square, No. 2, 300041 Timisoara, Romania
[4] Institute of Macromolecular Chemistry 'Petru Poni', 700487 Iasi, Romania
[5] Department of Pharmacology–Pharmacotherapy, Victor Babeș University of Medicine and Pharmacy, 2nd Eftimie Murgu Square, No. 2, 300041 Timisoara, Romania
[6] Deparment of Pharmacognosy, Faculty of Pharmacy, Victor Babeș University of Medicine and Pharmacy, Eftimie Murgu Square, No. 2, 300041 Timisoara, Romania
[7] Department of Toxicology, Faculty of Pharmacy, "Victor Babeș" University of Medicine and Pharmacy, Eftimie Murgu Square, No. 2, 300041 Timisoara, Romania
* Correspondence: alexandra.mioc@umft.ro; Tel.: +40-256-494-604

Abstract: Betulinic acid, BA, is a lupane derivative that has caught the interest of researchers due to the wide variety of pharmacological properties it exhibits towards tumor cells. Because of their prospective increased anti–proliferative efficacy and improved pharmacological profile, BA derivatives continue to be described in the scientific literature. The current work was conducted in order to determine the antiproliferative activity, under an in vitro environment of the newly developed 1,2,4–triazole derivatives of BA. The compounds and their reaction intermediates were tested on three cancer cell lines, namely RPMI–7951 human malignant melanoma, HT–29 colorectal adenocarcinoma, A549 lung carcinoma, and healthy cell line (HaCaT human keratinocytes). BA–triazole derivatives 4a and 4b revealed lower IC_{50} values in almost all cases when compared to their precursors, exhibiting the highest cytotoxicity against the RPMI–7951 cell line (IC_{50}: 18.8 μM for 4a and 20.7 μM for 4b). Further biological assessment of these compounds executed on the most affected cell line revealed a mitochondrial level induced apoptotic mechanism where both compounds inhibited mitochondrial respiration in RPMI–7951 cells. Furthermore, the triazole–BA derivatives caused a significant decrease of the anti–apoptotic Bcl–2 gene expression, while increasing the pro–apoptotic BAX gene's expression.

Keywords: betulinic acid–triazole derivatives; antiproliferative; cytotoxicity; melanoma; lung carcinoma; colorectal adenocarcinoma

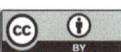

1. Introduction

Cancer chemotherapy has transformed cancer outcomes from terminal to treatable, or even curable; since its beginning, anticancer chemotherapy has evolved based on the continuous discovery in cancer cell biology so that today multitargeted therapy is being used [1]. However, the side effects of the anticancer drug therapy are often very severe, therefore the interests of oncologists have shifted from merely treating the tumor towards well–tolerated approaches [2]. Although belonging to traditional medicine, plant–derived compounds are currently recognized as reliable alternatives in the field of oncology considering their particular structures and mechanisms of action, which recommends them as alternatives to avoid the limitations of conventional chemotherapy [3]. There are many classes of phytocompounds that have been used as such or served as scaffolds for the development of semisynthetic derivatives with antitumor properties or able to act as drug sensitizers.

Pentacyclic triterpenes are biologically active phytochemicals found in higher plants, exhibiting a huge plethora of biological effects that include anti−inflammatory and antitumor activities and containing lupane, oleanane, and ursane as the main scaffolds [4]. Betulinic acid is a lupane derivative which gained immense interest in the medical field not only due to its plethora of pharmacological effects but mainly due to its selective cytotoxicity against tumor cells; nonetheless, it demonstrates two major drawbacks: the low water solubility, which affects its bioavailability, and its insufficient supply from natural sources [5]. Therefore, the chemical modulation of various positions in betulinic acid, together with the development of new preparation methods from more abundantly found compounds such as botulin, have paved the way to achieve semisynthetic derivatives able to overcome the above−mentioned bottlenecks. The main molecular positions susceptible to modulation are the C_3, C_{28} sites, ring A, as well as the C_{20-29} double bond; recent research emphasized that modifications on ring A and C_{20-29} double bond could significantly augment betulinic acid's biological effects (Figure 1) [6].

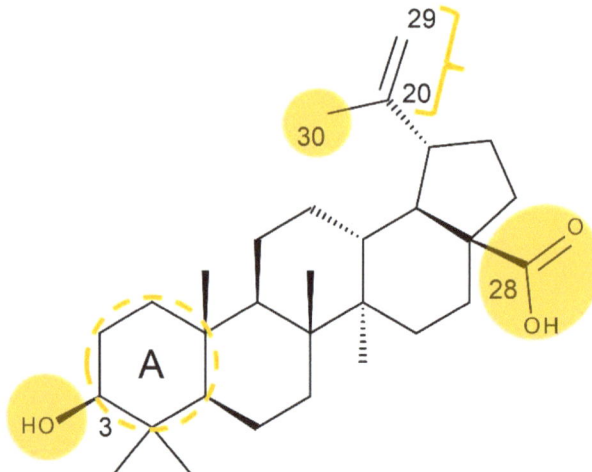

Figure 1. The main structural sites of betulinic acid susceptible to chemical modulation.

Among the many derivatization possibilities, the substitution with nitrogen−bearing heterocycles generates the most valuable agents within the medicinal chemistry; currently more than 75% of FDA approved marketed drugs bear nitrogen−containing heterocycles, while more such compounds will presumably soon reach the pharmaceutical market [7]. Such 1,2,3−triazole derivatives prepared from betulinic acid using click chemistry at C_3 were revealed as effective anti−leukemia agents with remarkably small IC_{50} values (within the micromolar range), thus showing a 5–7 fold increased potency compared to the parent compound (Figure 2) [8].

Similar compounds were also synthesized by Shi et al. with compound 30−[4−(4−fluorophenyl)−1H−1,2,3−triazol−1−yl] betulinic acid showing the highest potency as revealed by the IC_{50} value of 1.3 µM [9]. The Huisgen 1,3−cycloaddition was used to prepare 1,2,3−triazole derivatives at C_{30} via the corresponding azides in the structure of betulinic acid, simultaneously conjugated at C_3; the most active derivatives revealed IC_{50} values below 10 µM [10]. Functionalized triazole derivatives of betulinic acid were obtained by means of click cycloaddition through the modulation of the C_{28}−carboxyle group; the study revealed two series of lead compounds as anticancer agents against murine breast cancer and human pancreatic cancer [11]. Sousa et al. published in 2019 a comprehensive review emphasizing the main chemical processes able to functionalize betulinic acid and several related compounds [12]; various modulations were applied starting from simple transformations and click chemistry reactions and reaching complex molecules such as heterocycle−fused derivatives and polymer conjugates.

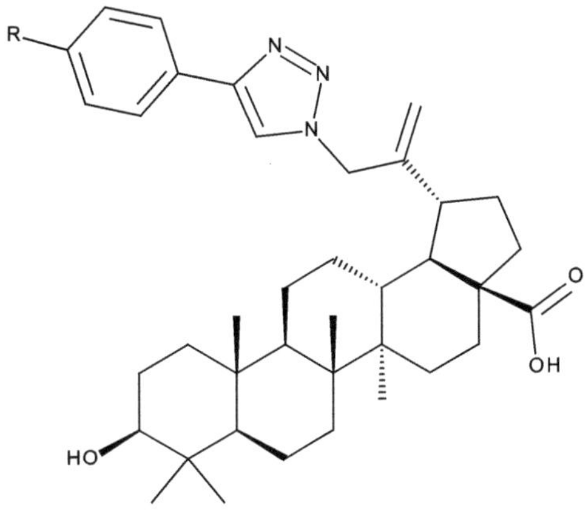

Figure 2. 1,2,3−triazole−substituted derivatives of BA acid synthesized via click chemistry acting as effective anti−leukemia agents.

The current study is a continuation of the previously published paper [13], which reported the cytotoxic activity of a C_3−acetylated 1,2,4−triazole derivative of BA; the compound revealed significant and selective cytotoxic effects against melanoma cells through mitochondrial apoptosis. Some studies reported that by inserting aryl groups as substituents in the triazole moiety grafted at C_{30} it may increase the antitumor activity of the resulting compounds [9,10]; on the contrary, when modulating the carboxyl group at C_{28}, the cytotoxic activity increased with the increase of the molecule's hydrophilic character imprinted partially by the triazole substituent. In order to clarify the impact of such C_{30}−substitutions on the compound's cytotoxic activity, the current study aims to synthesize some derivatives of betulinic acid bearing the 1,2,4−triazole ring supplementary substituted with an aryl group by the chemical modulation of C_{30}, followed by their physicochemical characterization. Subsequently, the semisynthetic derivatives will be biologically tested in terms of cell viability; moreover, since their previously published triazole analogue revealed a pro−apoptotic activity, we aimed to identify the underlying anticancer mechanism by performing DAPI staining, respirometry studies and rt−PCR assay.

2. Results

2.1. Chemistry

The synthetic preparation, together with the reaction media necessary to obtain BA−triazole derivatives (**4a, 4b**), are shown in Figure 3. Using modifications of previously reported methods [14,15], good yields (> 50%) were achieved for the triazole derivatives (**3a, 3b**) and the brominated acetyl−BA (**2**). In comparison to earlier steps, the alkylation of the thiol group on the triazole structure (**3a, 3b**) using BrBA in DMF/K_2CO_3 resulted in lower yields of BA−TZ derivatives (**4a, 4b**). Although the precursors were rather pure, TLC analysis showed that the reaction resulted in at least two additional major compounds among the many lipophilic side products. Despite this, the chromatographic separation (chloroform:acetate 1:1 eluent) remained feasible due to the substantial Rf value differences. The structure of all synthesized compounds was validated through ^{1}H and ^{13}C NMR spectroscopy. All spectral data is available in the Supplementary Materials File uploaded with the present manuscript.

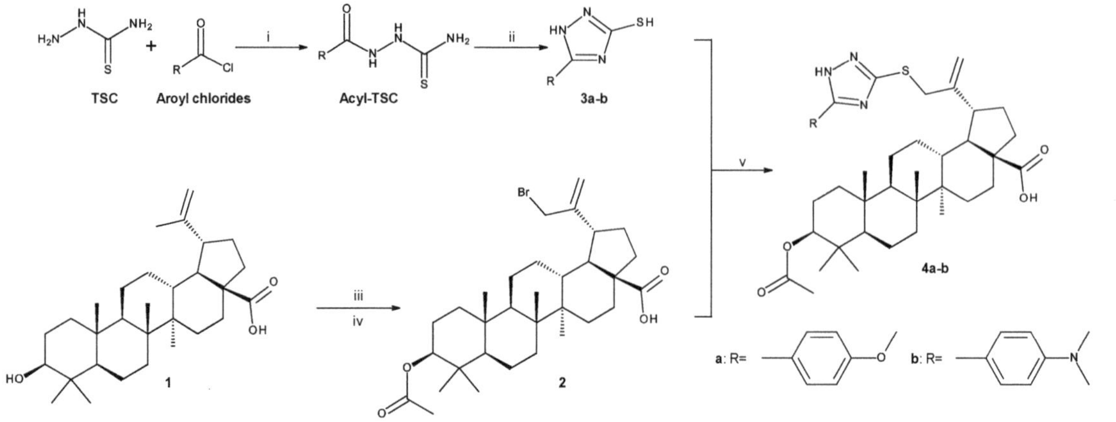

Figure 3. Synthesis pathways used to obtain BA−triazol derivatives; TSC = thiosemicarbazide, **1**—betulinic acid, **2**—3β−O−Acetyl−30−bromo−betulinic acid, **3a**—5−(4−methoxyphenyl)−1H−1,2,4−triazole−3−thiol, **3b** − 5−[4−(dimethylamino)phenyl]−1H−1,2,4−triazole−3−thiol, **4a**—3β−O−Acetyl−30−[5−(4−methoxyphenyl)−1H−1,2,4−triazol−3−ylsulfanyl]−betulinic acid, **4b**—3β−O−Acetyl−30−{5−[4−(dimethylamino)phenyl]−1H−1,2,4−triazol−3−yl)sulfanyl}−betulinic acid; reaction conditions: i. pyridine/DMF, 1h, 50 °C; ii. H$_2$O, NaOH, reflux; iii. acetic anhydride, pyridine, DMAP, r.t, 12 h; iv. NBS, CCl$_4$, r.t, 48 h; v. DMF, K$_2$CO$_3$, r.t, 72 h.

2.2. BA Triazole Derivatives Decrease Cell Viability of Malignant Melanoma Cells

Following a 48 h treatment period, the effect of **4a**, **4b**, as well as their precursors (0.08, 0.4, 2, 10, and 50 µM) in HaCaT healthy human keratinocytes, RPMI−7951 malignant melanoma, A549 lung carcinoma, and HT−29 colorectal adenocarcinoma cells was determined by employing the MTT assay, which enabled the calculation of IC$_{50}$ values (Table 1); the recorded viability in all tested cell lines is depicted in Figure 4. Among all the cell lines, malignant melanoma (RPMI−7951) proved to be the most sensitive toward the BA derivatives, in particular compound **4a**, which showed the maximum cytotoxic effect; thus, RPMI−7951 was chosen for further detailed study regarding the compounds **4a** and **4b** cytotoxic mechanism.

Table 1. IC$_{50}$ (µM) values of **4a**, **4b**, and their intermediates against normal and cancer cell lines; compounds displaying IC$_{50}$ values above 50 µM were considered not effective and, therefore, the specific values were not shown.

Compound	HaCaT	RPMI−7951	A549	HT−29
	IC$_{50}$ (µM/L) ± SD			
1	>50	30.8 ± 3.63	44.3 ± 6.81	>50
2	>50	29.7 ± 3.96	22.6 ± 3.01	26.4 ± 2.74
3a	>50	>50	>50	>50
3b	>50	>50	>50	>50
4a	>50	19.8 ± 2.25	28.3 ± 3.21	36.9 ± 4.57
4b	>50	20.7 ± 2.21	32.4 ± 3.68	31.3 ± 4.02
5FU	30.5 ± 2.8	19.5 ± 1.72	6.9 ± 0.92	>50

Available literature data as well as our own previous experiments revealed that 0.5% DMSO did not affect cell viability [16,17]. Subsequently we used DMSO−stimulated cells (at 0.5%) as negative control. All cytotoxic active compounds exhibited a dose dependent activity (Figure 4). The starting compound, BA (**1**), and its brominated derivative, compound **2**, had a significant activity on all tested cancer cell lines except HT−29, where BA was not effective, while the starting triazoles 3a and 3b did not exhibit IC_{50} values under 50 µM (Table 1). The BA−triazole derivatives (compounds **4a** and **4b**) displayed lower IC_{50} values against all tested cell lines, as opposed to their precursors, with one exception where compound **2** acted slightly stronger in HT−29 cells. Simultaneously, among all tested cell lines, **4a** and **4b** were the most effective against RPMI−7951 cells, exhibiting IC_{50} values of 19.8 ± 2.25 µM and 20.7 ± 2.21 µM, respectively. The cytotoxicity of compounds **4a** and **4b** was compared to the positive control 5−fluorouracil (5FU). While 5FU was inactive in A549 lung cancer cells, no compounds were revealed to surpass 5FU in HT−29 cells. However, in the case of RPMI−7951 melanoma cell line, compound **4a** exhibited a similar IC_{50} (19.8 µM) value when compared to the positive control 5FU (19.5 µM). These results suggested a high cytotoxic effect of compounds 4a and 4b against the RPMI−7951 melanoma cell line.

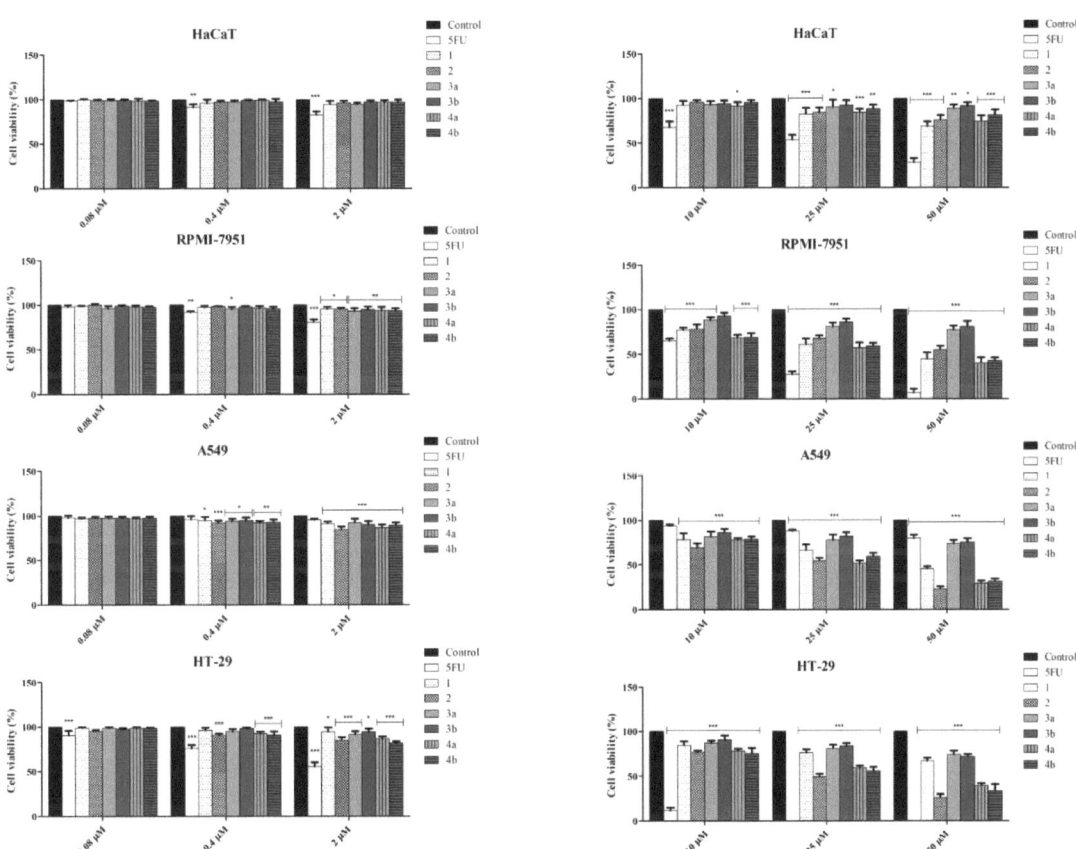

Figure 4. MTT assay assessed the cell viability of HaCaT, RPMI−7951, A549, and HT−29 cell lines after 48 h treatment with compounds **1–4b** at 6 different concentrations. Negative control: untreated cells. Positive control: 5FU. All results are expressed as percentages in cell viability (%) taking negative control (DMSO-stimulated cells) as reference. All experiments were performed in triplicate and data are presented as mean values ± SD. The statistical differences compared to negative control were identified through two-way ANOVA analysis followed by Bonferroni's multiple comparisons post-test (* $p < 0.05$, ** $p < 0.005$, and *** $p < 0.0001$).

2.3. BA Triazole Derivatives Induce Nuclear Alterations Associated with Apoptosis in Malignant Melanoma Cells

Considering the high antiproliferative effect at the lowest IC_{50}, the biological effects of compounds **4a** and **4b** were further investigated by assessing their effect on nuclear morphology using the DAPI staining. This particular dye that identifies nuclear modifications was employed, revealing that all tested compounds induced nuclei morphological changes, including shrinkage and fragmentation accompanied by the disruption of the cell membrane. All these changes were consistent with apoptotic processes; unlike necrotic processes where the nuclei stay relatively intact, in apoptosis the nucleus undergoes early degeneration and its morphological changes can be used as indicators of programmed cell death [18]. The morphological alterations in various degrees are presented by the yellow arrows in Figure 5, demonstrating changes that were consistent with apoptotic cell death, while apoptotic signs were not present on normal human keratinocytes (HaCaT).

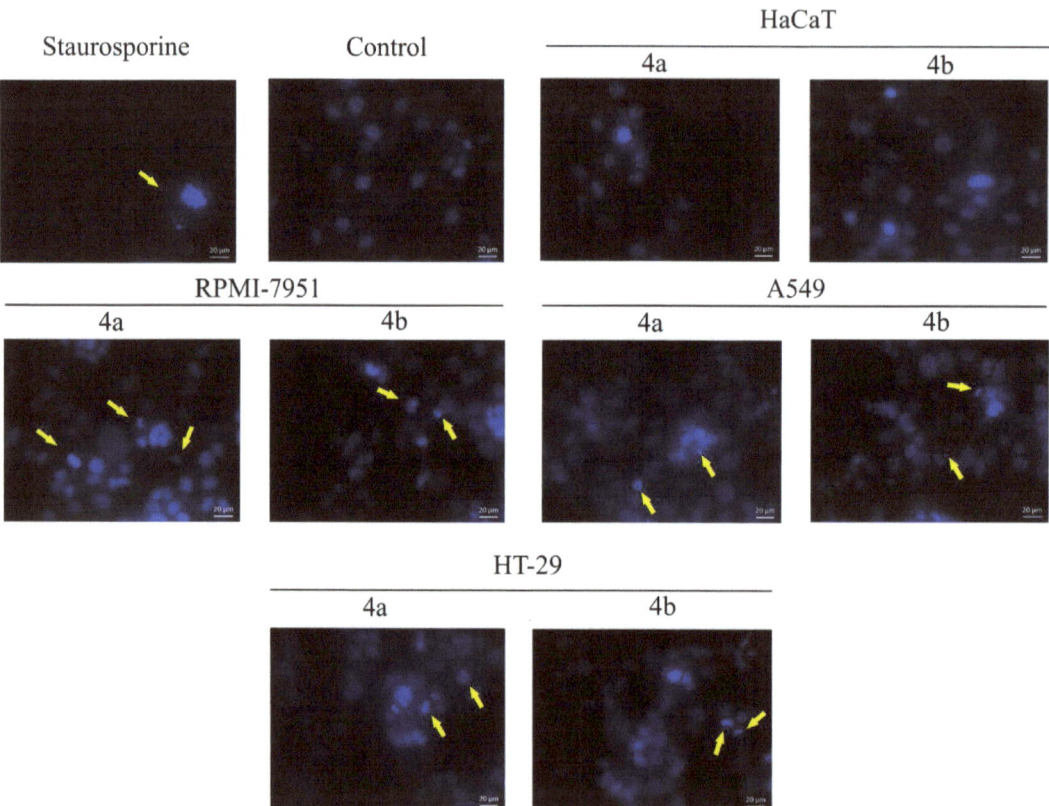

Figure 5. Morphological observation of HaCaT, RPMI−7951, A549, and HT−29 cell lines using DAPI assay, following treatment with **4a** and **4b** (tested at their respective IC_{50}) for 48 h. Positive control for nuclei apoptotic changes: staurosporine (5 μM). The apoptotic morphological changes are indicated by yellow arrows.

2.4. Compounds **4a** and **4b** Influence the Expression of Anti−Apoptotic (Bcl−2) and Pro−Apoptotic (BAX) Genes

In order to investigate the apoptotic activity of compounds **4a** and **4b** in RPMI−7951 melanoma cells, the gene expression fold change of Bcl−2 and BAX was assessed by using the quantitative real−time PCR method. Measurements were conducted after a 48 h incubation period with the tested compounds. The compounds were tested at 18.8 µM and 20.7 µM, respectively, with values that induced a 50% reduction in RPMI−7951 melanoma cell viability. The results revealed that both compounds caused the upregulation of BAX gene expression vs. control (Figure 6) thus indicating a pro−apoptotic effect. Specifically, the highest effect was observed for compound **4a** (3.892), followed by compound **4b** (2.594) vs. control (1). Upon evaluating the relative fold change expression in Bcl−2 mRNA, compound **4a** determined the strongest decrease (0.275), while compound **4b** decreased only to 0.505 vs. control (1) (Figure 5).

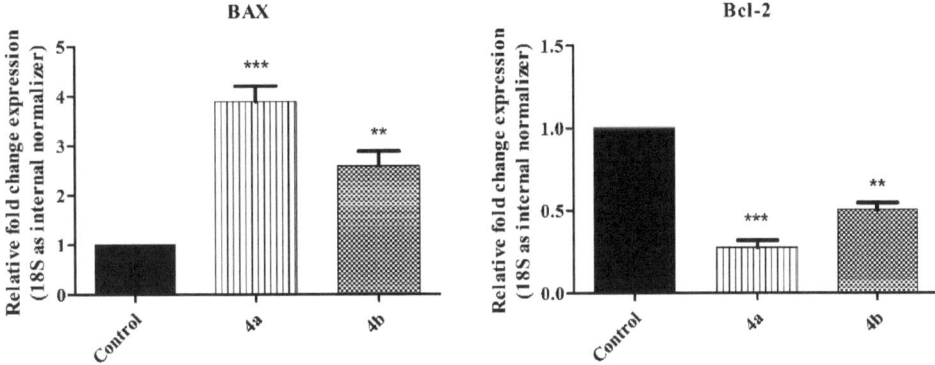

Figure 6. The difference in Bcl−2 and BAX mRNA expressions in RPMI−7951 cells following treatment with **4a** and **4b** (tested at IC$_{50}$: 18.8 µM and IC$_{50}$: 20.7 µM) for 48 h. The fold change expressions were compared to 18S RNA, while DMSO acted as the control. All experiments were performed in triplicate and the results were reported as mean values ± SD. Statistical differences vs. DMSO stimulated cells were determined using one−way ANOVA with Dunnett's post−test (** $p < 0.01$ and *** $p < 0.001$).

2.5. BA Triazole Derivatives Disrupt Mitochondrial Function of Melanoma Cells

The evaluation of mitochondrial function after the treatment with **4a** and **4b** at their IC$_{50}$ values revealed the inhibition of mitochondrial respiration of RPMI−7951 cells, while normal HaCaT cells' mitochondrial respiration remained unaffected (Figures 7 and 8). As presented in Figure 7, treatment of normal HaCaT cells with either compound did not affect the mitochondrial respiration. The expanded SUIT technique was performed to permeabilized HaCaT as well as RPMI−7951 cells; mitochondrial respiratory rates assessed at 37 °C demonstrated that all chemicals can severely impair RPMI−7951 mitochondrial activity (Figure 8), while having no evident effect on HaCaT mitochondria. In particular, one mitochondrial parameter reduced by semisynthetic derivatives was routine respiration, which was solely dependent on endogenous ADP. Later, digitonine was used to permeabilize the cell membrane in order to assess the expanded OXPHOS (oxidative phosphorylation) and enable the molecular transit between external environment and cytoplasm. Following that, both basal and LEAK respiration was dramatically reduced, suggesting that the compounds may reduce the basal respiration. Tested at 18.8 µM (the IC$_{50}$ value for **4a**) and 20.7 µM (the IC$_{50}$ value for **4b**), the compounds considerably suppressed the OXPHOS respiration reliant on glutamate and malate substrates for complex I (OXPHOSCI) and the OXPHOS when succinate, a complex II substrate, was added (OXPHOSCI + II). The electron transport system's maximum respiratory capacity in the complete noncoupled state (ETSCI + II) could be measured by quantifying the uncoupled state via FCCP titration. Compounds **4a** and **4b** were able to decrease the ETSCI + II and ETSCII, thus suggesting that they might lower the electron transport pathway capacity and impair ATP production. The mean values of the respiratory rates [pmol/(s × mL)] obtained after the treatment of RPMI−7951 cells with compounds **4a** and **4b** are presented in Table 2.

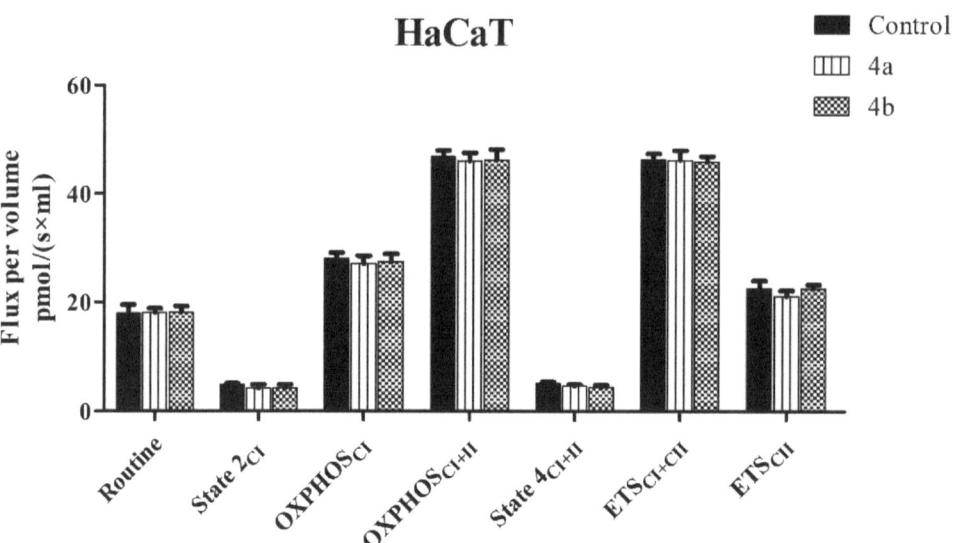

Figure 7. Rates of mitochondrial respiration measured in permeabilized HaCaT cells after treatment with compounds **4a** and **4b** (tested at IC$_{50}$: 18.8 µM and IC$_{50}$: 20.7 µM) for 48 h. All experiments were repeated five times and the results are reported as mean values ± SD. One–way ANOVA followed by Bonferroni's post–test were used in order to identify statistical differences vs. control ($p > 0.05$ implies no significant differences).

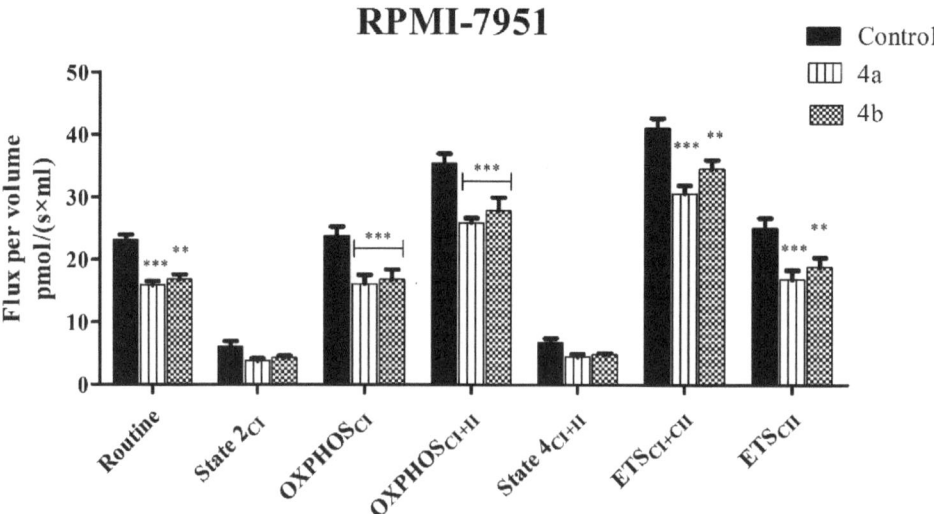

Figure 8. The rates of mitochondrial respiration in permeabilized RPMI–7951 cells after treatment with compounds **4a** and **4b** (tested at IC$_{50}$: 18.8 µM and IC$_{50}$: 20.7 µM, respectively) for 48 h. All experiments were repeated five times and the results are reported as mean values ± SD. One–way ANOVA followed by Bonferroni's post–test were used in order to identify statistical differences vs. control (** $p < 0.01$ and *** $p < 0.001$).

Table 2. Mitochondrial respiratory rates of RPMI−9751 cells treated with compounds **4a** and **4b**.

	RPMI−7951		
	Control	**4a**	**4b**
Routine	22.95	15.947	16.79
State 2CI	6.28	3.82	4.30
OXPHOSCI	24.22	15.96	16.83
OXPHOSCI + II	34.71	25.92	26.85
State 4CI + II	6.35	4.47	4.81
ETSCI + CII	42.08	30.52	31.36
ETSCII	24.87	16.49	17.83

2.6. Irritative Potential of BA Triazole Derivatives

The HET−CAM assay was involved in assessing the toxicological potential of compounds **4a**−**4b**. As presented in Figure 9, the investigated compounds did not interfere with the circulation process and did not produce any impairment on the vascular plexus.

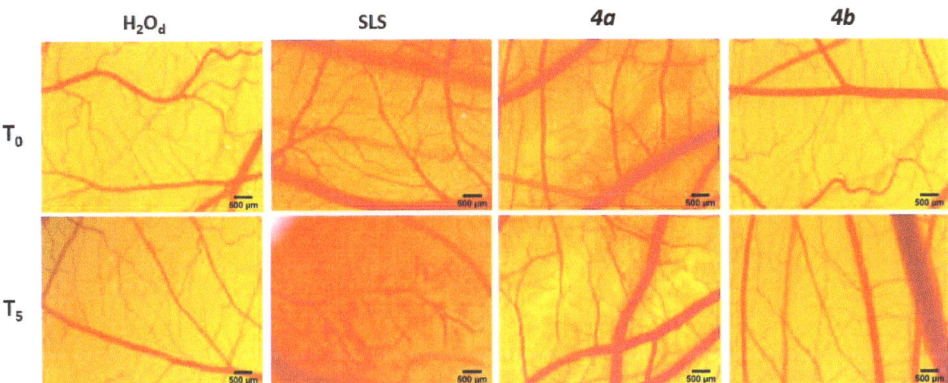

Figure 9. The irritation assessment using the HET−CAM method. Stereomicroscope images of the chorioallantoic membrane were taken before (T_0) and 300 s (T_5) after treatment with 300 μL compounds **4a** and **4b**, respectively (tested at IC_{50}: 18.8 μM and IC_{50}: 20.7 μM); distilled water was used as negative control while SLS 0.5% acted as positive control). Scale bars represent 500 μm.

The irritation potential was assessed on the Luepke scale that assigned scores between 0 and 21 according to the severity of the reaction as follows: non-irritant compounds classified between 0 and 0.9, a slight irritation was indicated by 1–4.9 values, 5–8.9 ranging values depicted moderate irritation, while strongly irritant compounds reached 9–21 values [19]. As presented in Table 3, the tested compounds did not show any irritation potential, and therefore, were suitable for mucosal and cutaneous use. These findings were noteworthy because pentacyclic triterpenes and their derivatives were known to be active in wound healing and re-epithelization. Compounds with no irritative potential, such as the BA structurally related triterpene, betulin, were currently being studied as topical formulations in phase III clinical trials for their accelerated re-epithelization effects and efficacy against epidermolysis bullosa [20,21].

Table 3. The irritation potential of tested compounds.

Compound Name	Irritation Score	Effect
H_2O_d	0	Non-irritant
SLS	15.3	Strong irritant
4a	0	Non-irritant
4b	0	Non-irritant

3. Discussions

Lately, a huge amount of interest has been raised by the potent and targeted antitumor effect of betulinic acid, a phytocompound identified by Pisha et al. in 1995 as an antimelanoma agent [22]. The precise underlying mechanisms have yet to be fully understood, although many possibilities have been proposed, including various signaling pathways involved in mitochondrial apoptotic death [23]. During research, poor water solubility and, subsequently, low bioavailability were revealed as the main flaws that hampered the therapeutic use of betulinic acid as an anticancer agent. There were multiple possibilities to improve the phytocompound's aqueous solubility, including structural modifications, which may simultaneously improve the overall antitumor efficacy [6].

The triazole moiety was involved in numerous functionalizations due to its polar character, as well as its ability to form non-covalent interactions with targeted ligands, thus exhibiting pharmacophore properties. However, the introduction of a triazole moiety at C_{30} in BA's molecule was only performed twice: by Shi et al. and Sidova et al. [9,10], by applying click chemistry on betulinic acid's C_{30}−bromo derivatives; both groups used the 1,2,3−triazole moiety. As far as we are aware, C_{30}−1,2,4−triazole derivatives were only developed by our group, using the unsubstituted triazole as a reaction partner for the brominated betulinic acid [13]. The resulted derivative revealed antitumor effects against melanoma cells exerted through apoptotic mechanisms.

Continuing our research, we tried to develop betulinic acid derivatives using aryl substituted−triazole moieties. The cytotoxic activities of both derivatives, as well as their parent compounds were tested by means of MTT assay, in order to quantitatively assess the change in cytotoxicity, induced by the chemical modulations, against various cancer cells. In our current study, we used a 50 µM threshold for IC_{50} values, above which we considered the cytotoxicity of any particular compound to be insignificant. In all tested settings, the starting triazoles (3a–b) did not exhibit IC_{50} values less than 50 µM. This is consistent with previous findings by our group on melanoma and colorectal cancer cell lines using structurally similar 1,2,4−triazole−3−derivatives [14,24], where the most active 1,2,4−triazole derivative exhibited an IC_{50} value 149.25 µM. Meanwhile, both BA−triazole derivatives (4a–b) increased cytotoxicity in all tested malignant cells, except for HT−29 cells, where the 30−brominated BA derivative was slightly more active. The RPMI melanoma cell line was the most affected by compound 4a and 4b's induced cytotoxic properties. These effects seem to be triggered by the presence of the triazole moiety that also revealed cytotoxic activity but to a lesser extent; therefore, we may assume that the triazole ring was included in the pharmacophore constellation of atoms in the molecule of betulinic acid. These results were supported by Sidova et al. who reported that the modification of the C_{30} position combined with the presence of an aromatic substituent on the triazole group was part of the pharmacophore being responsible for the compounds' cytotoxicity [10]. In this case, a 1,2,3−triazole − BA derivative with a p−dimethylamino−phenyl substituent on the triazole ring exhibited a highly similar cytotoxic behavior to our compound 4b against colon and lung cancer cell lines. The compound had an IC_{50} of 26.6 µM against the A549 cell line and 32.9 µM against HCT116 cells. Furthermore, when tested in colon cancer cells, the 3−acetyl−30−brominated BA revealed a higher cytotoxicity (IC_{50} = 15.9 µM) than most other 1,2,3−triazole derivatives, similar to our case, where the same compound (2) acted in a similar manner (IC_{50} = 15.9 µM) [10]. In addition, the presence of an acetyl group at C_3

provided the molecule with the necessary degree of lipophilicity to be able to penetrate cell membranes and exert their biological effects; the above–cited study revealed that hydroxyl groups may interfere with membrane permeability due to their hydrophilicity. Similarly, Shi et al. revealed that, within C_{30}–triazole substitutions, the cytotoxic activity was favored by the presence of large side chains with lipophilic or aromatic fragments, their antiproliferative effects being stronger than those reported for betulinic acid [9]. The introduction of triazole moieties in other positions on the triterpenic scaffold also produced improved cytotoxicity; as such, ursane and lupane triazole–hybrids obtained by the functionalization of the C_{28} carboxyl were identified as effective antitumor agents with IC_{50} values comparable to doxorubicin, while the supplementary C_3–acetyl substituent further increased the cytotoxic effect, the respective derivatives becoming more cytotoxic than doxorubicin [25]. Unfortunately, no other triazole derivatives of betulinic acid, other than the ones mentioned above, had been evaluated against human melanoma in the literature. Given that the triazole moiety was highly likely to enhance the compound's cytotoxicity, the lupane core structure of BA may have been responsible for the slightly increased cytotoxic activity against melanoma. This was consistent with previous findings according to which betulinic acid had similar or slightly higher antimelanoma efficacy versus its activity against various types of colon or lung cancer [26]. For example, data from two studies demonstrated that the IC_{50} values for BA against various types of colorectal and lung cancers ranged between 6.1–12.3 µg/mL for lung cancers and 3.8–16.4 µg/mL for colon cancers, while BA showed slightly lower IC_{50} values (1.5–1.6 µg/mL) against melanoma. BA exhibited the same cytotoxic activity against H460 non–small lung cancer cells (IC_{50} = 1.5 µg/mL) under the same environment [27,28]. With these considerations, we may state that the newly synthesized 1,2,4–triazole compounds were an effective anticancer, especially the antimelanoma agents, owing to their activity both to the triterpene scaffold and the new triazole substitution; their activity was also improved by the presence of the C_3–acetyl moiety that contributed to an adequate membrane penetration.

Keratinocytes are primary cells found in human epidermis that play a role in skin inflammatory response; the immortalized human keratinocytes HaCaT cells were established as the skin model since they do not alter the keratinocyte function [29], cellular responses, or differentiation capacity. Moreover, monolayer HaCaT cell cultures are currently used to test cellular toxicity and to conduct in vitro wound healing analysis [30]. In HaCaT cells, neither compounds **4a–b** nor their intermediates have IC_{50} values less than 50 µM, indicating no increased cytotoxicity. The C_{28}–benzotriazole esters of the three triterpenic acids showed similar outcomes, with all compounds exhibiting high levels of antitumor selectivity [31].

Very early studies on betulinic acid's antitumor mechanisms revealed its capacity to induce mitochondrial apoptosis [32]; many of its derivatives also revealed pro–apoptotic properties [33–35]. Therefore, we hypothesized that the BA triazole derivatives **4a** and **4b** synthesized in the current study, will act by similar mechanisms; subsequently, DAPI staining revealed apoptotic signs in all treated cancer cells. To further validate DAPI results, RPMI–7951 melanoma cells were subjected to quantitative real–time PCR in order to assess the variations in Bcl–2 and BAX gene expressions. Both compounds induced the upregulation of BAX accompanied by the downregulation of Bcl–2 genes, thus showing a clear pro–apoptotic activity. These results were consistent with similar reports regarding the parent structure, where BA was revealed as a strong inhibitor of several signaling pathways, being capable of selective apoptosis induction [36]. A novel triazole derivative of BA induced the scindation of Bcl–2 combined with BAX translocation, finally resulting in a decreased Bcl–2/BAX ratio in leukemia cells [37]. Our own research group already obtained C_{28}–triazole–substituted compounds starting from betulinic acid that acted in a similar manner on the Bcl–2/BAX ratio [31]; in addition, the C_{30}–triazole derivative of BA synthesized by our group [13] also revealed similar results, certifying for the first time that such compounds were able to induce apoptosis. Therefore, our findings were consistent with these previously published data and, due to similar structures to the above–mentioned triazole derivatives, we may assume that the currently reported compounds also caused the disruption of mitochondrial membrane potential.

Subsequently, the mitochondrial function was evaluated through high respirometry after the treatment of both malignant melanoma and normal cells with compounds **4a** and **4b**; the results revealed the inhibition of mitochondrial respiration in RPMI−7951 cells, while normal HaCaT cells mitochondrial respiration remained unaffected. These results were consistent with previous data that reported a decreased mitochondrial activity in A375 melanoma cells for betulinic acid alone; BA considerably reduced all respiratory parameters: routine, baseline, active, leak, and maximum uncoupled respiration [38]. A similar effect in terms of mitochondrial respiration was observed when benzotriazole esters of triterpenic acids were tested against the A375 melanoma cell line; all tested compounds were able to inhibit respiratory rates thus causing mitochondrial dysfunction and cell death [31]. As previously stated, mitochondrial malfunction and ATP production impairment had a beneficial impact in cancer cells, and any drugs that may have generated such alterations at the mitochondrial level could be regarded as prospective cancer therapy approaches.

The HET−CAM assay assessed the irritation potency and toxicity of **4a** and **4b,** which did not interfere with the circulation process and did not produce any impairment on the vascular plexus. The application of CAM assay was an easy way to study intact tissues including capillaries, arteries, and veins; various chemicals may have come in direct contact with CAM, triggering inflammatory reactions such as: hemorrhage, lysis, and coagulation. The test was a reliable opportunity to predict the irritant character of given compounds and could select irritating and non−irritating substances [39]. According to the Luepke score, the tested compounds did not show any irritation potential, and therefore, were suitable for mucosal and cutaneous use.

4. Materials and Methods
4.1. Reagents

All reagents for both chemical and biological procedures were purchased from Sigma Aldrich (Merck KGaA, Darmstadt, Germany) and further used without additional purification.

4.2. Chemistry
4.2.1. Instruments

The NMR spectrometry was conducted by using a Bruker NEO 400 MHz Spectrometer configured with a 5 mm QNP direct detection probe with z−gradients. All spectra were registered within standard parameters in DMSO−d_6 or CDCl$_3$ and calibrated on the solvent residual peak (1H: 2.51 ppm for DMSO−d_6 or 7.26 ppm for CDCl$_3$; ^{13}C: 39.5 ppm for DMSO−d_6 or 77.0 for CDCl$_3$). Melting points were recorded on a Biobase melting point instrument (Biobase Group, Shandong, China); thin−layer chromatography was conducted on 60 F254 silica gel−coated plates (Merck KGaA, Darmstadt, Germany). LC/MS spectra were recorded by using methanolic solutions on an Agilent 6120 Quadrupole LC/MS system (Santa Clara, CA, USA) equipped with a UV detector, an ESI ionization source and a Zorbax Rapid Resolution SB−C18 (1.8 μm; 50 2.1 mm) column in the negative ion mode; the samples were analysed at 0.4 mL/min, 25 °C, and l = 250 nm. The mobile phase contained a 1 mM isocratic combination of 85% methanol with 15% ammonium formate.

4.2.2. General Synthesis for 5−Substituted−1H−1,2,4−Triazole−3−Thiols

The synthesis of 5−R−1,2,4−triazole−3−thiol was accomplished according to previously published protocols [14]. A total of 20 mmoles of thiosemicarbazide were dissolved in 50 mL DMF under magnetic stirring, followed by the addition of 22 mmoles pyridine and 20 mmoles aroyl chloride. Magnetic stirring was continued at room temperature for 30 min before the temperature was raised to 50 °C and maintained for approximately 1 h; the end-point of the reaction was validated by TLC. The resulting aroyl−thiosemicarbazides were precipitated with aqueous HCl, filtered, and dried. 5−substituted−1H−1,2,4−triazole−3−thiols were obtained by cyclizing 10 mmoles of obtained aroyl−tiosemicarbazide in ethanolic NaOH at reflux, until TLC control indicated the end of the reaction. The resulting 5−substituted−1H−1,2,4−triazole−3−thiols were precipitated using HCl.

5−(4−*methoxyphenyl*)−1H−1,2,4−*triazole*−3−*thiol* (**3a**); white powder, m.p. 234−237 °C (uncorrected), yield 60%; ^{1}H NMR (400.13 MHz, DMSO−d_6, δ, ppm): 13.70 (s, 1H), 13.56 (s, 1H), 7.85 (d, J = 8.6 Hz, 2H), 7.07 (d, J = 8.6 Hz, 2H), 3.81 (s, 3H); ^{13}C NMR (100.6 MHz, DMSO−d_6, δ, ppm): 165.6, 161.0, 150.1, 127.3, 117.8, 114.5, 55.4. LC−MS Rt = 0.427 min, m/z = 206 [M−H+]−.

5−[4−(*dimethylamino*)*phenyl*]−1H−1,2,4−*triazole*−3−*thiol* (**3b**); white powder, m.p. 282−287 °C (uncorrected), yield 70%; ^{1}H NMR (400.13 MHz, DMSO−d6, δ, ppm): 13.39 (br s, 2H), 7.72 (d, J = 8.9 Hz, 2H), 6.76 (d, J = 8.9 Hz, 2H), 2.96 (s, 6H); ^{13}C NMR (100.6 MHz, DMSO−d_6, δ, ppm): 165.1, 151.4, 150.9, 126.7, 112.4, 111.7, 39.7 (overlapped with the residual solvent peak). LC−MS Rt = 0.49 min, m/z = 219 [M−H+]−.

4.2.3. Synthesis Procedure for 3β−O−Acetyl−30−Bromobetulinic Acid

BA was subjected to acetylation according to the modified version of the procedure previously described by Petrenko et al. [15], which involved the reaction between **1** (1 Eq) and acetic anhydride (4 Eq) in a medium of pyridine, while also adding DMAP (0.1 Eq); the mixture was stirred for 12 h at room temperature. The resulting mixture was initially diluted with water and further extracted with CHCl$_3$. Anhydrous MgSO$_4$ was used to dry the organic phase, followed by the removal of the remaining solvent in a rotary evaporator. Afterward, 1.78 g of recently recrystallized NBS (10 mmoles) was added to 2.5 g of 3−O−Acetyl−betulinic acid (5 mmoles) that had been solubilized in 50 mL CCl$_4$. The reaction continued under stirring for 48 h at room temperature followed by filtration, solvent removal, and chromatographic separation over silica using a 40:1 volume ratio of CHCl$_3$ and ethyl acetate. The spectral data collected for *3β−O−Acetyl−30−bromobetulinic acid* were reported by our group in a previously published paper [13] and were aligned with the existing literature [10].

4.2.4. General Synthesis for 30−Triazole Substituted BA Derivatives

In total 5 mL DMF were added to 0.3 mmoles anhydrous K$_2$CO$_3$ and 0.2 mmoles 3β−O−Acetyl−30−bromobetulinic acid and magnetically stirred for 10 min at 25 °C; after the addition of 0.2 mmoles 5−R−1H−1,2,4−triazole−3−thiol, the mixture continued to be stirred for another 72 h at 25 °C. In the next step, 50 mL of water were added to the mixture, which was then extracted with CHCl$_3$ (4 × 15 mL). The organic phase was dried using anhydrous MgSO$_4$, the solvent was removed, and the crude product was then chromatographed using 2:1 CHCl$_3$: ethyl acetate (v/v).

3β−O−Acetyl−30−[5−(4−methoxyphenyl)−1H−1,2,4−triazol−3−yl)−sulfanyl]−betulinic acid (**4a**); white crystalline powder, yield 22%; ^{1}H NMR (400.13 MHz, CDCl$_3$, δ, ppm): 8.01 (d, J = 8.5 Hz, 2H), 6.84 (d, J = 8.8 Hz, 2H), 5.09, (s, 1H), 4.97 (s, 1H), 4.44 (dd, J = 6.0 Hz, J= 9.6 Hz, 1H), 3.91 (AB spin system, J = 14.0 Hz, 2H) 3.82 (s, 3H), 3.01 (td, J = 4.3 Hz, J = 11.3 Hz, 1H), 2.28 (d, J = 11.9 Hz, 1H), 2.17−2.09 (m, 2H), 2.04 (s, 3H), 1.92 (dd, J = 8.2 Hz, J = 12.9 Hz, 1H), 1.72 (t, J = 11.1 Hz, 1H), 1.57−1.14 (m, 15H), 0.97−0.72 (m, 21H); ^{13}C NMR (100.6 MHz, CDCl$_3$, δ, ppm): 180.8, 171.3, 161.9, 155.9, 155.8, 149.5, 128.7, 128.4, 114.5, 112.2, 81.1, 56.3, 55.4, 50.7, 50.3, 43.8, 42.4, 40.7, 38.3, 37.8, 37.1, 36.8, 34.2, 32.7, 32.0, 29.7, 27.9, 27.0, 23.7, 21.4, 21.0, 18.2, 16.5, 16.2, 16.0, 14.7. LC−MS Rt = 1.85 min, m/z = 703 [M−H+]−.

3β−O−Acetyl−30−{5−[4−(dimethylamino)phenyl]−1H−1,2,4−triazol−3−yl)sulfanyl}−betulinic acid (**4b**); pale yellow crystalline powder, yield 25%; ^{1}H NMR (400.13 MHz, CDCl$_3$, δ, ppm): 7.86 (d, J = 8.7 Hz, 2H), 6.73 (d, J = 8.1 Hz, 2H), 5.08, (s, 1H), 4.96 (s, 1H), 4.44 (dd, J = 5.9 Hz, J= 9.8 Hz, 1H), 3.87 (s, 2H), 3.02−2.99 (m, 7H), 2.28 (d, J = 12.0 Hz, 1H), 2.20−2.10 (m, 2H), 2.04 (s, 3H), 1.93 (dd, J = 7.8 Hz, J = 13.1Hz, 1H), 1.72 (t, J = 11.2 Hz, 1H), 1.57−1.00 (m, 15H), 0.94−0.73 (m, 21H); ^{13}C NMR (100.6 MHz, CDCl$_3$, δ, ppm): 180.7, 171.2, 157.7, 157.3, 151.4, 149.9, 129.0, 128.0, 112.3, 111.7, 81.1, 56.4, 55.4, 50.6, 50.3, 44.0, 43.5, 42.4, 40.7, 40.5, 38.3, 37.8, 37.1, 36.9, 34.2, 32.6, 32.1, 29.7, 27.9, 26.9, 23.7, 21.4, 21.0, 18.2, 16.5, 16.2, 16.0, 14.7. LC−MS Rt = 1.97 min, m/z = 716 [M−H+]−.

4.3. Cell Culture

Immortalized human keratinocytes HaCaT (CLS Cell Lines Service GmbH, Eppelheim, Germany), human malignant melanoma RPMI−7951, human colorectal adenocarcinoma HT−29, and human lung carcinoma A549 (ATCC® HTB−66™, HTB−38™, and CCL−185™, American Type Culture Collection ATCC, Lomianki, Poland) cell lines were selected for this study. DMEM, EMEM, McCoy's 5A Medium, and F−12K Medium (Kaighn's Modification of Ham's F−12 Medium), respectively, were used to culture BaCaT, RPMI−7951, HT−29, and A549 cells; 10% FBS and 1% penicillin/streptomycin mixture (10,000 IU/mL) were added to all media. All experimental procedures were conducted under standard conditions consisting in incubation at 37 °C under 5% CO_2 atmosphere.

4.4. Cellular Viability

The 3−(4,5−dimethylthiazol−2−yl)−2,5−diphenyltetrazolium bromide (MTT) was used to assess cell viability. Briefly, the different types of cells were seeded in 96−well plates (1 × 10^4 cells/well) followed by stimulation with 0.08, 0.4, 2, 10, 25, and 50 μM of the tested compounds (**1−4b**) previously solubilized in 0.5% DMSO. An amount of 10 μL/well MTT reagent were added to the plates after a 48 h stimulation period; the plates were then maintained at 37 °C for 3 h, followed by the addition of solubilization buffer (100 μL/well). The absorbance values were read at 570 nm using a xMark™ Microplate Spectrophotometer, Bio−Rad. All experiments were conducted in triplicate allowing for the presentation of data as mean values ± SD.

4.5. Immunofluorescence Assay

The 4, 6'−Diamidino−2−Phenylindole (DAPI) staining was used to assess the indicative signs of apoptosis; briefly, RPMI−7951 cells (1 × 10^6 cells/well) were stimulated for 48 h with tested compounds (**4a, 4b**) using concentrations matching their respective IC_{50} values. Cells were fixated with 4% paraformaldehyde, permeabilized with 2% Triton X−100 in PBS and then washed 3 times with cold PBS, the cells were blocked for 1h at 25 °C using 30% FCS in 0.01% Triton X. In the final step, the cells were treated with 300 nM DAPI and microscopically assessed by using the Olympus IX73 inverted microscope (Olympus, Tokyo, Japan) equipped with CellSens V1.15 software.

4.6. Mitochondrial Respiration Assessment

Mitochondrial respiration was evaluated at 37 °C by high resolution respirometry (HRR, Oxygraph−2k Oroboros Instruments GmbH, Innsbruck, Austria) using a previously described modified substrate uncoupler−inhibitor titration (SUIT) protocol [40]. Malignant cells (RPMI−7951, HT−29, A549) were cultured until reaching 80−85% confluence and treated for 48 h with compounds **4a** and **4b** (at their respective IC_{50} values). Cells were then washed with PBS, trypsinized, counted, and resuspended (1 × 10^6/mL cells) in mitochondrial respiration medium (MIRO5: EGTA 0.5 mM, taurine 20 mM, K−lactobionate 60 mM, $MgCl_2$ 10 mM, D−sucrose 110 mM, HEPES 20 mM, 3mM KH_2PO_4, and BSA 1 g/l, pH 7.1). Cells were introduced in the respirometric device in the presence of MIRO5 and maintained under the oxygen flux for 15 min when routine respiration was recorded followed by basal respiration ($State2_{CI}$), after the addition of digitonine (35 μg/1 × 10^6 cells, a cell membrane permeabilizer) and CI substrates: glutamate (10 mM) and malate (5 mM).

The addition of ADP (5 mM) allowed for the measurement of the active respiration reliant on CI (OXPHOSCI), and the addition of succinate (10 mM), a CII substrate, allowed for the measurement of the active respiration reliant on both CI and CII (OXPHOSCI + CII). The assessment of LEAK respiration dependent on CI and CII (State4CI + II) was enabled by the consecutive suppression of complex V with oligomycin (1 g/mL). Subsequently, successive titrations with *p*−(trifluoromethoxy) phenylhydrazone carbonyl cyanide − FCCP (1 M/step) led to the measurement of the maximal respiratory capacity of the electron transport system (ETSCI + II), whereas the addition of rotenone (0.5 M, a CI inhibitor) ensured the measurement of the maximal respiratory capacity of the ETS that was dependent solely on CI (ETSCI). In the last phase of the process, mitochondrial respiration was suppressed by adding antimycin A (2.5 M), a CIII inhibitor, and residual oxygen consumption was then measured (ROX) and used to adjust all acquired values.

4.7. Quantitative Real−Time PCR

RPMI−795 cells were treated with compounds **4a** and **4b** (at their respective IC$_{50}$ value) for 48 h. The Quick−RNA™ purification kit (Zymo Research Europe, Freiburg im Breisgau, Germany) and the TRIzol reagent (Thermo Fisher Scientific, Inc., Waltham, MA, USA) were used to isolate the total RNA. Total RNA transcription was conducted using a Maxima® First Strand cDNA Synthesis Kit (Thermo Fisher Scientific, Inc., Waltham, MA, USA). Quant Studio 5 real−time PCR system (Thermo Fisher Scientific, Inc., Waltham, MA, USA) was used to conduct the quantitative real−time PCR analysis, in the presence of Power SYBR−Green PCR Master Mix (Thermo Fisher Scientific, Inc.). The primer pairs used were acquired from Thermo Fisher Scientific Inc. (Waltham, MA, USA) and were as follows: 18 S (forward: 5′GTAACCCGTTGAACCCCATT3′ and reverse: 5′CCA−TCC−AAT−CGG−TAGTAG−CG3′), BAX (forward: 5′GGCCGGGTTGTCGCCCTTTT3′ and reverse: 5′CCGCTCCCGGAG GAAGTCCA3′) and Bcl−2 (forward: 5′CGGGAGATGTCGCCCCTGGT3′ and reverse: 5′−GCATGCTGGGGCCGTACAGT−3′). Normalized, relative expression data were calculated using the comparative threshold cycle ($2^{-\Delta\Delta Ct}$) method.

4.8. Evaluation of Compounds **4a**, **4b** *Irritation Potential Using the HET−CAM Assay*

The HET−CAM in vivo protocol was applied in order to assess the safety profile for use in living tissues; the protocol involved using the developing chorioallantoic membrane in embryonated chicken (Gallus domesticus) eggs and followed the ICCVAM recommendations [41] tailored to our own circumstances. According to a modified version of the conventional methodology [42], the eggs were incubated at 37 °C and 50% humidity. On the third day of incubation, 5–6 mL of albumen was extracted, followed by the construction of a hole in the top of the eggs. On the developing chorioallantoic membrane of the chick embryo, 300 μL of both the control and test chemicals 4a and 4b were administered at their respective IC$_{50}$ values. The CAM alterations were monitored using stereomicroscopy (Discovery 8 Stereomicroscope, Zeiss), recording significant pictures (Axio CAM 105 color, Zeiss) before the application and after five minutes of contact with the materials. During the 5 min, the effect on three parameters, namely hemorrhage, lysis, and coagulability of the vascular plexus, was detected. Every experiment was conducted in triplicate. The results were expressed as irritation factor values, calculated using the given formula, and compared to distillate water as a negative control and SLS 0.5% as a positive control with an IF of 15.3 (according to the Luepke scale: 0–0.9 non−irritant, 1–4.9 weak irritant, 5–8.9 moderate irritant, and 9–21 strong irritant [19].

$$IS = 5 \times \frac{301 - Sec\ H}{300} + 7 \times \frac{301 - Sec\ L}{300} + 9 \times \frac{301 - Sec\ C}{300}$$

where H = hemorrhage; L = vascular lysis; C = coagulation; Sec H = start of hemorrhage reactions (s); Sec L = onset of vessel lysis on CAM (s); Sec C = onset of (s).

4.9. Statistical Analysis

The statistical differences vs. control of the cellular viability and quantitative rtPCR results were determined using one−way ANOVA analysis followed by Dunnett post−test. For the high−resolution respirometry studies, the statistical differences vs. control of mitochondrial respiratory rates were determined using two−way ANOVA analysis followed by Bonferroni's multiple comparisons post−test (GraphPad Prism version 6.0.0, GraphPad Software, San Diego, CA, USA). The difference between groups was considered statistically significant if $p < 0.05$ and was marked with * (* $p < 0.05$, ** $p < 0.01$, and *** $p < 0.001$). The IC$_{50}$ values were calculated using the GraphPad Prism software (San Diego, CA, USA).

5. Conclusions

The current paper described the synthesis and cytotoxicity investigation of two novel aryl substituted−1,2,4−triazole derivatives of betulinic acid against RPMI−7951 (human malignant melanoma), HT−29 (human colorectal adenocarcinoma), A549 (human lung carcinoma), as well as healthy human keratinocytes HaCaT cell line. Among all cell lines subjected to cytotoxicity screening, the two compounds were proven to induce the highest cytotoxic effects against melanoma cells (IC$_{50}$: 18.8 µM for 4a and 20.7 µM for 4b) and were more cytotoxically active than their parent compounds as well. Bot derivatives also induced apoptotic related nuclear changes, induced a pro−apoptotic fold change expression in the Bcl−2/BAX gene ratio, and impaired mitochondrial function. While the antiproliferative biological evaluation indicated that C$_{30}$ substitution using 1,2,4−triazole was highly advantageous for the overall antiproliferative potential, especially against melanoma, the synthetic procedure needs future adjustments in order to produce higher yields. Nonetheless, BA−1,2,4−triazole derivatives stand as promising scaffolds for the development of novel heterocyclic triterpenoids with antimelanoma activity.

Supplementary Materials: The following supporting information can be downloaded at: https://www.mdpi.com/article/10.3390/pr11010101/s1. Figure S1: 1H NMR spectra of compound 2; Figure S2: 13C NMR spectra of compound 2; Figure S3: 1H NMR spectra of compound 3a; Figure S4: 13C NMR spectra of compound 3a; Figure S5: 1H NMR spectra of compound 3b; Figure S6: 13C NMR spectra of compound 3b; Figure S7: 1H NMR spectra of compound 4a; Figure S8: 13C NMR spectra of compound 4a; Figure S9: 1H NMR spectra of compound 4b; Figure S10: 13C NMR spectra of compound 4b.

Author Contributions: Conceptualization: G.N. and M.M.; methodology: G.N., M.M., A.M. (Alexandra Mioc), M.B.-P., R.R., R.G., A.M. (Andreea Milan), A.P., Ș.A., A.S., C.D. and C.Ș.; validation: A.M. (Alexandra Mioc) and M.M.; investigation: G.N. and M.M.; writing—original draft preparation: G.N., M.M., A.M. (Alexandra Mioc), M.B.-P., R.R., R.G., A.M. (Andreea Milan), A.P., Ș.A., A.S. and C.D.; writing—review and editing: C.Ș.; visualization: G.N., R.R. and R.G.; supervision: M.M. and C.Ș.; project administration: M.M. and C.Ș.; funding acquisition: M.M. and C.Ș. All authors have read and agreed to the published version of the manuscript.

Funding: This research was funded by the Romanian UEFISCDI national grant PN-III-P1-1.1-PD-2019-1078 (M.M.) and an Internal grant at "Victor Babes" University of Medicine and Pharmacy, Grant 1EXP/1233/30.01.2020 LUPSKINPATH (C.Ș.).

Institutional Review Board Statement: Not applicable.

Informed Consent Statement: Not applicable.

Data Availability Statement: Data is contained within the article and Supplementary Files.

Conflicts of Interest: The authors declare no conflict of interest.

References

1. Amjad, M.T.; Chidharla, A.; Kasi, A. *Cancer Chemotherapy*; StatPearls Publishing: Tampa, FL, USA, 2022.
2. Schirrmacher, V. From Chemotherapy to Biological Therapy: A Review of Novel Concepts to Reduce the Side Effects of Systemic Cancer Treatment (Review). *Int. J. Oncol.* **2019**, *54*, 407–419. [CrossRef]
3. Dehelean, C.A.; Marcovici, I.; Soica, C.; Mioc, M.; Coricovac, D.; Iurciuc, S.; Cretu, O.M.; Pinzaru, I. Plant-Derived Anticancer Compounds as New Perspectives in Drug Discovery and Alternative Therapy. *Molecules* **2021**, *26*, 1109. [CrossRef]
4. Ghante, M.H.; Jamkhande, P.G. Role of Pentacyclic Triterpenoids in Chemoprevention and Anticancer Treatment: An Overview on Targets and Underling Mechanisms. *J. Pharmacopunct.* **2019**, *22*, 55–67. [CrossRef]
5. Lou, H.; Li, H.; Zhang, S.; Lu, H.; Chen, Q. A Review on Preparation of Betulinic Acid and Its Biological Activities. *Molecules* **2021**, *26*, 5583. [CrossRef]
6. Zhong, Y.; Liang, N.; Liu, Y.; Cheng, M.-S. Recent Progress on Betulinic Acid and Its Derivatives as Antitumor Agents: A Mini Review. *Chin. J. Nat. Med.* **2021**, *19*, 641–647. [CrossRef]
7. Kerru, N.; Gummidi, L.; Maddila, S.; Gangu, K.K.; Jonnalagadda, S.B. A Review on Recent Advances in Nitrogen-Containing Molecules and Their Biological Applications. *Molecules* **2020**, *25*, 1909. [CrossRef]

8. Majeed, R.; Sangwan, P.L.; Chinthakindi, P.K.; Khan, I.; Dangroo, N.A.; Thota, N.; Hamid, A.; Sharma, P.R.; Saxena, A.K.; Koul, S. Synthesis of 3-O-Propargylated Betulinic Acid and Its 1,2,3-Triazoles as Potential Apoptotic Agents. *Eur. J. Med. Chem.* **2013**, *63*, 782–792. [CrossRef]
9. Shi, W.; Tang, N.; Yan, W.D. Synthesis and Cytotoxicity of Triterpenoids Derived from Betulin and Betulinic Acid via Click Chemistry. *J. Asian Nat. Prod. Res.* **2015**, *17*, 159–169. [CrossRef]
10. Sidova, V.; Zoufaly, P.; Pokorny, J.; Dzubak, P.; Hajduch, M.; Popa, I.; Urban, M. Cytotoxic Conjugates of Betulinic Acid and Substituted Triazoles Prepared by Huisgen Cycloaddition from 30-Azidoderivatives. *PLoS ONE* **2017**, *12*, e0171621. [CrossRef]
11. Suman, P.; Patel, A.; Solano, L.; Jampana, G.; Gardner, Z.S.; Holt, C.M.; Jonnalagadda, S.C. Synthesis and Cytotoxicity of Baylis-Hillman Template Derived Betulinic Acid-Triazole Conjugates. *Tetrahedron* **2017**, *73*, 4214–4226. [CrossRef]
12. Sousa, J.L.C.; Freire, C.S.R.; Silvestre, A.J.D.; Silva, A.M.S. Recent Developments in the Functionalization of Betulinic Acid and Its Natural Analogues: A Route to New Bioactive Compounds. *Molecules* **2019**, *24*, 355. [CrossRef] [PubMed]
13. Nistor, G.; Mioc, M.; Mioc, A.; Balan-Porcarasu, M.; Racoviceanu, R.; Prodea, A.; Milan, A.; Ghiulai, R.; Semenescu, A.; Dehelean, C.; et al. The C30-Modulation of Betulinic Acid Using 1,2,4-Triazole: A Promising Strategy for Increasing Its Antimelanoma Cytotoxic Potential. *Molecules* **2022**, *27*, 7807. [CrossRef] [PubMed]
14. Mioc, M.; Soica, C.; Bercean, V.; Avram, S.; Balan-Porcarasu, M.; Coricovac, D.; Ghiulai, R.; Muntean, D.; Andrica, F.; Dehelean, C.; et al. Design, Synthesis and Pharmaco-Toxicological Assessment of 5-Mercapto-1,2,4-Triazole Derivatives with Antibacterial and Antiproliferative Activity. *Int. J. Oncol.* **2017**, *50*, 1175–1183. [CrossRef]
15. Petrenko, N.I.; Elantseva, N.V.; Petukhova, V.Z.; Shakirov, M.M.; Shul'ts, E.E.; Tolstikov, G.A. Synthesis of Betulonic Acid Derivatives Containing Amino-Acid Fragments. *Chem. Nat. Compd.* **2002**, *38*, 331–339. [CrossRef]
16. Chen, B.-H.; Chang, H.B. Inhibition of Lung Cancer Cells A549 and H460 by Curcuminoid Extracts and Nanoemulsions Prepared from Curcuma Longa Linnaeus. *Int. J. Nanomed.* **2015**, *10*, 5059. [CrossRef]
17. Mioc, M.; Pavel, I.Z.; Ghiulai, R.; Coricovac, D.E.; Farcaş, C.; Mihali, C.-V.; Oprean, C.; Serafim, V.; Popovici, R.A.; Dehelean, C.A.; et al. The Cytotoxic Effects of Betulin-Conjugated Gold Nanoparticles as Stable Formulations in Normal and Melanoma Cells. *Front. Pharmacol.* **2018**, *9*, 429. [CrossRef]
18. Eidet, J.R.; Pasovic, L.; Maria, R.; Jackson, C.J.; Utheim, T.P. Objective Assessment of Changes in Nuclear Morphology and Cell Distribution Following Induction of Apoptosis. *Diagn. Pathol.* **2014**, *9*, 92. [CrossRef]
19. Luepke, N.P. Hen's Egg Chorioallantoic Membrane Test for Irritation Potential. *Food Chem. Toxicol. Int. J. Publ. Br. Ind. Biol. Res. Assoc.* **1985**, *23*, 287–291. [CrossRef] [PubMed]
20. Barret, J.P.; Podmelle, F.; Lipový, B.; Rennekampff, H.-O.; Schumann, H.; Schwieger-Briel, A.; Zahn, T.R.; Metelmann, H.-R. Accelerated Re-Epithelialization of Partial-Thickness Skin Wounds by a Topical Betulin Gel: Results of a Randomized Phase III Clinical Trials Program. *Burns* **2017**, *43*, 1284–1294. [CrossRef]
21. Schwieger-Briel, A.; Ott, H.; Kiritsi, D.; Laszczyk-Lauer, M.; Bodemer, C. Mechanism of Oleogel-S10: A Triterpene Preparation for the Treatment of Epidermolysis Bullosa. *Dermatol. Ther.* **2019**, *32*, e12983. [CrossRef]
22. Pisha, E.; Chai, H.; Lee, I.-S.; Chagwedera, T.E.; Farnsworth, N.R.; Cordell, G.A.; Beecher, C.W.W.; Fong, H.H.S.; Kinghorn, A.D.; Brown, D.M.; et al. Discovery of Betulinic Acid as a Selective Inhibitor of Human Melanoma That Functions by Induction of Apoptosis. *Nat. Med.* **1995**, *1*, 1046–1051. [CrossRef] [PubMed]
23. Kumar, P.; Bhadauria, A.S.; Singh, A.K.; Saha, S. Betulinic Acid as Apoptosis Activator: Molecular Mechanisms, Mathematical Modeling and Chemical Modifications. *Life Sci.* **2018**, *209*, 24–33. [CrossRef] [PubMed]
24. Mioc, M.; Avram, S.; Bercean, V.; Kurunczi, L.; Ghiulai, R.M.; Oprean, C.; Coricovac, D.E.; Dehelean, C.; Mioc, A.; Balan-Porcarasu, M.; et al. Design, Synthesis and Biological Activity Evaluation of S-Substituted 1H-5-Mercapto-1,2,4-Triazole Derivatives as Antiproliferative Agents in Colorectal Cancer. *Front. Chem.* **2018**, *6*, 373. [CrossRef] [PubMed]
25. Alam, M.M. 1,2,3-Triazole Hybrids as Anticancer Agents: A Review. *Arch. Pharm.* **2022**, *355*, 2100158. [CrossRef]
26. Csuk, R. Betulinic Acid and Its Derivatives: A Patent Review (2008–2013). *Expert Opin. Ther. Pat.* **2014**, *24*, 913–923. [CrossRef]
27. Zuco, V.; Supino, R.; Righetti, S.C.; Cleris, L.; Marchesi, E.; Gambacorti-Passerini, C.; Formelli, F. Selective Cytotoxicity of Betulinic Acid on Tumor Cell Lines, but Not on Normal Cells. *Cancer Lett.* **2002**, *175*, 17–25. [CrossRef]
28. Kessler, J.H.; Mullauer, F.B.; de Roo, G.M.; Medema, J.P. Broad in vitro Efficacy of Plant-Derived Betulinic Acid against Cell Lines Derived from the Most Prevalent Human Cancer Types. *Cancer Lett.* **2007**, *251*, 132–145. [CrossRef]
29. Beilin, A.K.; Gurskaya, N.G.; Evtushenko, N.A.; Alpeeva, E.V.; Kosykh, A.V.; Terskikh, V.V.; Vasiliev, A.V.; Vorotelyak, E.A. Immortalization of Human Keratinocytes Using the Catalytic Subunit of Telomerase. *Dokl. Biochem. Biophys.* **2021**, *496*, 5–9. [CrossRef]
30. Şenkal, S.; Burucku, D.; Hayal, T.B.; Kiratli, B.; Şisli, H.B.; Sagrac, D.; Asutay, B.; Sumer, E.; Şahin, F.; Dogan, A. 3D Culture Of HaCaT Keratinocyte Cell Line as an in vitro Toxicity Model. *Trak. Univ. J. Nat. Sci.* **2022**, *23*, 211–220. [CrossRef]
31. Mioc, M.; Mioc, A.; Prodea, A.; Milan, A.; Balan-Porcarasu, M.; Racoviceanu, R.; Ghiulai, R.; Iovanescu, G.; Macasoi, I.; Draghici, G.; et al. Novel Triterpenic Acid—Benzotriazole Esters Act as Pro-Apoptotic Antimelanoma Agents. *Int. J. Mol. Sci.* **2022**, *23*, 9992. [CrossRef] [PubMed]
32. Fulda, S. Betulinic Acid for Cancer Treatment and Prevention. *Int. J. Mol. Sci.* **2008**, *9*, 1096–1107. [CrossRef]
33. Santos, R.C.; Salvador, J.A.R.; Cortés, R.; Pachón, G.; Marín, S.; Cascante, M. New Betulinic Acid Derivatives Induce Potent and Selective Antiproliferative Activity through Cell Cycle Arrest at the S Phase and Caspase Dependent Apoptosis in Human Cancer Cells. *Biochimie* **2011**, *93*, 1065–1075. [CrossRef] [PubMed]

34. Zhang, L.; Hou, S.; Li, B.; Pan, J.; Jiang, L.; Zhou, G.; Gu, H.; Zhao, C.; Lu, H.; Ma, F. Combination of Betulinic Acid with Diazen-1-Ium-1,2-Diolate Nitric Oxide Moiety Donating a Novel Anticancer Candidate. *Onco. Targets. Ther.* **2018**, *11*, 361–373. [CrossRef] [PubMed]
35. Nedopekina, D.A.; Gubaidullin, R.R.; Odinokov, V.N.; Maximchik, P.V.; Zhivotovsky, B.; Bel'skii, Y.P.; Khazanov, V.A.; Manuylova, A.V.; Gogvadze, V.; Spivak, A.Y. Mitochondria-Targeted Betulinic and Ursolic Acid Derivatives: Synthesis and Anticancer Activity. *Medchemcomm* **2017**, *8*, 1934–1945. [CrossRef] [PubMed]
36. Cháirez-Ramírez, M.H.; Moreno-Jiménez, M.R.; González-Laredo, R.F.; Gallegos-Infante, J.A.; Rocha-Guzmán, N.E. Lupane-Type Triterpenes and Their Anti-Cancer Activities against Most Common Malignant Tumors: A Review. *EXCLI J.* **2016**, *15*, 758–771. [CrossRef]
37. Khan, I.; Guru, S.K.; Rath, S.K.; Chinthakindi, P.K.; Singh, B.; Koul, S.; Bhushan, S.; Sangwan, P.L. A Novel Triazole Derivative of Betulinic Acid Induces Extrinsic and Intrinsic Apoptosis in Human Leukemia HL-60 Cells. *Eur. J. Med. Chem.* **2016**, *108*, 104–116. [CrossRef]
38. Coricovac, D.; Dehelean, C.A.; Pinzaru, I.; Mioc, A.; Aburel, O.-M.; Macasoi, I.; Draghici, G.A.; Petean, C.; Soica, C.; Boruga, M.; et al. Assessment of Betulinic Acid Cytotoxicity and Mitochondrial Metabolism Impairment in a Human Melanoma Cell Line. *Int. J. Mol. Sci.* **2021**, *22*, 4870. [CrossRef]
39. Budai, P.; Kormos, É.; Buda, I.; Somody, G.; Lehel, J. Comparative Evaluation of HET-CAM and ICE Methods for Objective Assessment of Ocular Irritation Caused by Selected Pesticide Products. *Toxicol. Vitr.* **2021**, *74*, 105150. [CrossRef]
40. Petrus, A.; Ratiu, C.; Noveanu, L.; Lighezan, R.; Rosca, M.; Muntean, D.; Duicu, O. Assessment of Mitochondrial Respiration in Human Platelets. *Rev. Chim.* **2017**, *68*, 768–771. [CrossRef]
41. Interagency Coordinating Committee on the Validation of Alternative Methods (ICCVAM). ICCVAM-Recommended Test Method Protocol: Hen' s Egg Test—Chorioallantoic Membrane (HET-CAM) Test Method. 2010, B30–B38. Available online: https://ntp.niehs.nih.gov/iccvam/docs/protocols/ivocular-hetcam.pdf (accessed on 1 October 2022).
42. Maghiari, A.L.; Coricovac, D.; Pinzaru, I.A.; Macașoi, I.G.; Marcovici, I.; Simu, S.; Navolan, D.; Dehelean, C. High Concentrations of Aspartame Induce Pro-Angiogenic Effects in Ovo and Cytotoxic Effects in HT-29 Human Colorectal Carcinoma Cells. *Nutrients* **2020**, *12*, 3600. [CrossRef]

Disclaimer/Publisher's Note: The statements, opinions and data contained in all publications are solely those of the individual author(s) and contributor(s) and not of MDPI and/or the editor(s). MDPI and/or the editor(s) disclaim responsibility for any injury to people or property resulting from any ideas, methods, instructions or products referred to in the content.

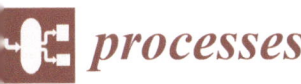

Article

Anti-Inflammatory and Anti-Diabetic Activity of Ferruginan, a Natural Compound from *Olea ferruginea*

Abdur Rauf [1,*], Umer Rashid [2], Zafar Ali Shah [1], Gauhar Rehman [3], Kashif Bashir [4], Johar Jamil [5], Iftikhar [1], Abdur Rahman [3], Abdulrahman Alsahammari [6], Metab Alharbi [6], Abdulmajeed Al-Shahrani [7] and Giovanni Ribaudo [8,*]

1. Department of Chemistry, University of Swabi, Swabi, Anbar 23430, Pakistan
2. Department of Chemistry, COMSATS University Islamabad, Abbottabad Campus, Islamabad 22060, Pakistan
3. Department of Zoology, Abdul Wali Khan University, Mardan 23200, Pakistan
4. Department of Health and Biological Sciences, Abasyn University, Peshawar 25000, Pakistan
5. Department of Microbiology, University of Swabi, Swabi, Anbar 23430, Pakistan
6. Department of Pharmacology and Toxicology, College of Pharmacy, King Saud University, P.O. Box 2455, Riyadh 11451, Saudi Arabia
7. Laboratory Department, Almadah General Hospital, Ministry of Health, Riyadh 10336, Saudi Arabia
8. Dipartimento di Medicina Molecolare e Traslazionale, Università Degli Studi di Brescia, Viale Europa 11, 25123 Brescia, Italy
* Correspondence: abdurrauf@uoswabi.edu.pk (A.R.); giovanni.ribaudo@unibs.it (G.R.)

Abstract: Inflammation is a complex response of the human organism and relates to the onset of various disorders including diabetes. The current research work aimed at investigating the anti-inflammatory and anti-diabetic effects of ferruginan, a compound isolated from *Olea ferruginea*. Its in vitro anti-inflammatory activity was determined by using the heat-induced hemolysis assay, while the anti-diabetic effect of the compound was studied by the yeast cell glucose uptake assay. Ferruginan exhibited a maximum of 71.82% inhibition of inflammation and also increased the uptake of glucose by yeast cells by up to 74.96% at the highest tested concentration (100 µM). Moreover, ferruginan inhibited α-amylase dose-dependently, by up to 75.45% at the same concentration. These results indicated that ferruginan possesses promising anti-inflammatory and anti-diabetic properties in vitro, even if at high concentrations. To provide preliminary hypotheses on the potentially multi-target mechanisms underlying such effects, docking analyses were performed on α-amylase and on various molecular targets involved in inflammation such as 5′-adenosine monophosphate-activated protein kinase (AMPK, PDB ID 3AQV), cyclooxygenase (COX-1, PDB ID 1EQG, and COX-2, 1CX2), and tumor necrosis factor alpha (TNF-α, PDB ID 2AZ5). The docking studies suggested that the compound may act on α-amylase, COX-2, and AMPK.

Keywords: *Olea ferruginea*; *Oleaceae*; ferruginan; anti-inflammatory; anti-diabetic; molecular docking

---

1. Introduction

Diabetes mellitus (DM) comprehends a group of metabolic diseases related to impaired insulin secretion, insensitivity of the target tissues to insulin, or a combination of these phenomena. The hallmark feature of DM is uncontrolled hyperglycemia, which causes severe complications. Additionally, the occurrence of diabetes is aggressively increasing worldwide, and this condition appears to be related to inflammation [1].

Natural products, especially those derived from plants, have been used for therapeutic applications towards several diseases from the ancient ages, and there are several examples of natural compounds being used or investigated as therapeutic agents also in more recent times [2–4]. In particular, *Olea* is a genus that comprehends forty common species belonging to the *Oleaceae* family. *Olea ferruginea* is one of the most widespread species of the *Olea* genus, which is found in Afghanistan, Pakistan, and Kashmir, as well as in the Mediterranean region [5].

A variety of compounds and preparations isolated from *Olea* plants have been traditionally used to treat various diseases, and native peoples use its stem bark to treat fevers. The bark and oil of this plant have been utilized to treat diabetes, headache, and asthma [5]. *O. ferruginea* also finds application as an antimalarial, anti-leprosy, and antitumor agent in traditional medicine, and the *O. ferruginea* fruit oil can treat arthritis and bone fractures [6]. More specifically, the fruits of *O. ferruginea* are a source of antioxidants, antidiabetic, and antihypertensive agents. Traditionally, *O. ferruginea* has shown antimalarial, anti-leprosy, and antitumor activity [6].

The *Olea* genus is a rich source of many natural compounds such as flavonoids and other phenolic substances including secoiridoid glycosides, lignans, and other compounds [7]. Secoiridoid and triterpenoids were previously identified in *O. ferruginea*, and their cytotoxic and alkaline phosphatase inhibitory activities were studied. A flavanone and a secoiridoid glycosidic lignin ester were also reported as components in the *Olea* genus [8]. Oleanolic acid, a biologically active compound isolated from the chloroform extract of *O. ferruginea* R., was shown to exhibit antitumor, antimicrobial, hepatoprotective, and antiallergic potential [9,10], while neuroprotective effects were observed in a focal brain hypoxia rat model [11]. *Olea europaea* and other species have also potent antiviral activity against several viruses [8]. More in general, the leaves of *Olea* species have been traditionally used in Mediterranean and European regions for treating hypertension, bacterial infections, and hyperglycemia in diabetic patients [12]. Similarly, the *Olea* fruit has been reported to have antihyperglycemic action in cell cultures and animal models [8].

On such basis, the present study aimed at investigating ferruginan from *O. ferruginea* for its in vitro anti-inflammatory and anti-diabetic activity.

2. Results

2.1. Extraction and Characterization of Ferruginan

The ethyl acetate fraction of *O. ferruginea* extract was subjected to normal-phase liquid chromatography, which yielded purified ferruginan (Figure 1). We obtained 1.02 g of compound from 7.00 kg of dried plant material (extraction yield: $1.46 \times 10^{-2}\%$ w/w). Ferruginan identity was initially checked by precoated TLC visualized under UV light. The structure of the isolated compound was identified previously by our research group through UV analysis, advanced NMR analysis, and mass spectrometry, and the spectra were in agreement with reported literature data [6]. In particular, the UV spectrum showed maximum absorption at 230 and 283 nm, and the structure of ferruginan was fully supported by 2D-NMR spectral data such as HSQC, HMBC, and COSY spectra, which were closely related to those reported [6,13].

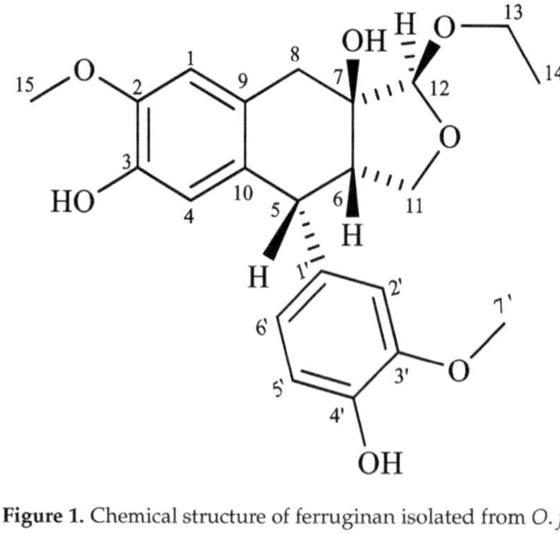

Figure 1. Chemical structure of ferruginan isolated from *O. ferruginea*.

It must be noted that ferruginan was previously investigated as a cytotoxic agent and showed mild cytotoxic activity in MCF-7 cells (IC$_{50}$ = 10.41 µg/mL) [6]. Moreover, our group evaluated ferruginan as a potential leishmanicidal and antioxidant compound [6,13].

In the present study, the anti-inflammatory and anti-diabetic actions of ferruginan isolated from *O. ferruginea* were investigated using in vitro models, and such studies were paralleled by preliminary computational simulations.

2.2. In Vitro Anti-Inflammatory Activity

The role of ferruginan on membrane stabilization was evaluated by measuring the inhibition of the lysis of human red blood cells' (HRBCs) membrane at high temperature. This method is adopted to evaluate the anti-inflammatory effect of a molecule. The hemoglobin level in the samples was measured, and the experiment showed that ferruginan inhibited inflammation. For comparison, the standard drug diclofenac sodium was used as a reference in the experiment. Various concentrations of the compound were used, i.e., 10, 20, 30, 40, 50, 80, and 100 µM, which showed 10.96%, 21.89%, 38.74%, 50.61%, 59.75%, 65.91%, and 71.82% of inhibition, respectively. An IC$_{50}$ value of 53.91 µM was calculated for ferruginan. Concerning the positive control, diclofenac sodium was used at 10, 20, 30, 40, 50, 80, and 100 µM concentrations, which showed 32.66%, 64.23%, 73.80%, 77.38%, 78.57%, 80.95%, and 85.71% of inhibition, respectively. Figure 2 shows the results of the test, demonstrating that the activity of ferruginan paralleled that of the standard. The minimum rate of inhibition for ferruginan was measured at 10 µM (10.96%), while the maximum rate of inhibition was shown at 100 µM and was 71.82%.

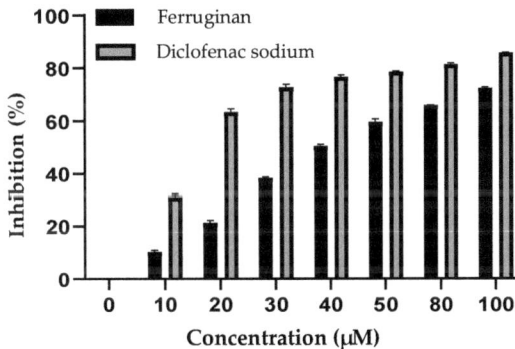

Figure 2. Effect of ferruginan, in comparison with diclofenac sodium (standard), in the heat-induced hemolysis assay. Experiments were performed in triplicate, and values are reported as mean ± SD.

2.3. In Vitro Anti-Diabetic Activity

To study the effects of ferruginan on glucose uptake in yeast cells in a 5 mM glucose solution, various concentrations of the compound (from 5 µM to 100 µM) were tested. Impaired glucose uptake by cells is one of the hallmarks of diabetes, and insulin-sensitizing antihyperglycemic agents act by facilitating the action of insulin in promoting glucose distribution. The studied compound increased glucose uptake from 6.71% to 74.96% in yeast cells at 5 µM and 100 µM, respectively, showing an EC$_{50}$ value of 47.12 µM and indicating that the observed effect was dose-dependent. The standard drug metronidazole has also a pronounced effect on glucose uptake by yeast cells. According to the assay, there was an increase from 17.09% and 85.71% in glucose uptake at 5 µM and 100 µM of metronidazole, respectively. The results of the test are reported in Figure 3, which shows that the activity of the tested compound paralleled that of the standard.

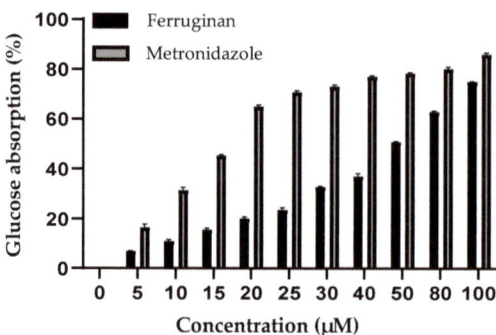

Figure 3. Results of the glucose yeast uptake assay (5 mM glucose) for ferruginan and metronidazole (standard). Experiments were performed in triplicate, and values are reported as mean ± SD.

2.4. α-Amylase Inhibition Assay

Noteworthy results were produced by ferruginan also in the α-amylase inhibition assay. More specifically, the activity of the compound was determined at increasing concentrations, i.e., 10, 20, 40, 60, 80, and 100 µM, for which the recorded inhibition percentage was 12.51%, 15.32%, 31.90%, 50.12%, 67.68%, and 75.45%, respectively. The compound expressed an IC$_{50}$ value of 43.47 µM. Acarbose was used as a reference and, at 100 µM, inhibited the enzyme activity by 87.85%. The results of dose-dependent enzyme inhibition are reported in Figure 4, together with a representative model of the interaction of acarbose and ferruginan with the protein.

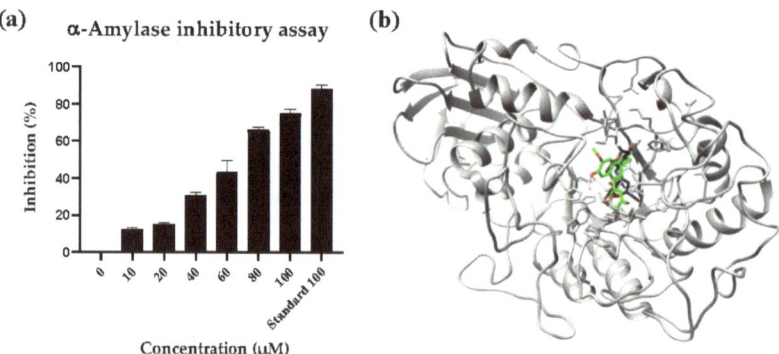

Figure 4. Effect of ferruginan on α-amylase activity at various concentrations. Acarbose was used as a standard; the experiments were performed in triplicate, and the values are reported as mean ± SD (**a**). Representative model showing the interaction of ferruginan (green, docked pose −7.6 kcal/mol), in comparison with co-crystallized acarbose (black), with α-amylase (1B2Y, artwork produced with UCSF Chimera) (**b**).

2.5. Molecular Docking towards Targets Involved in Inflammation

In the subsequent step of this study, we aimed at exploring the mechanism(s) of action through which ferruginan may exert the observed biological effects, by means of computational tools.

Target pathway prediction tools were utilized to hypothesize the involved molecular mechanisms. According to the ligand-based study carried out using PathwayMap [14], ferruginan was predicted to target several pathways. Nevertheless, the five mechanisms for a which a higher score was computed were "signal transduction" (in particular, cAMP pathway, score 0.174), "endocrine system" (in particular, insulin secretion, score 0.158), "cell proliferation" (score 0.135), "amino acid metabolism" (in particular, lysine degradation, score 0.121), and "cardiovascular disease" (score 0.101).

Then, in our preliminary docking study, we considered four molecular targets known to be involved mainly in inflammation but also in diabetes to perform the docking studies. More in detail, 5′-adenosine monophosphate-activated protein kinase (AMPK), cyclooxygenase-1 (COX-1), cyclooxygenase-2 (COX-2), and tumor necrosis factor alpha (TNF-α) were thus selected. The tree-dimensional (3D) crystal structures of all the target macromolecules were obtained from the Protein Data Bank (PDB). The PDB codes of the downloaded enzymes are the following: 3AQV (for AMPK), 1EQG (For COX-1), 1CX2 (COX-2), and 2AZ5 (for TNF-α) [15–18]. After the preparation of the downloaded models, their native ligands were redocked into the binding pockets of their respective proteins to validate the docking protocols, and procedures leading to RMSD values lower than 2.0 Å were used for further studies.

The docking simulations showed that in the binding site of AMPK, the native ligand interacts with Val96 via hydrogen bond interactions, while Tyr95 (π-π stack) and Met93 (π-sulfur) form hydrophobic interactions. Ferruginan forms three hydrogen bonds with Val96, Glu100, and Asp103, while Tyr95 establishes π–π stacking as a hydrophobic interaction. The binding energy value computed for ferruginan was −7.67 kcal/mol. Overall, the two compounds establish a similar interaction pattern with the target and bind to the same region of the protein, as depicted in Figure 5.

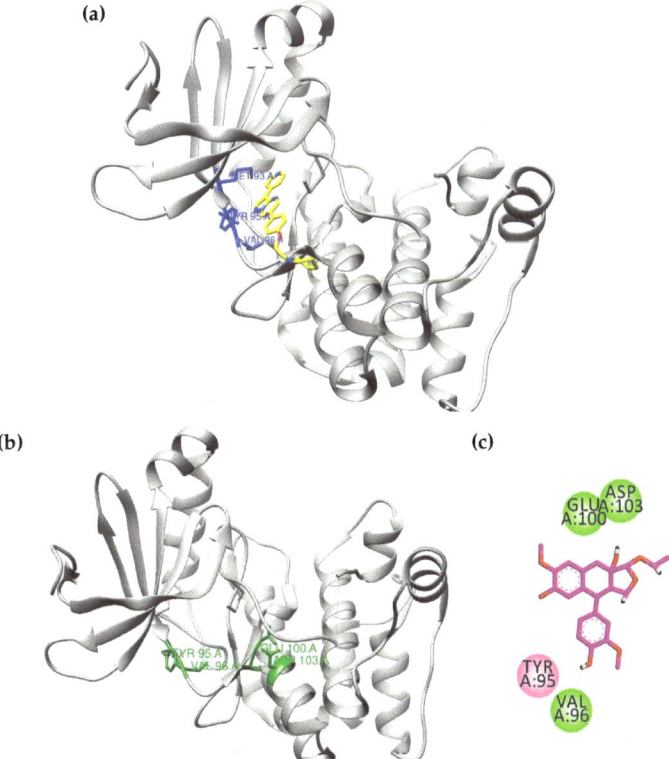

Figure 5. Predicted interaction pattern, in terms of involved residues, for (**a**) the native ligand and (**b**) ferruginan in the binding site of AMPK. The involved residues are highlighted, and the amino acids targeted by ferruginan are also reported in panel (**c**).

For investigating its role in the context of the inflammatory response, ferruginan was also docked into the binding sites of COX-1 and COX-2. In the binding site of COX-1, hydrogen bond interactions with Leu352 were highlighted, while Val349, Ile523, and Ala52 appeared to interact via π–σ interactions (Figure 6a). In the binding site of COX-2, the hydroxyl group appeared oriented towards the COX-2 specific pocket and to form hydrogen bond interactions with His90 and Ser353. A weak π–alkyl interaction was also observed between the phenyl ring and Val523, an important residue of this pocket. Tyr385 was also shown to interact with the compound via a hydrogen bond (Figure 6b). The computed binding energy values in the binding site of COX-1 and COX-2 were −4.81 kcal/mol and −7.36 kcal/mol, respectively. Eventually, in the binding site of TNF-α, ferruginan was found to interact with amino acid residues via hydrogen bond interactions. The residues involved in the interaction were identified as Ser60, Gly121, and Tyr151 (Figure 6c). The computed binding energy value for ferruginan in this site corresponded to −6.16 kcal/mol.

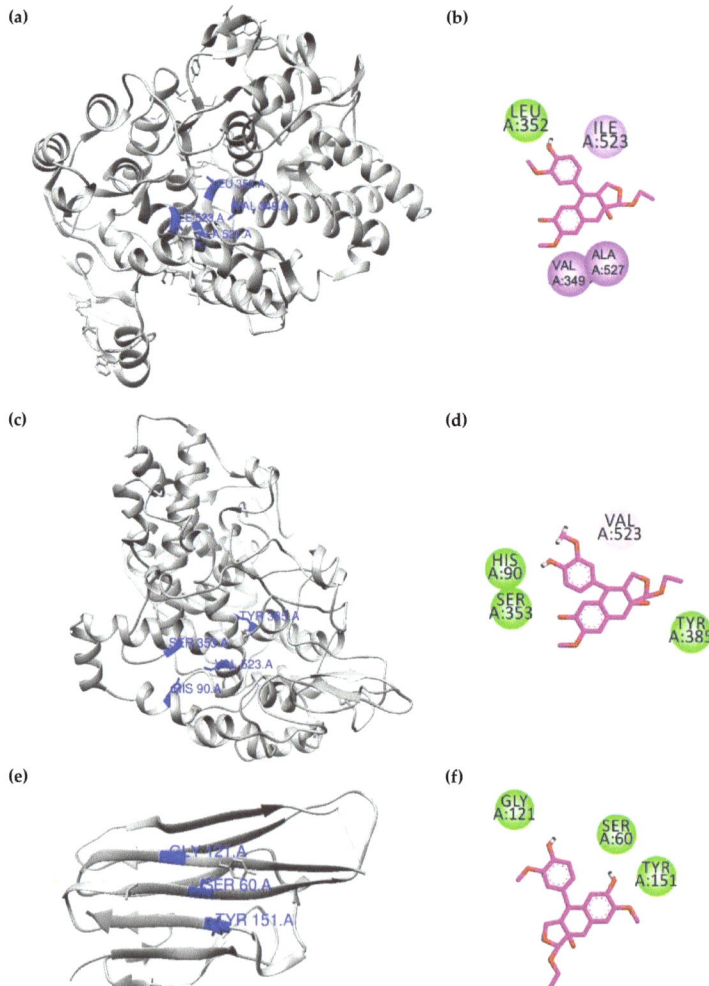

Figure 6. Predicted interaction pattern, in terms of involved residues, for ferruginan with COX-1 (**a,b**), COX-2 (**c,d**), and TNF-α (**e,f**). The targeted amino acids are highlighted, and 2D interaction maps are reported.

3. Discussion

O. ferruginea is a medicinal plant traditionally used to treat different diseases and conditions such as teeth problems, fever, skeleton disorders, debility, and even cancer cell proliferation [10]. Its bark possesses antidiabetic and cytotoxic potential. It has also been reported as a possible tool to treat asthma, rheumatism, wounds, and malaria, and its dried fruits are used for lowering the blood glucose level [19].

Inflammation is a complex response of the body that acts against various damages in cells, tissues, and organs caused by stimuli such as mechanical injuries, allergens, burns, microbial infections, and other toxic substances which activate macrophages, leukocytes, mast cells, and complement factors [20]. Diabetes is related to inflammation, and the treatment of DM in the current scenario is mainly based on parenteral insulin and oral anti-diabetic drugs. Due to the serious side effects of oral hypoglycemic agents, there is a need to search newer anti-diabetic agents having minimum side effects and high therapeutic efficacy [21]. In Pakistan, medicinal plants are mostly used locally by the rural population, since the soil is rich in this natural resource, especially in northern areas, where lush green mountains still host unidentified wild plants. It is of primary relevance to gain a deep knowledge concerning herbs and their constituents, especially considering their therapeutic activity and potential synergistic effects with other drugs [22].

Ferruginan is a compound that, according to its physico-chemical properties calculated using SwissADME, can be defined as drug-like. This molecule is predicted to be moderately soluble in water. As reported in Supplementary Information, ferruginan falls within the ideal chemical space in terms of lipophilicity, size, polarity, solubility, degree of instauration, and flexibility for a drug-like compound (Figure S1) [23].

The effect of ferruginan from *O. ferruginea* on HRBC membrane stabilization was tested by measuring the hemoglobin level in the samples after inhibiting HRBC membrane hemolysis at high temperatures. Ferruginan counteracted inflammation by reducing the hemolysis of HRBCs at high temperature dose-dependently. For comparison, diclofenac sodium was used as a standard drug [24]. The maximum degree of inhibition for ferruginan was reached at 100 μM (71.82%).

Then, to study the effect of the compound on glucose uptake by yeast cells in a 5 mmol glucose solution, various concentrations of the isolated molecule (from 5 μM to 100 μM) were tested. In fact, the utilization of carbohydrates is greatly affected by DM, which leads to an imbalance in the metabolism of lipids [25]. The compound dose-dependently increased the uptake of glucose to a maximum of 74.96% at 100 μM. The standard drug metronidazole, which was used as a reference, had an even more marked effect on glucose uptake, leading to an increase of up to 85.71% in yeast cells at a 100 μM concentration.

Moreover, ferruginan inhibited α-amylase, an enzyme that breaks polysaccharides to produce glucose and maltose, dose-dependently and by up to 75.45% at 100 μM, in a range similar to that of the control compound acarbose. This evidence further supports the potential role of ferruginan as an anti-diabetic agent.

Then, we performed ligand-based target prediction studies which highlighted that inflammation and glucose degradation pathways may indeed be involved in the activity of ferruginan. Moreover, preliminary docking data showed that ferruginan binds to the same pocket occupied by acarbose in the enzyme.

In general, the causes and risk factors of diabetes are genetic and environmental conditions. The deregulation of the immunological and inflammatory systems increases the vulnerability to type 1 and type 2 diabetes, according to evidence from the past 10 years. On this basis, by means of computational tools, we explored the mechanism of action of ferruginan isolated from *O. ferruginea*. For this purpose, we selected four molecular targets for the docking studies. AMPK is considered a key target to design drugs against obesity, metabolic syndrome, and type 2 diabetes. Detailed views of the predicted interaction patterns of ferruginan with the studied targets are reported in Supplementary Information (Figures S2–S5).

These computational studies carried out on various macromolecular targets involved in the abovementioned diseases suggested that ferruginan may preferentially act through the interaction with COX-2 and AMPK, for which the most promising calculated binding values were retrieved. More specifically, the docking scores computed for ferruginan were overall not optimal. Nevertheless, it must be considered that the compound indeed showed the higher number of hydrogen bonds with these two proteins compared to other targets (Figures 5 and 6).

4. Materials and Methods

4.1. Plant Collection and Processing

The aerial parts of *O. ferruginea* Royle plants were collected from the Agriculture Research Institute Tarnab, Peshawar, Khyber Pakhtunkhwa, Pakistan, in the month of May, and the samples were identified by Dr. Muhammad Ilyas at the Department of Botany, University of Swabi. The plant was washed with tap water to remove any dust particles and then was shade-dried. The dried plant material (7.00 kg) was finally grinded to powder and stored for further processing.

4.2. Extraction and Isolation

For the crude methanolic extract preparation, *O. ferruginea* powder (7.00 kg) was suspended in methanol and kept for 7 days at room temperature with occasional mixing and shaking. After that, all insoluble components were filtered. The filtrate was evaporated through a rotary evaporator at 45 °C to obtain a semi-solid crude extract (87.00 g). Then, 22.54 g of the extract was dissolved in ethyl acetate and then subjected to further purification. More in detail, silica gel column chromatography was performed after dry loading of the sample by using hexane and ethyl acetate (75:25) as a mobile phase, affording ferruginan as an isolated compound (1.02 g). The analytical profile of the extracted compound was in agreement with data reported previously [6,13].

4.3. In Vitro Anti-Inflammatory Activity

The in vitro anti-inflammatory activity assay was performed to evaluate the heat-induced hemolysis activity. This test examines the stabilization and lysis of the plasma membrane of red blood cells. The assay was carried out by the method reported in [24], with minor modifications. The potency of the compound was tested at high temperature, measuring the inhibition of RBC membrane lysis through the assay. The experimental protocol was approved by the Research grants and Experimentation Ethics Committee of the Department of Zoology, Abdul Wali Khan University, Mardan, on the use of human tissue samples and blood. Fresh blood was collected from healthy volunteers in EDTA tubes and centrifuged at 3000 rpm for 15 min. The supernatant was discarded, while the pellet was washed with an isosaline solution. The process was repeated 3 times until a clear supernatant appeared. The pellet containing human red blood cells (HRBCs) was used to prepare a 10% suspension in an isotonic saline solution. Diclofenac sodium in phosphate-buffered saline (PBS, pH 7.4) was used as a control in this test. The control reaction mixture contained 100 µL of the 10% blood suspension, 20 µL of distilled water, and 880 µL of PBS solution. The standard reaction mixture contained 100 µL of the 10% blood suspension and various concentrations of diclofenac sodium (DS) in PBS solution (10 µg DS + 890 µL PBS, 20 µg DS + 880 µL PBS, 30 µg DS + 870 µL PBS, and 80 µg DS + 820 µL PBS). The test sample reaction mixture contained 100 µL of the 10% blood suspension and various concentrations of the compound in PBS solution (10 µM compound + 890 µL PBS, 20 µM compound + 880 µL PBS, 30 µM compound +870 µL PBS, and 80 µM compound + 820 µL PBS). Incubation was performed at 54 °C for 30 min, then the samples were centrifuged at 5400 rpm for 5 min. All samples were analyzed in triplicate, and absorbance was analyzed through a spectrophotometer (UV5100B, PIOWAY, Nanjing, China) at 560 nm. The formula used for the determination of the percentage of inhibition of HRBC lysis is reported below:

$$\%\text{inhibition} = \frac{\text{Abs(control)} - \text{Abs(sample)} \times 100}{\text{Abs(control)}} \quad (1)$$

All the tests were performed in triplicate, and the mean ± SD was calculated.

4.4. In Vitro Anti-Diabetic Activity

The in vitro anti-diabetic activity was tested by determining the glucose uptake using the yeast cells assay. The assay was performed as per the method described in [17] with slight modifications. Yeast cells have affinity for glucose uptake and thus they are used as a model for diabetes. Baker's yeast was washed by repeated centrifugation in distilled water till the appearance of a clear supernatant. Then, a 10% colloidal suspension from the pellet was added to distilled water. Different concentrations of the compound were incubated with 1 mL of the solution containing glucose (5 mM). All samples were incubated at 37 °C for 10 min, and then the yeast suspension was added to start the reaction. The samples were vortexed and incubated further for 1 h at 37 °C, then they were finally centrifuged at 3000 rpm for 5 min. The amount of glucose uptake was determined through a spectrophotometer (UV5100B, PIOWAY, China) at 520 nm. The percentage increase in glucose uptake in the yeast cells was measured using Formula (1). All the tests were performed in triplicate, and the mean ± SD was calculated.

4.5. α-Amylase Inhibition Assay

Different concentrations of the compound and the reference standard drug were incubated with 2 U/mL of porcine pancreatic amylase (500 µL) in phosphate buffer for 20 min at 37 °C. Then, 250 µL of 1% starch was added, and the reaction was incubated for 1 h at 37 °C. Afterwards, 1 mL of dinitro salicylate reagent was added, and the mixture was boiled for 10 min. The absorbance was then measured at 540 nm, and the values were compared to those obtained for the control to calculate the inhibitory activity. Formula (1) was used for the calculations. All the tests were performed in triplicate, and the mean ± SD was calculated.

4.6. Molecular Modeling

The physico-chemical parameters were computed using SwissADME [23], and the target prediction studies were performed using PathwayMap [14].

For the docking studies, the 3D crystal structures of all the target macromolecules were obtained from PDB (https://www.rcsb.org/ accessed on 23 December 2022). The PDB codes of the downloaded enzymes are: 3AQV (AMPK), 1EQG (COX-1), 1CX2 (COX-2), and 2AZ5 (TNF-α). For α-amylase, shown in Figure 4, the 1B2Y model was used. The ligand and downloaded targets were prepared by using previously reported procedures [18,19]. The docking studies were carried out by using Molecular Operating Environment (MOE 2016.0802). The downloaded proteins were prepared and 3D protonated by using the "Prepare" module of MOE. Energy minimization was carried out by using AMBER 10EHT forcefield. For the docking simulations, docking grids were determined within 10 Å from the co-crystallized ligands. For all the ligands, 10 conformations were generated, and the top-ranked conformations based on the docking score were selected. Ligand interaction and visualization were carried out via Discovery Studio Visualizer (BIOVIA, Dassault Systèmes, San Diego, CA, USA) and UCSF Chimera, which were also used for the analysis of the docking results [26].

5. Conclusions

The present study on ferruginan extracted from *O. ferruginea* demonstrates that this natural compound has anti-inflammatory and anti-diabetic multi-target potential, as proved by a set of in vitro assays, including the α-amylase inhibition test, supported by computational data. Ligand-based target prediction and preliminary docking studies suggest that ferruginan may act on various molecular targets involved in diabetes and inflammation. On the other hand, it must be observed that the compound showed promising bioactivity, according to the tests performed on inflammation, glucose uptake, and α-amylase inhibition, only at rather high concentrations. This suggests that optimization of the small molecule is mandatory, as higher potency is needed for a future development as a drug candidate. Moreover, it must be stressed that while this study paved the way for the investigation of the bioactivity of ferruginan through computational and experimental evidence, further in vitro and in vivo studies are needed to fully assess the pharmacological potential and safety of this natural compound.

Supplementary Materials: The following supporting information can be downloaded at: https://www.mdpi.com/article/10.3390/pr11020545/s1, Figures S1–S5: computational studies and interaction pattern of native ligands and docked compounds.

Author Contributions: Conceptualization, A.R. (Abdur Rauf) and U.R.; methodology, Z.A.S. and I.; software, G.R. (Giovanni Ribaudo); validation, K.B., J.J., and A.R. (Abdur Rahman); formal analysis, A.A.; investigation, M.A., A.A.-S.; resources, A.A.; data curation, G.R. (Gauhar Rehman); writing—original draft preparation, A.R. (Abdur Rauf), A.A.-S.; writing—review and editing, G.R. (Giovanni Ribaudo); visualization, M.A.; supervision, A.R. (Abdur Rauf); project administration, A.A.; funding acquisition, M.A. All authors have read and agreed to the published version of the manuscript.

Funding: This research was founded by Researchers Supporting Project number (RSP2023R491), King Saud University, Riyadh, Saudi Arabia.

Institutional Review Board Statement: The experimental protocol was approved by the Research grants and Experimentation Ethics Committee of the Department of Zoology Abdul Wali Khan University, Mardan, on the use of human tissue samples and blood (AWKUM/Zoo/2022/2788).

Informed Consent Statement: Not applicable.

Data Availability Statement: The data associated with this paper are provided in the main text of this paper.

Acknowledgments: G.R. acknowledges funding from the University of Brescia.

Conflicts of Interest: The authors declare no conflict to interest.

References

1. Johannsen, D.L.; Ravussin, E. The Role of Mitochondria in Health and Disease. *Curr. Opin. Pharmacol.* **2009**, *9*, 780–786. [CrossRef] [PubMed]
2. Diniz do Nascimento, L.; De Moraes, A.A.B.; Da Costa, K.S.; Galúcio, J.M.P.; Taube, P.S.; Costa, C.M.L.; Cruz, J.N.; Andrade, E.H.D.A.; De Faria, L.J.G. Bioactive Natural Compounds and Antioxidant Activity of Essential Oils from Spice Plants: New Findings and Potential Applications. *Biomolecules* **2020**, *10*, 988. [CrossRef] [PubMed]
3. Rana, A.; Samtiya, M.; Dhewa, T.; Mishra, V.; Aluko, R.E. Health Benefits of Polyphenols: A Concise Review. *J. Food Biochem.* **2022**, *46*, e14264. [CrossRef] [PubMed]
4. Atanasov, A.G.; Zotchev, S.B.; Dirsch, V.M.; Supuran, C.T. Natural products in drug discovery: Advances and opportunities. *Nat. Rev. Drug Discov.* **2021**, *20*, 200–216. [CrossRef]
5. Sarker, S.D.; Nahar, L. An Introduction to Natural Products Isolation. *Methods Mol. Biol.* **2012**, *864*, 1–25. [CrossRef]
6. Shah, Z.A.; Mujawah, A.A.H.; Ullah, I.; Rauf, A.; Rashid, U.; Khalil, A.A.; Shah, S.M.M.; Pervaiz, A.; Shaheen, F.; Al-Awthan, Y.S.; et al. Antioxidant and Cytotoxic Activity of a New Ferruginan A from Olea Ferruginea: In Vitro and In Silico Studies. *Oxidative Med. Cell. Longev.* **2022**, *2022*, 8519250. [CrossRef]
7. Amin, A.; Khan, M.A.; Shah, S.; Ahmad, M.; Zafar, M.; Hameed, A. Inhibitory Effects of Olea Ferruginea Crude Leaves Extract against Some Bacterial and Fungal Pathogen. *Pak. J. Pharm. Sci.* **2013**, *26*, 251–254.
8. Anwar, S.; Saleem, H.; Khurshid, U.; Ansari, S.Y.; Alghamdi, S.; Al-Khulaidi, A.W.A.; Malik, J.A.; Ahemad, N.; Awadh Ali, N.A. Comparative Phytochemical Composition, Oleuropein Quantification, Antioxidant and Cytotoxic Properties of *Olea Europaea* L. Leaves. *Nat. Prod. Res.* **2022**, 1–7. [CrossRef]
9. Ayeleso, T.; Matumba, M.; Mukwevho, E. Oleanolic Acid and Its Derivatives: Biological Activities and Therapeutic Potential in Chronic Diseases. *Molecules* **2017**, *22*, 1915. [CrossRef]
10. Mehmood, A.; Murtaza, G. Phenolic Contents, Antimicrobial and Antioxidant Activity of Olea Ferruginea Royle (Oleaceae). *BMC Complement. Altern. Med.* **2018**, *18*, 173. [CrossRef]

11. Sun, N.; Li, D.; Chen, X.; Wu, P.; Lu, Y.-J.; Hou, N.; Chen, W.-H.; Wong, W.-L. New Applications of Oleanolic Acid and Its Derivatives as Cardioprotective Agents: A Review of Their Therapeutic Perspectives. *Curr. Pharm. Des.* **2019**, *25*, 3740–3750. [CrossRef] [PubMed]
12. Yu, M.; Gouvinhas, I.; Rocha, J.; Barros, A.I.R.N.A. Phytochemical and Antioxidant Analysis of Medicinal and Food Plants towards Bioactive Food and Pharmaceutical Resources. *Sci. Rep.* **2021**, *11*, 10041. [CrossRef]
13. Zafar, S.; -Ur-Rehman, F.; Shah, Z.A.; Rauf, A.; Khan, A.; Humayun Khan, M.; Ur Rahman, K.; Khan, S.; Ullah, A.; Shaheen, F. Potent Leishmanicidal and Antibacterial Metabolites from *Olea Ferruginea*. *J. Asian Nat. Prod. Res.* **2019**, *21*, 679–687. [CrossRef] [PubMed]
14. Jiménez, J.; Sabbadin, D.; Cuzzolin, A.; Martínez-Rosell, G.; Gora, J.; Manchester, J.; Duca, J.; De Fabritiis, G. PathwayMap: Molecular Pathway Association with Self-Normalizing Neural Networks. *J. Chem. Inf. Model.* **2019**, *59*, 1172–1181. [CrossRef] [PubMed]
15. He, M.M.; Smith, A.S.; Oslob, J.D.; Flanagan, W.M.; Braisted, A.C.; Whitty, A.; Cancilla, M.T.; Wang, J.; Lugovskoy, A.A.; Yoburn, J.C.; et al. Small-Molecule Inhibition of TNF-α. *Science* **2005**, *310*, 1022–1025. [CrossRef]
16. Kurumbail, R.G.; Stevens, A.M.; Gierse, J.K.; McDonald, J.J.; Stegeman, R.A.; Pak, J.Y.; Gildehaus, D.; Iyashiro, J.M.; Penning, T.D.; Seibert, K.; et al. Structural Basis for Selective Inhibition of Cyclooxygenase-2 by Anti-Inflammatory Agents. *Nature* **1996**, *384*, 644–648. [CrossRef]
17. Selinsky, B.S.; Gupta, K.; Sharkey, C.T.; Loll, P.J. Structural Analysis of NSAID Binding by Prostaglandin H$_2$ Synthase: Time-Dependent and Time-Independent Inhibitors Elicit Identical Enzyme Conformations. *Biochemistry* **2001**, *40*, 5172–5180. [CrossRef]
18. Handa, N.; Takagi, T.; Saijo, S.; Kishishita, S.; Takaya, D.; Toyama, M.; Terada, T.; Shirouzu, M.; Suzuki, A.; Lee, S.; et al. Structural Basis for Compound C Inhibition of the Human AMP-Activated Protein Kinase A2 Subunit Kinase Domain. *Acta Cryst. D Biol. Crystallogr.* **2011**, *67*, 480–487. [CrossRef]
19. Liaqat, S.; Islam, M.; Saeed, H.; Iqtedar, M.; Mehmood, A. Investigation of Olea Ferruginea Roylebark Extracts for Potential in Vitro Antidiabetic and Anticancer Effects. *Turk. J. Chem.* **2021**, *45*, 92–103. [CrossRef]
20. Shams, W.A.; Rehman, G.; Onoja, S.O.; Ali, A.; Khan, K.; Niaz, S. In Vitro Antidiabetic, Anti-Inflammatory and Antioxidant Potential of the Ethanol Extract of Uromastyx Hardwickii Skin. *Trop. J. Pharm. Res.* **2021**, *18*, 2109–2115. [CrossRef]
21. Sagbo, I.J.; van de Venter, M.; Koekemoer, T.; Bradley, G. In Vitro Antidiabetic Activity and Mechanism of Action of *Brachylaena Elliptica* (Thunb.) DC. *Evid.-Based Complement. Altern. Med.* **2018**, *2018*, 4170372. [CrossRef] [PubMed]
22. Sekhon-Loodu, S.; Rupasinghe, H.P.V. Evaluation of Antioxidant, Antidiabetic and Antiobesity Potential of Selected Traditional Medicinal Plants. *Front. Nutr.* **2019**, *6*, 53. [CrossRef] [PubMed]
23. Daina, A.; Michielin, O.; Zoete, V. SwissADME: A Free Web Tool to Evaluate Pharmacokinetics, Drug-Likeness and Medicinal Chemistry Friendliness of Small Molecules. *Sci. Rep.* **2017**, *7*, 42717. [CrossRef] [PubMed]
24. Rehman, G.; Hamayun, M.; Iqbal, A.; Ul Islam, S.; Arshad, S.; Zaman, K.; Ahmad, A.; Shehzad, A.; Hussain, A.; Lee, I. In Vitro Antidiabetic Effects and Antioxidant Potential of *Cassia nemophila* Pods. *BioMed Res. Int.* **2018**, *2018*, 1824790. [CrossRef]
25. Diedisheim, M.; Carcarino, E.; Vandiedonck, C.; Roussel, R.; Gautier, J.-F.; Venteclef, N. Regulation of Inflammation in Diabetes: From Genetics to Epigenomics Evidence. *Mol. Metab.* **2020**, *41*, 101041. [CrossRef]
26. Pettersen, E.F.; Goddard, T.D.; Huang, C.C.; Couch, G.S.; Greenblatt, D.M.; Meng, E.C.; Ferrin, T.E. UCSF Chimera?A Visualization System for Exploratory Research and Analysis. *J. Comput. Chem.* **2004**, *25*, 1605–1612. [CrossRef]

Disclaimer/Publisher's Note: The statements, opinions and data contained in all publications are solely those of the individual author(s) and contributor(s) and not of MDPI and/or the editor(s). MDPI and/or the editor(s) disclaim responsibility for any injury to people or property resulting from any ideas, methods, instructions or products referred to in the content.

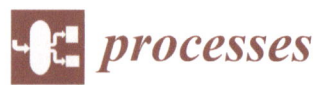

Article

Computational and *In Vitro* Assessment of a Natural Triterpenoid Compound Gedunin against Breast Cancer via Caspase 3 and Janus Kinase/STAT Modulation

Talib Hussain [1], Muteb Alanazi [2], Jowaher Alanazi [1], Tareq Nafea Alharby [2], Aziz Unnisa [3], Amir Mahgoub Awadelkareem [4], AbdElmoneim O. Elkhalifa [4], Mohammad M. Algahtani [5], SMA Shahid [6] and Syed Mohd Danish Rizvi [7,*]

[1] Department of Pharmacology and Toxicology, College of Pharmacy, University of Ha'il, Ha'il 81442, Saudi Arabia; mdth_ah@yahoo.com (T.H.); js.alanzi@uoh.edu.sa (J.A.)
[2] Department of Clinical Pharmacy, College of Pharmacy, University of Ha'il, Ha'il 81442, Saudi Arabia; ms.alanazi@uoh.edu.sa (M.A.); tn.alharby@uoh.edu.sa (T.N.A.)
[3] Department of Pharmaceutical Chemistry, College of Pharmacy, University of Ha'il, Ha'il 81442, Saudi Arabia; khushiazeez@yahoo.co.in
[4] Department of Clinical Nutrition, College of Applied Medical Sciences, University of Hail, Ha'il 81442, Saudi Arabia; mahgoubamir22@gmail.com (A.M.A.); ao.abdalla@uoh.edu.sa (A.O.E.)
[5] Department of Pharmacology and Toxicology, College of Pharmacy, King Saud University, Riyadh 11451, Saudi Arabia; mohgahtani@ksu.edu.sa
[6] Department of Biochemistry, College of Medicine, University of Ha'il, Ha'il 81442, Saudi Arabia; sm.shahid@uoh.edu.sa
[7] Department of Pharmaceutics, College of Pharmacy, University of Ha'il, Ha'il 81442, Saudi Arabia
* Correspondence: sm.danish@uoh.edu.sa

Citation: Hussain, T.; Alanazi, M.; Alanazi, J.; Alharby, T.N.; Unnisa, A.; Awadelkareem, A.M.; Elkhalifa, A.O.; Algahtani, M.M.; Shahid, S.; Rizvi, S.M.D. Computational and *In Vitro* Assessment of a Natural Triterpenoid Compound Gedunin against Breast Cancer via Caspase 3 and Janus Kinase/STAT Modulation. *Processes* 2023, *11*, 1452. https://doi.org/10.3390/pr11051452

Academic Editors: Alina Bora, Luminita Crisan and Elwira Sieniawska

Received: 26 March 2023
Revised: 27 April 2023
Accepted: 5 May 2023
Published: 11 May 2023

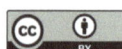

Copyright: © 2023 by the authors. Licensee MDPI, Basel, Switzerland. This article is an open access article distributed under the terms and conditions of the Creative Commons Attribution (CC BY) license (https://creativecommons.org/licenses/by/4.0/).

Abstract: Breast cancer is the most prevalent type of malignancy among females as per the report of the World Health Organization. There are several established chemotherapeutic regimes for the clinical management of different solid cancers; however, the after-effects of these therapeutics serve as a significant limiting factor. The natural triterpenoid compound, gedunin is one of the principal phytoconstituent found in *Azadirachta indica*. In this study, we have investigated the anticancer potential of gedunin against human breast cancer MDA-MB-231 and MCF-7 cells. Based on computational studies, gedunin exhibited significantly higher binding affinity of −7.1 and −6.2 Kcal/mol towards Janus kinase (JAK) and STAT proteins, respectively. Further, the anticancer potential of gedunin against human breast cancer was studied using hormone-independent and -dependent MCF-7 and MDA-MB-231 cell lines, respectively. The results indicated that gedunin inhibited the growth and multiplication of both MCF-7 and MDA-MB-231 cells. The nuclear fragmentation and ROS were qualitatively enhanced in the treated MCF-7 and MDA-MB-231 cells in comparison to untreated cells. The caspase-3 level was significantly enhanced with a concomitant decline in JAK1 and STAT3 mRNA expression. Based on these results, gedunin might be considered as a potential therapeutic lead against hormone-dependent and -independent breast cancer MCF-7 and MDA-MB-231 cells, respectively. However, further detailed mechanistic studies are warranted to conclusively establish the anti-breast cancer effects.

Keywords: natural compound; anticancer; breast cancer; caspase-3; Janus kinase1/STAT3

1. Introduction

Breast cancer, as per the World Health Organization, represents the most common carcinoma among females globally. The latest report by Global Cancer Observatory found that 2,261,419 new cases of breast carcinomas were reported during 2020, constituting nearly 11.7% of all the diagnosed 19,292,789 cases of various cancers globally. Subsequently, the report also stated that breast cancer was the reason behind 6.9% of deaths from

9,958,133 cancer-associated demises globally in 2020 [1]. At the molecular biology level, breast cancer exhibits considerable heterogeneity and is thus differentiated into various subtypes based on the presence and absence of various receptors. Exhaustive investigations costing billions of dollars have resulted in a better understanding of breast carcinoma's proliferation, invasiveness, and metastasis. These have further led to the development of frequently used adjuvant chemotherapeutic regimes, including docetaxel/cyclophosphamide, adriamycin/cyclophosphamide, and adriamycin/cyclophosphamide with combinatorial administration of paclitaxel. However, these regimes also have adverse clinical side effects [2]. Apart from the chemotherapy, endocrine therapy had long been recognized as a powerful and important adjuvant treatment for women with hormone receptor–positive, early-stage breast cancer. Many randomized clinical trial data demonstrated the benefit of ovarian function suppression, tamoxifen, and aromatase inhibitors alone, in combination, and sequentially, of different durations, and according to menopausal state and risk. Moreover, recent data provided evidence of the role of adjuvant CDK-4/-6 inhibitor/endocrine therapy combinations for those with high- and intermediate-risk disease [3]. Indeed, it has previously been reported that a combination of anticancer chemotherapeutics exerts superior therapeutical efficacy by improving the survival rate and reducing treatment-associated pain compared to a single chemotherapeutic [4]. Nevertheless, the adverse effects of these combinatorial chemotherapeutics cannot be overlooked since these, apart from cancer cells, also adversely affects normal healthy cells [5]. Intriguingly, breast cancer chemotherapy was recently found to be associated with the instigation of several complications, including cardiopathy, in patients [6].

Since ancient times, plants are not only a source of nutrition but have also been extensively used in the treatment of various ailments. The plants and their various isolated secondary metabolites have been substantially investigated for their anticancer potential apart from various other pharmacological characteristics [7]. One such natural compound is gedunin belonging to limonoid falling in various genera of the *Meliaceae* family, such as *Carapa*, *Cabralea*, *Azadirachta*, and *Guarea* [8]. In the epicarp of the fruit *Azadirachta indica A. Juss*, gedunin was abundantly reported [9]. Indeed, various pharmacological attributes have been previously associated with gedunin, which include anti-inflammatory, anti-allergic, anticancer, and antimalarial properties, among others [10]. Concerning breast cancer, previously anticancer effects of plants and their parts, along with purified compounds usually considered nutritive, are reported to be biologically active and possess pharmacological properties [10,11]. Limonoid is a particularly important bioactive phytocompound found abundantly in several member genera of the family *Meliaceae*. Among several other bioactive compounds extracted from *Azadirachta indica* or Indian neem, as presented in Figure 1, gedunin ($C_{28}H_{34}O_7$) is a member of the tetranotriterpenoid family, which has been explored for its anticancer effects against different cancer cell lines from colon, prostate, and ovarian origin [12–14]. Gedunin chemically acts as a reactive-thiol electrophile that activates the heat shock response by a mechanism closely similar to celastrol. Gedunin is readily soluble in organic solvents such as ethanol and DMSO; however, it is known for its poor solubility in water. Gedunin has also been previously documented for several pharmacological properties, including anti-allergic, neuroprotective effects, anti-inflammatory, antimalarial, and anticancer attributes [15]. Multiple studies have demonstrated that gedunin holds the therapeutic potential for the treatment of various cancers and its underlying mechanistic action is extensively studied. Furthermore, previous preclinical studies have shown that gedunin is capable of treating carcinomas of various organs such as lung, brain, colon, pancreas, stomach, ovary, prostate, and stem cells [9]. However, subsequent studies are warranted to provide a better understanding relating to the specific mechanism behind anticancer effects of gedunin. Gedunin is frequently used in the Indian medicine system for treating infectious diseases such as malaria [16].

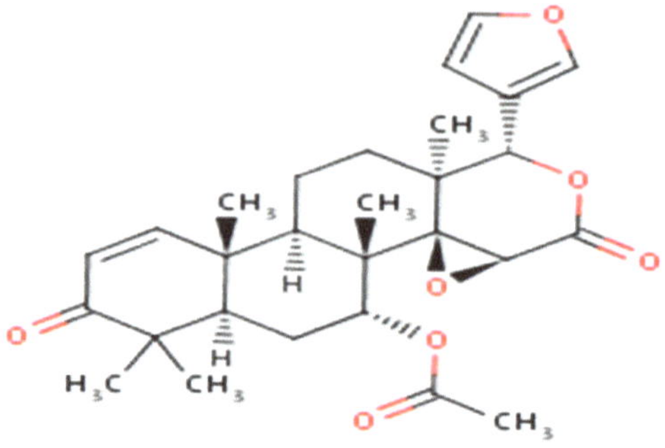

Figure 1. Chemical structure of gedunin. (Adopted from ChEBI; CHEBI:65954).

On the molecular basis, several altered signaling pathways have been associated with nearly all reported cancers. Janus kinase (JAK) signal transducer and activator of transcription (STAT) signaling play a pivotal role during embryo development by regulating various homeostatic cellular functions, including hematopoiesis, maintenance of cells, and inflammatory response. The pathway is responsible for transducing signals from growth factors, interleukins, and cytokines, which are functionally active through various transmembrane receptors. Previously, it was demonstrated that JAK1 serves to be an essential kinase required for cytokine-based activation of STAT protein in breast cancer cells [17]. Furthermore, recently, it has also been demonstrated that hyper- and constitutive-expression of STAT3 is involved in developing chemo-resistance, progression, and metastasis of breast cancer. Intriguingly, upstream and downstream STAT3 target-associated novel pathways have also been recently deciphered in breast carcinoma [18]. However, the anticancer effects of gedunin against human breast adenocarcinoma MCF-7 cells remain unexplored. Therefore, based on present evidence, the authors hypothesize that gedunin may exert an antiproliferative effect on human breast cancer MCF-7 cells by altering the expression of the JAK/STAT signaling pathway.

2. Results

2.1. Molecular Docking Results

3D structures of gedunin and gemcitabine were downloaded from the Pub Chem database. These compounds were docked to the JAK1 and STAT3 proteins to predict the mechanism of breast cancer cell suppression, as shown in Figure 2a–d. This report selected the commercial anticancer drug gemcitabine as a reference compound. Our docking studies have predicted that the binding energy of gedunin towards JAK1 and STAT3 are −7.1 and −6.2 kcal/mol, respectively, which are nearer to the binding energies of gemcitabine to JAK1 and STAT3 (−6.6 and −5.0 kcal/mol, respectively) as shown in Figures 3 and 4. More negative binding energy correlates with the better stability of the protein–ligand complex. Thus, it can be inferred from the results that gedunin showed better interactions with the targeted JAK1 and STAT3 proteins than gemcitabine. Moreover, further analysis showed the details of amino acids of JAK1 and STAT3 involved in hydrophobic interactions and hydrogen bonding with gedunin and gemcitabine.

The residues involved in hydrophobic interaction of JAK1 with gemcitabine are Phe^{1046} (A), Arg^{1041} (A), and Phe^{1044} (A). However, Gln^{1098} (B), Asp^{1042} (A), His^{885} (A), Ser^{1043} (A), and Val^{1045} (A) are engaged in hydrogen bonding (bond lengths 2.93, 3.05, 2.80, 3.01, and 3.30). Furthermore, the amino acids involved in hydrophobic interactions of STAT3 with gemcitabine are Tyr^{446} (A), Gln^{361} (A), Leu^{358} (B), Gln^{361} (B), His^{447} (B), and Tyr^{446} (B). However, Glu^{357} (B) and Gln^{448} (B) are engaged in hydrogen bond interactions (bond lengths 2.98 Å, 3.01 Å, and 3.25 Å) (Figure 3a,b).

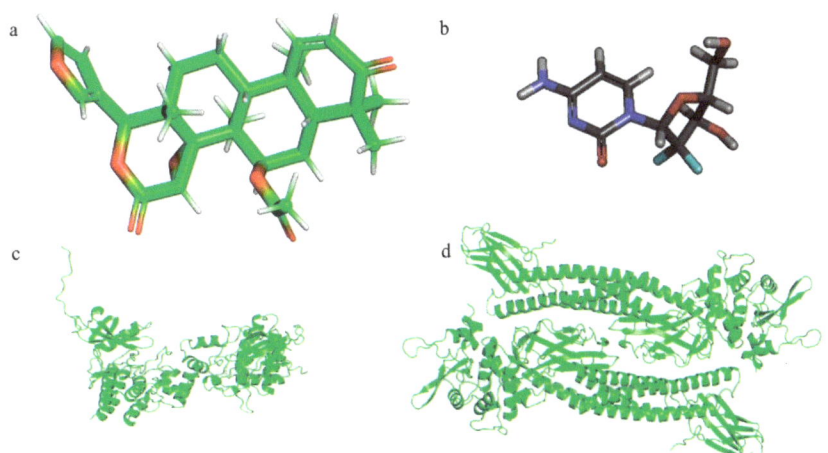

Figure 2. 3D chemical structures of (**a**) gedunin, (**b**) gemcitabine, (**c**) JAK1, and (**d**) STAT3.

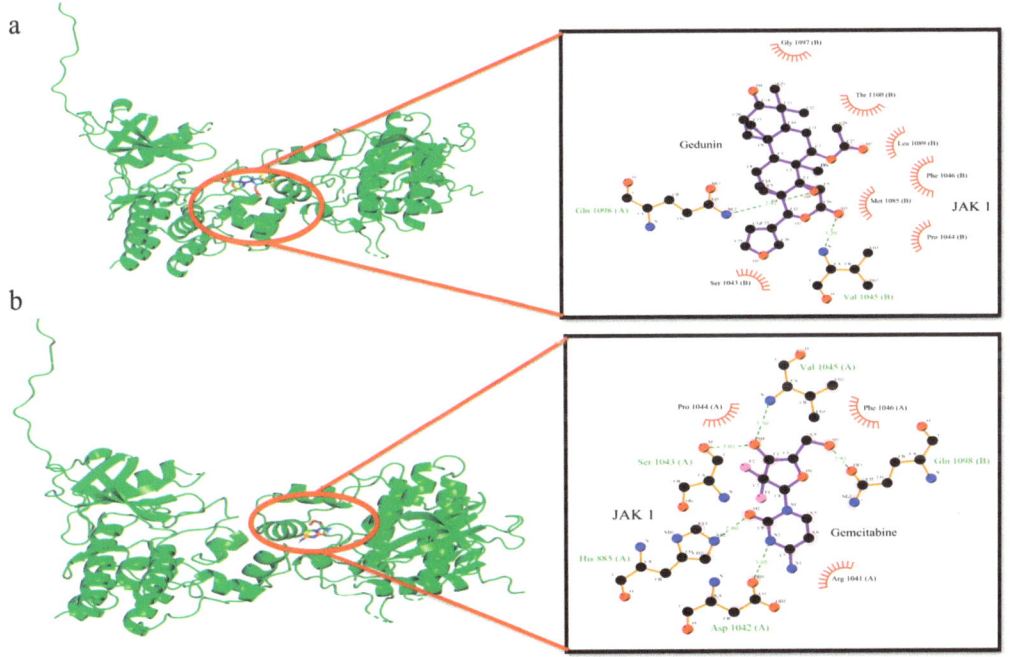

Figure 3. 2D interaction complex of (**a**) gedunin and (**b**) gemcitabine with JAK1 protein; where red shows the target protein, purple shows the ligand molecule, and red circle shows the enlarged view of the residues of gedunin with respective target proteins.

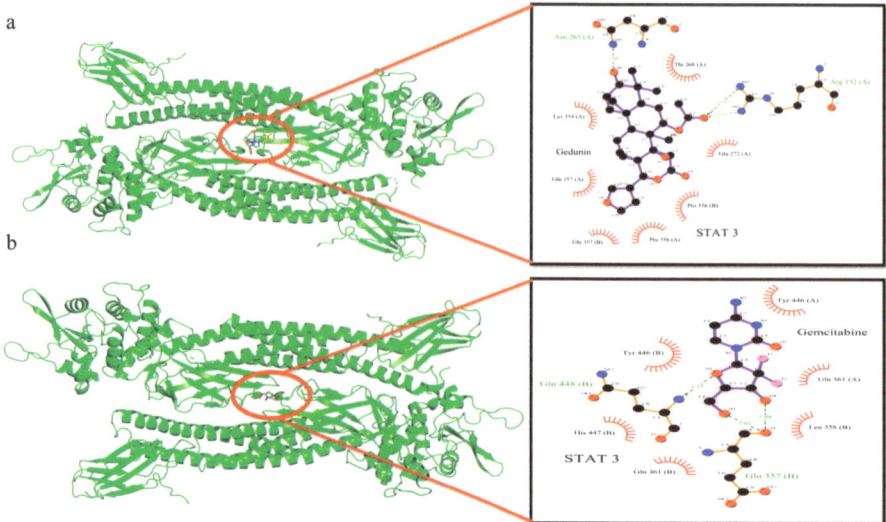

Figure 4. 2D interaction complex of (**a**) gedunin and (**b**) gemcitabine with STAT3 protein; where red shows the target protein, purple shows the ligand molecule, and red circle shows the enlarged view of the residues of gedunin with respective target proteins.

Gedunin has been hypothesized to interact with JAK1 and STAT3 proteins. It was found that the JAK1 residues involved in hydrophobic interaction with gedunin are Gly^{1097}, Thr^{1100}, Leu^{1089}, Phe^{1046}, Met^{1085}, Pro^{1044}, Ser^{1043}, and Val^{1045}, Gln^{1098}, which are engaged in hydrogen bonding (bond lengths 3.20 Å and 2.81 Å), whereas the amino acids of STAT3 involved in hydrophobic interactions with gedunin are Thr^{268} (A), Glu^{272} (A), Pro^{356} (B), Pro^{356} (A), Gln^{357} (B), Gln^{357} (A), and Lys^{354} (A). However, Arg^{152} (A) and Asn^{265} (A) engage in hydrogen bond interactions (bond lengths 3.31 Å, 2.93 Å, and 2.59 Å), as shown in Figure 3a,b and Figure 4a,b. The binding energies of gedunin and gemcitabine with breast cancer targets (JAK1 and STAT3) and the interacting amino acids have been summarized in Table 1.

Table 1. Binding energies of gedunin and gemcitabine with breast cancer targets (JAK1 and STAT3) and the interacting amino acids.

Compound	Binding Energy (Kcal/mol)	Hydrogen Bonds (Bond Length in Å)	Hydrophobic Interactions
JAK1–gedunin	−7.1	Gln^{1098} engage in hydrogen bonding (bond lengths 3.20 and 2.81)	Gly^{1097}, Thr^{1100}, Leu^{1089}, Phe^{1046}, Met^{1085}, Pro^{1044}, Ser^{1043}, and Val^{1045}
JAK1–gemcitabine	−6.6	Gln^{1098} (B), Asp^{1042} (A), His^{885} (A), Ser^{1043} (A), and Val^{1045} (A) engage in hydrogen bonding (bond lengths 2.93, 3.05, 2.80, 3.01, and 3.30).	Phe^{1046} (A), Arg^{1041} (A), and Phe^{1044} (A)
STAT3–gedunin	−6.2	Arg^{152} (A) and Asn265 (A) engage in hydrogen bond interactions (bond lengths 3.31, 2.93, and 2.59).	Thr^{268} (A), Glu^{272} (A), Pro^{356} (B), Pro^{356} (A), Gln^{357} (B), Gln^{357} (A), and Lys^{354} (A).
STAT3–gemcitabine	−5.0	Glu357 (B), and Gln448 (B) engage in hydrogen bond interactions (bond lengths 2.98, 3.01, and 3.25).	Tyr446 (A), Gln361 (A), Leu358 (B), Gln361 (B), His447 (B), and Tyr446 (B).

2.2. Gedunin Impeded the Growth of MCF-7 and MDA-MB-231 Cells

To investigate the plausible cytotoxic effects of gedunin on MCF-7 cells, 3-(4,5-dimethylthiazol-2-yl)-2,5-diphenyl-2H-tetrazolium bromide or MTT assay was performed after incubating MCF-7 cells with various doses of gedunin (5, 15, and 20 µM) for 24 h. The results showed that gedunin exerted substantial cytotoxic effects by suppressing the growth of MCF-7 cells by 83.13 ± 3.70%, 61.09 ± 3.87%, and 33.06 ± 4.23% at the indicated concentration of 5µM, 10µM, and 15µM, respectively (Figure 5a). Furthermore, the viability of MCF-7 was reduced to 70.13 ± 4.03% (5 µM), 46.75 ± 4.56% (10 µM), and 27.40 ± 2.03% (15 µM) after 48 h of incubation with gedunin (Figure 5c). Gedunin further reduced the viability of hormone independent MDA-MB-231 cells to 88.98 ± 3.14%, 54.01 ± 3.17%, and 29.75 ± 3.81% (Figure 5b) at above stated concentrations. The viability of MDA-MB-231 cells was also further reduced to 79.65 ± 4.56% (5 µM), 48.35 ± 5.55% (10 µM), and 24.75 ± 4.72% (15 µM) after 48 h of incubation with gedunin (Figure 5d). Gemcitabine used as a positive control in our study also significantly impeded the viability of both the stated human-derived breast cancer cell lines. The IC_{50} of gedunin was found to be 11.80 ± 1.047 µM and 10.67 ± 1.02 µM % for breast cancer MCF-7 and MDA-MB-231 cells, respectively (Figure 6a,b). Furthermore, we also inspected the toxicity of gedunin against human normal cell line HEK-293. As shown in Figure 6c, gedunin exerts insignificant cytotoxic effects on HEK-293 cells, which confirm its non-toxic nature.

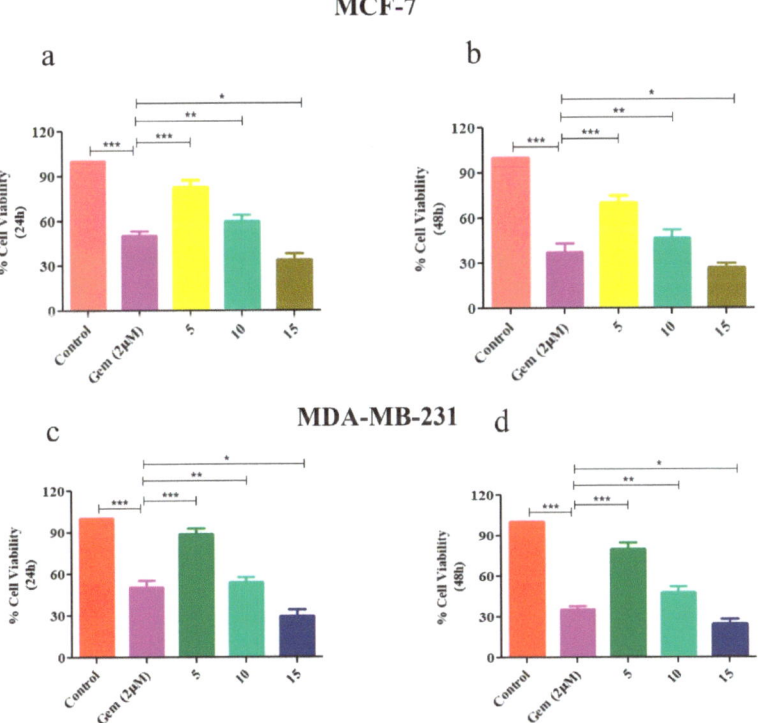

Figure 5. Gedunin suppressed the proliferation of breast cancer cells. Cell viability percentage of gedunin-treated after (**a**) 24 h and (**b**) 48 h in MCF-7 cells. The viability of MDA-MB-231 cells after treatment with gedunin after (**c**) 24 h and (**d**) 48 h. A significant difference determined by the *p* value < 0.05 was labeled with asterisk (*); *p* value < 0.01 was labeled with double asterisks (**); and *p* value < 0.001 was labeled with double asterisks (***).

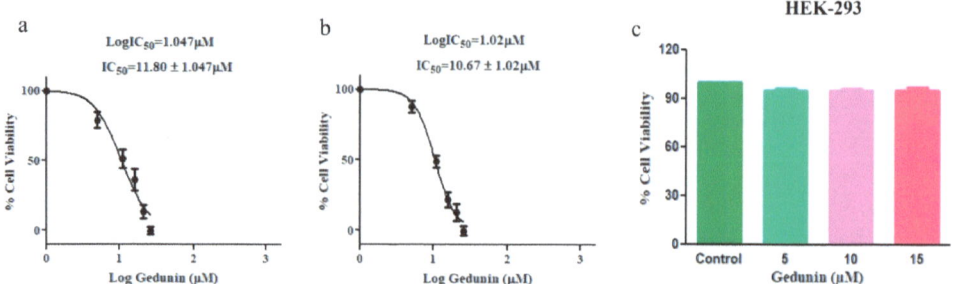

Figure 6. IC$_{50}$ calculation for gedunin against (**a**) MCF-7 cells, (**b**) MDA-MB-231 cells, and (**c**) non-significant cytotoxicity of gedunin on HEK-293 cells.

2.3. Gedunin-Induced Nuclear Condensation and Fragmentation

4′,6-Diamidino-2-phenylindole also known as DAPI staining was performed to determine whether gedunin-mediated cell growth inhibition in breast cancer cells resulted from the induction of apoptosis. After 24 h treatment with gedunin at different concentrations (5, 10, and 15 µM), changes in nuclear morphology for both the cell lines (MCF-7 and MDA-MB-231) were observed. Fluorescence micrographs presented in Figure 7 showed bright-blue fluorescence and condensed nuclei with the increasing concentration of gedunin in both MCF-7 and MDA-MB-231 cells, indicating the onset of apoptosis. Gemcitabine-treated MCF-7 and MDA-MB-231 cells also exhibited increased nuclear condensation as seen in Figure 7. However, no substantial condensation was observed in untreated hormone-dependent and independent breast cancer cells demonstrating diffusely stained intact nuclei. The results, finally, suggested that gedunin-induced apoptosis in MCF-7 cells in a dose-dependent manner.

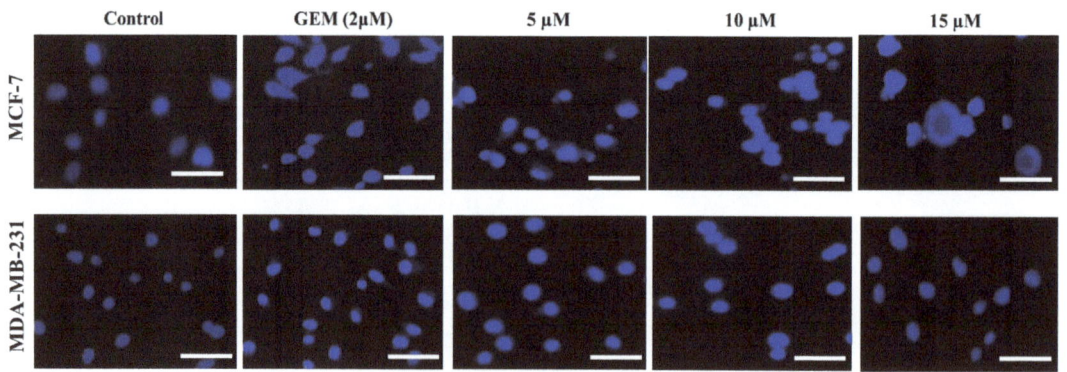

Figure 7. Efficacy of gedunin in altering the homeostatic nuclear morphology in MCF-7 and MDA-MB-231 cells as evaluated through DAPI stain. Scale bar = 20 µm; magnification: 30×.

Furthermore, the level of nuclear fragmentation and condensation induced by gedunin at different concentrations was quantified using ImageJ software, NIH, Maryland, USA. Gedunin succeeded in enhancing the levels of nuclear fragmentation and condensation by 33.38 ± 3.74 (5 µM), 54.35 ± 3.05 (10 µM), and 78.42 ± 4.61 (15 µM) after 24 h of incubation with MCF-7 cells (Figure 8a). Furthermore, in MDA-MB-231 cells, gedunin-mediated nuclear condensation and fragmentation was found to be escalated by 35.38 ± 4.32 (5 µM), 57.68 ± 4.68 (10 µM), and 73.42 ± 3.24 (15 µM) after 24 h (Figure 8b). Furthermore, gemcitabine also showed its competence in elevating the levels of nuclear fragmentation and condensation in both human-derived breast cancer cell lines.

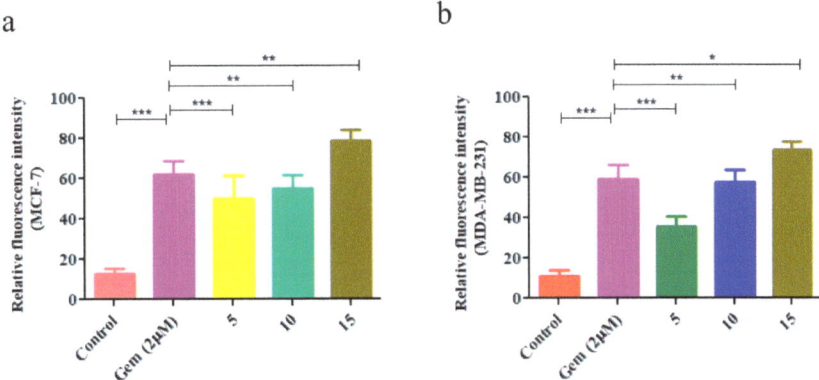

Figure 8. Quantification of gedunin-mediated nuclear condensation and fragmentation. (**a**) MCF-7 and (**b**) MDA-MB-231 cells as evaluated through DAPI stain. A significant difference determined by the p value < 0.05 was labeled with asterisk (*); p value < 0.01 was labeled with double asterisks (**), and p value < 0.001 was labeled with double asterisks (***).

2.4. Gedunin Treatment Elevated Caspase-3 Activity

Caspases are essential for transmitting the signals during apoptosis, and these are represented by a group of proteases mediating the essential functions of proteolytic cleavage of various proteins. The investigators tried to substantiate whether gedunin-instigated apoptosis altered the expression of caspase-3 comparatively with untreated control MCF-7 cells. The activity of caspase-3 was elevated by 37.40 ± 4.66% (at 5 µM gedunin concentration), 55.79 ± 5.46% (at 10 µM gedunin concentration), and 113.42 ± 3.77% (at 15 µM gedunin concentration) within the MCF-7 cells (Figure 9a). In case of MDA-MB-231 breast cancer cell lines, caspase-3 activity was found to be increased by 41.69 ± 4.45%, 59.12 ± 4.62%, and 107.25 ± 5.29% at 5 µM, 10 µM, and 15 µM concentrations of gedunin, respectively (Figure 9c). Thus, it can be concluded that the treatment of gedunin significantly increases the activity of caspase-3 in both MCF-7 and MDA-MB-231 cells. Furthermore, gemcitabine acted as a positive control and also elevated caspase-3 activity within MCF 7 (79.91 ± 3.662) and MDA-MB-231 cells (67.25 ± 3.42) in comparison with respective untreated control.

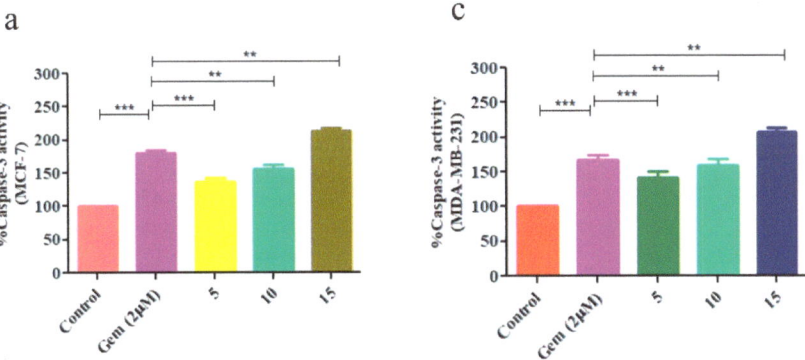

Figure 9. *Cont.*

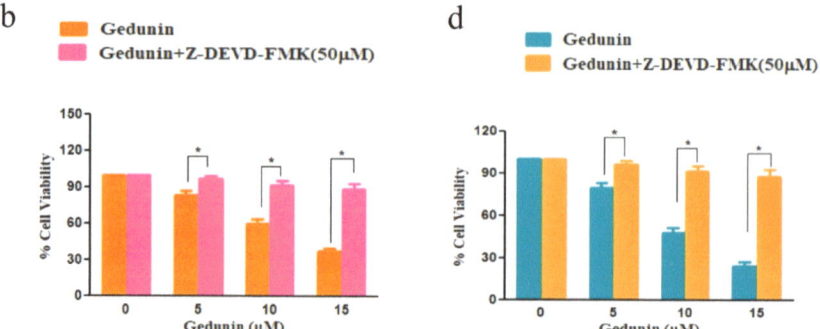

Figure 9. Gedunin mediated the activation of caspase-3 in (**a**) MCF-7 (**c**) MDA-MB-231 cells. Pretreatment with caspase-3 inhibitor significantly ameliorated the cytotoxic effects induced by gedunin in both MCF-7 and MDA-MB-231 cells (**b**,**d**). A significant difference determined by the p value < 0.05 was labeled with asterisk (*); p value < 0.01 was labeled with double asterisks (**), and p value < 0.001 was labeled with double asterisks (***).

2.5. Caspase-3 Inhibitor Alleviated Gedunin-Mediated Cytotoxicity

To confirm the activation of caspase-3 in MCF-7 and MDA-MB-231 breast cancer cells by gedunin and its role in cytotoxicity, the cells pre-treated with caspase-3 inhibitor (Z-DEVD-FMK) were further treated with 5, 10, and 15 μM concentrations of gedunin. It was observed that caspase-3 inhibitor pre-treatment substantially impeded the gedunin-mediated cytotoxicity against both MCF-7 and MDA-MB-231 cells (Figure 9b,d), indicating a key role of caspase-3 activation during gedunin-induced effect. However, pretreatment of caspase inhibitors did not completely attenuate the cell viability in both MCF-7 and MDA-MB-231 cells, which indicated plausible role of the caspase-independent pathways as well. Thus, it is reasonable to say that gedunin might induce effects on breast cancer cells via both caspase-dependent and independent manner.

2.6. Gedunin-Instigated Intracellular ROS

Enhanced ROS production levels could be linked with the activation of apoptotic pathways in the cancer cells [19]. Thus, we investigated the effect of ROS generation after treatment with different concentrations of gedunin for 24 h in breast cancer cells. As shown in Figure 10a,b, a substantial increase in ROS level by 17.32 ± 3.12% was seen as compared to control cells following treatment with 5 μM of gedunin. Intriguingly, ROS generation was further enhanced by 54.01 ± 3.14% and 101.08 ± 4.79% in MCF-7 cells at the concentrations of 10 μM and 15 μM, respectively. Similarly, ROS levels increased by 26.38 ± 2.89% (5 μM) in comparison with untreated MDA-MB-201 control cells. ROS levels further escalated by 58.68 ± 4.84% (10 μM) and 117.75 ± 3.53% (15 μM) (Figure 10c,d). Importantly, gedunin also succeeded in instigating the production of intracellular ROS. As shown in Figure 10c,d, gemcitabine also increased intracellular ROS level by 71.42 ± 4.90% in MCF-7 cells whereas in MDA-MB-231 cells the levels of ROS increased by 77.75 ± 3.53% in comparison with respective untreated control. The stated observations indicated that gedunin treatment augmented ROS production in hormone-dependent and independent breast cancer cells.

2.7. NAC Pretreatment Abrogated Gedunin-Instigated Intracellular ROS

N-acetyl-l-cysteine (NAC; a potent ROS inhibitor) was used to ascertain the role of gedunin in augmenting ROS within MCF-7 and MDA-MB-231 cells. Initially, both the cells were treated with NAC for 15 min, followed by the treatment with various concentrations of gedunin (5, 10, and 15 μM) for another 24 h, using MTT assay. It was demonstrated that pretreatment with NAC significantly decreased the amount of gedunin-induced ROS in breast cancer cells. Moreover, NAC pre-treatment also subdued ROS production in both MCF-7 and MDA-MB-231 cells treated with gemcitabine. Thus, our results suggested that increased generation of intracellular ROS is crucial for apoptosis induced by the treatment of gedunin (Figure 10e,f). However, it was intriguing to note that NAC did not entirely ameliorate the inhibitory action of gedunin on the growth of MCF-7 and MDA-MB-231 cells, which suggested the involvement of various other ROS-independent pathways in gedunin-treated breast cancer cells.

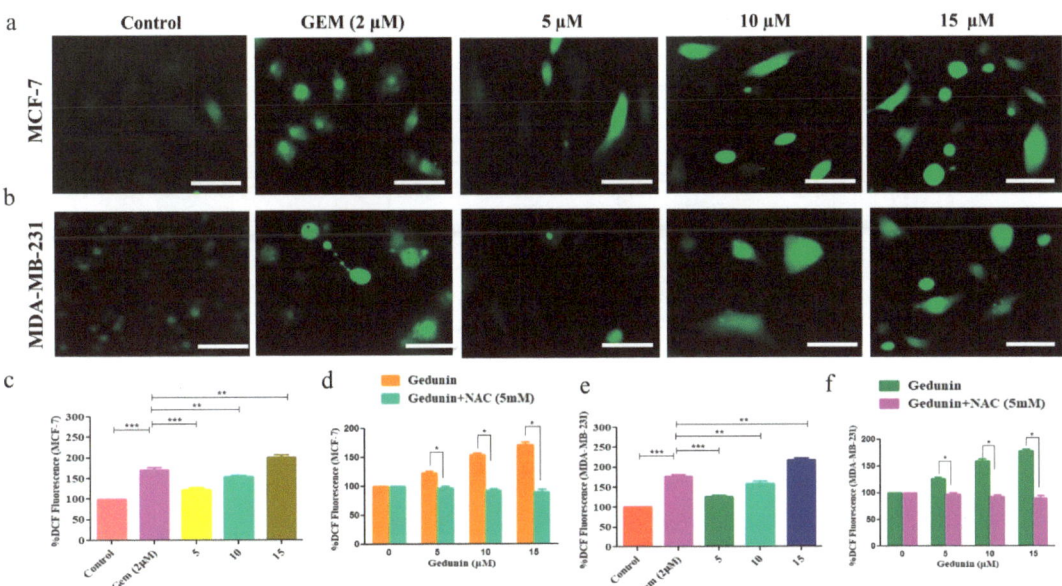

Figure 10. Gedunin-mediated effects on (**a,b**) instigation of intracellular ROS within human breast adenocarcinoma MCF-7 and MDA-MB-231 cells, (**c,d**) percent DCHF-DA fluorescence in gedunin-treated MCF-7 and MDA-MB-231 cells, and (**e,f**) the effects of NAC pretreatment in ameliorating gedunin-mediated ROS. Scale bar = 20 µm; magnification: 30×. A significant difference determined by the p value < 0.05 was labeled with asterisk (*); p value < 0.01 was labeled with double asterisks (**) and p value < 0.001 was labeled with double asterisks (***).

2.8. Gedunin Reduced JAK1/STAT3 Expression

Among different cellular pathways that reported their abrupt regulation, the JAK/STAT pathway was found to be crucial for proliferation, cellular differentiation, and immune system responsiveness [20]. Gedunin-mediated modulation of the JAK1/STAT3 signaling pathway in both the breast cancer cells was investigated. The observations indicated that gedunin exposure impeded JAK1/STAT3 signaling by reducing JAK1 and STAT3 mRNA expression. Gedunin suppressed JAK1 mRNA expression to $0.88 \pm 0.04\%$ (5 µM), $0.50 \pm 0.04\%$ (10 µM), and $0.39 \pm 0.05\%$ (15 µM) ($p < 0.05$) and mRNA level of STAT3 to $0.92 \pm 0.02\%$, $0.71 \pm 0.05\%$, and $0.36 \pm 0.03\%$ ($p < 0.05$), respectively (Figure 11a,b), in MCF-7 cells. Furthermore, gedunin succeeded in reducing the expression of JAK1 mRNA to $0.78 \pm 0.07\%$, $0.57 \pm 0.06\%$, and $0.35 \pm 0.09\%$ at 5 µM, 10 µM, and 15 µM concentration of gedunin in MDA-MB-231 cells, respectively. Similarly, STAT3 mRNA expression was reduced to $0.76 \pm 0.07\%$, $0.49 \pm 0.05\%$, and $0.25 \pm 0.05\%$ at 5 µM, 10 µM, and 15 µM concentration of gedunin in MDA-MB-231 cells, respectively (Figure 11c,d).

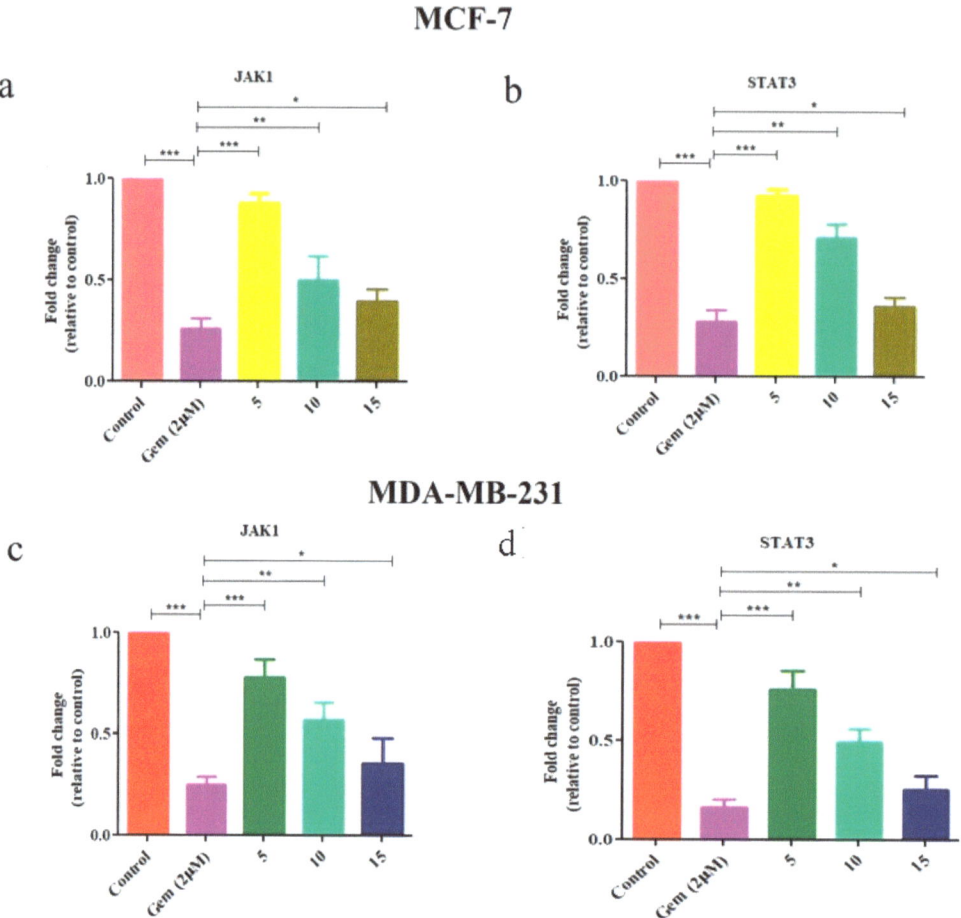

Figure 11. The effect of gedunin in modulating the expression of JAK1 and STAT3 genes in (**a,b**) MCF-7 and (**c,d**) MDA-MB-231 cells. A significant difference determined by the p value < 0.05 was labeled with asterisk (*); p value < 0.01 was labeled with double asterisks (**); and p value < 0.001 was labeled with double asterisks (***).

2.9. Gedunin Regulated the Gene Expression of JAK1/STAT3-Associated Genes

Intriguingly, constitutive STAT3 gene expression has been reported to promote the proliferation, survival, and migration of cancer cells. Furthermore, an increase in STAT3 also plays a crucial role in limiting the responsiveness of cancer cells to the individual's immune response [21]. An earlier published report has demonstrated that docetaxel can bind to Bcl-2, overexpressed in several different cancer cells, including breast and prostate cancer cells. Bcl-X_L is also downregulated by docetaxel [22]. Anti-apoptotic proteins, including Bcl-2, Bcl-X_L, and Mcl-1, are often elevated after activation of STAT3, which subsequently assist cancer cell survival [23,24]. We observed that there was a significant reduction in the level of expression of these stated anti-apoptotic markers (Bcl-X_L and Bcl-2) after gedunin exposure at the indicated concentrations of 5, 10, and 15 μM to 0.81 ± 0.04%, 0.66 ± 0.03%, and 0.44 ± 0.07%; 0.90 ± 0.02%, 0.74 ± 0.06%, and 0.57 ± 0.03% (Figure 12a–c), whereas the same in case of MDA-MB-231 cells was found to be 0.87 ± 0.04%, 0.61 ± 0.04%, and 0.37 ± 0.05%; 0.83 ± 0.05%, 0.71 ± 0.05%, and 0.41 ± 0.05%, respectively (Figure 12d–f). Concomitantly, gedunin enhanced the expression of Bax to 1.25 ± 0.03, 1.65 ± 0.05, and 1.99 ± 0.08 folds and was also seen in MCF-7 cells, whereas the same in case of MDA-MB-231 cells was found to be 1.32 ± 0.06, 1.53 ± 0.07, and 2.08 ± 0.06 folds, respectively (Figure 12d).

Enhanced proliferation of cancer cells is usually associated with enhanced c-myc and cyclin D1 expression [25]. The qPCR results revealed that cyclin D1 and c-myc mRNA expression was lowered to 0.82 ± 0.03%, 0.64 ± 0.04%, and 0.33 ± 0.03% ($p < 0.05$) and 0.84 ± 0.02%, 0.61 ± 0.05%, and 0.23 ± 0.04% ($p < 0.01$), respectively, in MCF-7 cells (Figure 13). In case of MDA-MB-231, the reduction was calculated to be 0.79 ± 0.07%, 0.59 ± 0.06%, and 0.38 ± 0.08%; 0.84 ± 0.06%, 0.62 ± 0.05%, and 0.37 ± 0.08%, respectively. Gedunin-mediated modulation of cell cycle regulatory genes within MCF-7 cells were also investigated. mRNA expression of p21^{Cip1} was significantly increased by 1.22 ± 0.04, 1.54 ± 0.02, and 1.76 ± 0.03 ($p < 0.001$) folds post-gedunin exposure whereas the same in case of MDA-MB-231 cells was found to be 1.64 ± 0.05, 1.94 ± 0.06, and 2.53 ± 0.11 folds, respectively. STAT3 downregulation is also associated with regulating protein expression such as p53, which is important for apoptosis induction [26,27]. The results indicated that gedunin declined p53 expression by 1.14 ± 0.02, 1.37 ± 0.04, and 2.16 ± 0.05 ($p < 0.001$) folds in MCF-7 cells. In case of MDA-MB-231, the reduction in p53 expression was calculated to be 1.32 ± 0.03, 1.60 ± 0.09 and 2.06 ± 0.04 folds, respectively (Figure 13e,f).

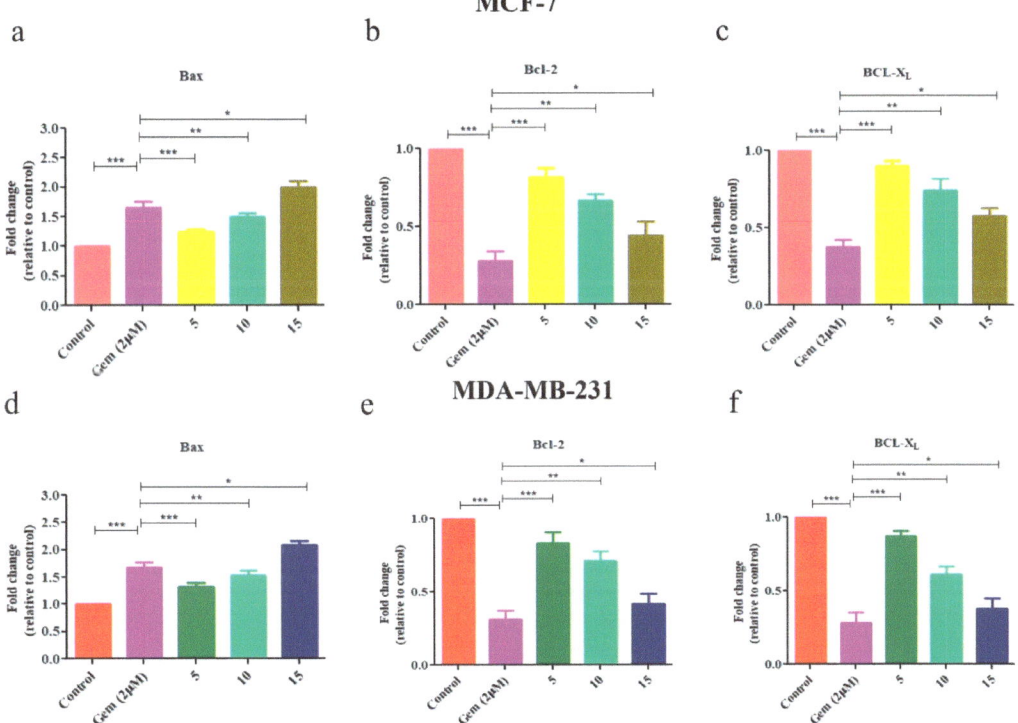

Figure 12. The modulation of JAK/STAT-associated gene expression in gedunin-treated human breast adenocarcinoma (**a–c**) MCF-7 and (**d–f**) MDA-MB-231 cells. A significant difference determined by the p value < 0.05 was labeled with asterisk (*); p value < 0.01 was labeled with double asterisks (**); and p value < 0.001 was labeled with double asterisks (***).

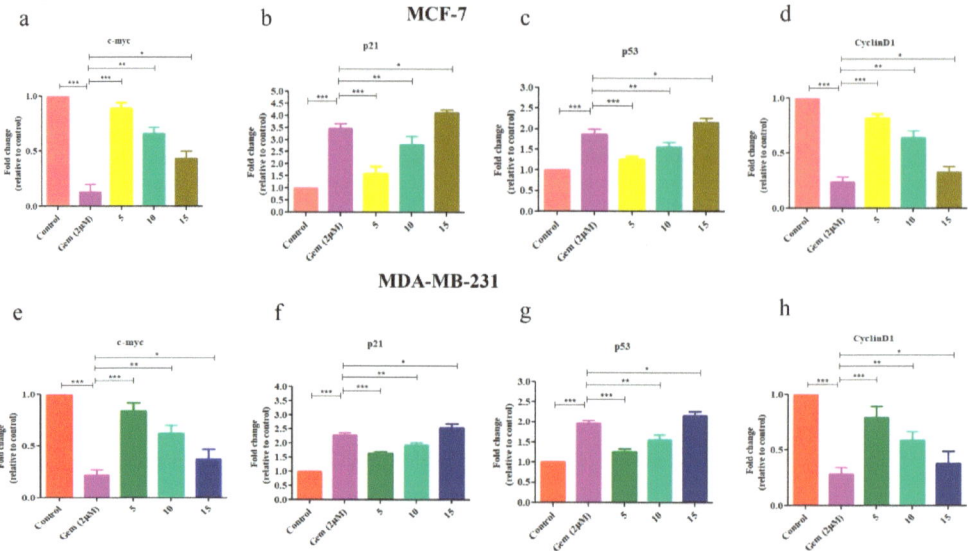

Figure 13. The modulation of JAK/STAT-associated gene expression in gedunin-treated human breast adenocarcinoma (**a–d**) MCF-7 and (**e–h**) MDA-MB-231 cells. A significant difference determined by the *p* value < 0.05 was labeled with asterisk (*); *p* value < 0.01 was labeled with double asterisks (**) and *p* value < 0.001 was labeled with double asterisks (***).

3. Discussion

Several natural compounds are usually associated with considerable anticancer efficacy because their intrinsic capabilities restrain several carcinomas' proliferation, angiogenesis, growth and metastasis. Furthermore, these natural compounds usually exhibit reduced cytotoxic effects against normal cells, reducing the chances of adverse side effects upon treatment. These attributes have compelled the exhaustive investigation of natural products for their anticancer potential because of their competence in inhibiting growth and metastasis despite instigating considerable side effects [26]. Despite the critical pharmacological relevance of gedunin, its anticancer efficacy against human breast adenocarcinoma MCF-7 cells and triple negative MDA-MB-231 cells remains unexplored. Thus, the authors hypothesized that in light of the pharmacological activities, gedunin might impede the proliferation of MCF-7 and MDA-MB-231 cells by modulating the expression of the JAK/STAT pathway.

In the present investigation, the efficacy of gedunin in modulating JAK1 and STAT3 protein was evaluated through molecular docking studies to elucidate the modulation of JAK/STAT signaling during breast cancer. The observation during the in silico studies indicated that gedunin could be an effective inhibitor of the JAK/STAT pathway due to the considerable binding efficiency of gedunin against JAK1 and STAT3 proteins. The binding efficiency of gedunin was comparable with the standard breast cancer chemotherapeutic gemcitabine. Thus, this observation served to be an initial indicator that gedunin may be involved in altering the expression of the JAK/STAT pathway, which in turn was implicated generally with cancer development and progression of breast cancer. Our preliminary in vitro observation also indicated that gedunin exerted a significant cytotoxic effect against MCF-7 and MDA-MB-231 cells exhibiting a dose and time-dependent effect. Notably, the onset of cellular death in response to several chemotherapeutics may be through autophagy, apoptosis, and necrosis. However, instigating apoptosis or cell death through either of the other stated pathway is plausibly considered a therapeutical intervention against several carcinomas [28]. An essential attribute during the instigation of apoptotic pathways was the condensation of the nucleus and the generation of apoptotic bodies [29]. Moreover, the qualitative data of DAPI staining was also supported by quantitative data suggesting that these findings were in line with the reported observation. They elucidated that gedunin instigated the condensation of the nucleus upon exposure, with gedunin exhibiting a dose-dependent effect against breast adenocarcinoma MCF-7 and triple negative MDA-MB-231 cells.

Activating caspases during apoptosis is a peculiar characteristic defining the site-specific cleavage of aspartate residues [30]. Thus, the level of **Caspase-3 activity was estimated post-gedunin treatment in MCF-7 and MDA-MB-231 cells. The activation of caspase-3 was evident by its higher activity post-gedunin treatment, indicating apoptosis instigation by gedunin. This was further reaffirmed by the ameliorative effect of caspase-3 inhibitor in alleviating the induction of apoptosis after MCF-7 and MDA-MB-231 cells were exposed to gedunin. Cancer cells are also accredited with enhanced levels of basal ROS, which act as a dual-edged sword by supporting pro-oxidants' actions.

Nevertheless, ROS instigation resulting in the onset of apoptosis is regarded as a productive strategy for the clinical management of different carcinomas. The results presented in the report also explicitly indicated that gedunin exposure was competent in inducing ROS generation within the MCF-7 cells. Importantly, gedunin-induced ROS augmentation was significantly ameliorated in NAC-pretreated MCF-7 and MDA-MB-231 cells. Also, NAC pretreatment considerably ameliorated gedunin-mediated cytotoxicity. These results indicated that ROS instigation was essential in gedunin-mediated cytotoxicity against MCF-7 and MDA-MB-231 cells.

As previously stated, JAK/STAT **signaling is reported to be closely associated with the progression and development of metastatic carcinomas. Due to its substantial involvement in the progression of breast cancer, several antagonistic or inhibitor molecules targeting JAK/STAT pathways have been developed [29]. Indeed, the constitutive expression of JAK/STAT signaling is implicated with the downstream activation of several genes involved in modulating apoptotic pathways, including Bcl-XL, Bax, and Bcl-2 [31]. The gene expression analysis observations established that gedunin reduced the expression of anti-apoptotic genes with a concomitant increase in their apoptotic counterparts. Significantly, consecutive expression of STAT3 is further associated with enhanced proliferation, metastasis, and drug resistance of several carcinomas [32]. Thus, the elucidation of STAT3 inhibitor is a valued strategy for preventing different associated carcinomas. During our investigation, it was also found that gedunin reduced the mRNA expression of STAT3 protein, which could be attributed to reduced proliferation and instigation of apoptosis in breast adenocarcinoma MCF-7 and MDA-MB-231 cells in the present study.

In summary, our present article has demonstrated the anticancer efficacy of gedunin against MCF-7 and MDA-MB-231 breast cancer cells via attenuating the JAK1/STAT3 signaling pathway. It was observed that gedunin substantially instigated apoptotic cell death by modulating the mRNA expression of BcL-2, BclXL, and Bax genes involved in apoptosis. Therefore, it is concluded that gedunin could be an adjunct therapeutic for the treatment and management of breast cancer.

Although gedunin holds the potential to treat various human cancers and its anti-cancer efficacy is associated with the alteration of various signaling pathways, the low hydrophobicity of gedunin reduces its bioavailability and pharmacokinetic profile [33]. Moreover, the employment of advanced research techniques such as liposomal drug delivery and nanoformulation could ameliorate the efficacy of gedunin as a cancer therapeutic along with the combination with various chemotherapeutic drugs. Therefore, subsequent studies are needed to better understand the underlying mechanism and also substantiate the safety of gedunin for human consumption by conducting pre-clinical and clinical trials. Furthermore, it is difficult to produce gedunin in larger amounts and also cannot be easily chemically synthesized, which poses a limitation on its usage. Thus, it is recommended to encourage the production of gedunin at commercial levels for research analysis [34]. The molecular mechanistic action of gedunin against breast cancer cells has been summarized in Figure 14.

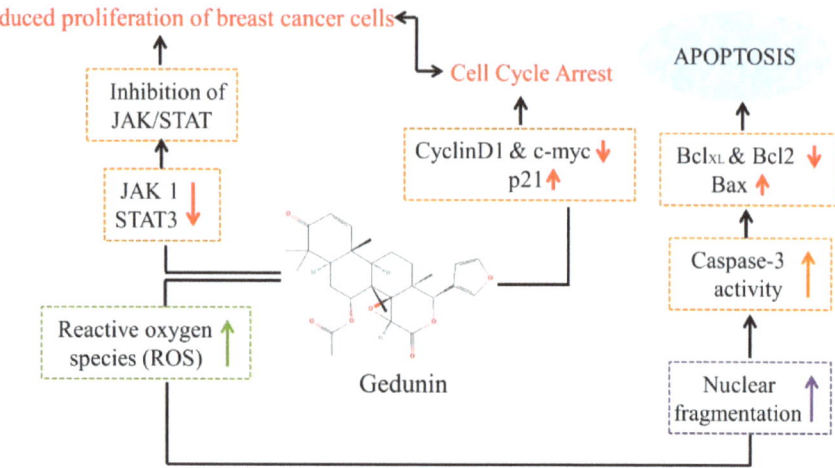

Figure 14. Schematic flowchart representation of gedunin against breast cancer cells.

4. Materials and Methods

4.1. Materials

3-(4,5-Dimethylthiazol-2-yl)-2,5-diphenyl-2H-tetrazolium bromide (MTT) dye (catalogue no: RM1131) was commercially obtained from Himedia, India. 2′,7′-Dichlorofluorescin diacetate (DCF-DA) (catalogue no: 21884), acridine orange (catalogue no: MB071), ethidium bromide (catalogue no: TC262-5G), and Z-DEVD-FMK; ** caspase-3 inhibitor (catalogue no: 264156-M), gemcitabine hydrochloride (cas no. 122111-03-9) were procured from Sigma. Gedunin (purity > 95%) was obtained from Santa Cruz Biotechnology, USA. Minimum essential medium **Eagle (MEM) with Earle's salt (catalogue no: AT154], fetal bovine serum (FBS) (catalogue no: 26140087), and the antibiotic–antimycotic solution were commercially obtained from Gibco. The caspase-3 colorimetric assay kit used was purchased from BioVision (San Francisco, CA, USA).

4.2. Cell Culture Maintenance

Human-derived estrogen, progesterone, and glucocorticoid receptor positive MCF-7 cells, MDA-MB-231, and human normal cell line HEK-293 were procured from the cell repository of the National Center of Cell Sciences, Pune. They were allowed to proliferate in minimum essential medium (MEM) with Earle's modification and DMEM-high glucose media under humidified atmosphere constituted by 5% CO_2 maintained at 37 °C. The media was supplemented with 10% fetal bovine serum (FBS) and 1% **antibiotic-antimycotic solution. Cells were monitored regularly and were passaged once the flask attained <85% confluence.

4.3. Methods

4.3.1. In Silico Investigations

Retrieval of 3D Protein Structure

The crystal structure of JAK1 and STAT3 with PDB ID: 4I5C and 6TLC, respectively, used during the present study were taken from Brookhaven Protein Data Bank (www.rcsb.org/pdb; accessed on 28 January 2023). The structures of JAK1 and STAT3 (x = 0.26, y = 32.3, z = 33.52) transcription factors employed for docking were devoid of any heteroatoms, including the non-receptor atoms, namely water, ions, etc. The binding pocket coordinates for JAK1 (x = 9.844, y = 31.334, z = 9.614) and STAT3 (x = 0.26, y = 32.3, z = 33.52) were set as default, and the grid box of proteins was put within a cubic box of magnitudes 40 × 40 × 40 Å [35].

Retrieval of 3D Structure Ligands

Required ligands were searched on a database of Pub Chem (http://pubchem.ncbi.nlm.nih.gov). The structural and functional details of the different organic compounds were retrieved from the database of PubChem, having a unique CID or compound identification number. The structural details about the desired ligands were collected using the Simplified Molecular Input Line Entry Specification string, which was further deposited in CORINA (http://www.molecular-networks.com/products/Corina) software. This software utilizes the SMILES string to create a 3D structure of the desired molecules, which can then be retrieved in PDB format for AutoDock Vina 4.0. We have utilized the Linux subsystem command line and used MMFF94 force filed for energy minimization (EM); after EM, we prepared the ligand molecules by using mgltools 1.5.6.

Docking Complex Visualization

The visualization of best-docked position was selected out of nine possible confirmations on the basis of interacting residues including hydrogen bonds with large binding energy (kcal/mol). Thereafter, LigPlot was employed to visualize the protein–ligand interaction of docked complexes in two dimensions [36], and PyMol was utilized to generate all the binding pockets [37,38]. The interactions among protein and ligand are mediated by hydrogen bonds or may arise due to hydrophobic interactions. Hydrogen bonds are represented by dashed lines within the interacting atoms. Contrastingly, hydrophobic interactions in these regions are shown by an arc with spokes radiating towards the atoms within the ligand interacting with the protein whereas the atoms contacted are represented with spokes radiating backwards.

4.3.2. In Vitro Assessments

Cytotoxic Effects of Gedunin against Breast Cancer

To investigate the cytotoxic potential of gedunin against breast cancer MCF-7 cells and HEK-293 cells, an MTT-based colorimetric assay was undertaken, as described previously [39]. Concisely, 5×10^3 MCF-7 and MDA-MB-231 cells were exposed to varying gedunin concentrations (5, 10, and 15 µM) for 24 h and 48 h under standard conditions of tissue culture. Subsequently, the treated cells were exposed to MTT dye (5 mg/mL) for an additional 4 h. Finally, the formazan crystals were read for their absorbance intensity at 570 nm by solubilizing them with tissue grade DMSO (100 µL) through a microplate reader BioRad (Hercules, CA, USA). The results were elucidated in terms of cell viability percentage (%) in contrast with untreated using the formula

Cellular viability % = (Absorbance of treated MCF-7 and MDA-MB-231 cells)/(Absorbance of untreated MCF-7 and MDA-MB-231 control cells) × 100

Assessment of Nuclear Morphology

Changes within the nuclear morphology, such as condensation of the nucleus in breast adenocarcinoma MCF-7 and MDA-MB-231 cells, were assessed using DAPI staining, as earlier reported [40]. Precisely 5×10^4 cells/well was exposed to varying stated concentrations of gedunin for 12 h. Subsequently, after washing the cells with $1\times$ PBS, these were fixed using chilled methanol for around 10 min. The treated and untreated cells were exposed to permeabilizing buffer constituted by TritonX100 (0.25% v/v) and stained with DAPI. Eventually, DAPI-associated blue fluorescence was visualized and recorded using Carl Zeiss GmbH microscope (Model: LSM780NLO, Oberkochen, Baden-Württemberg, Germany).

Evaluation of Gedunin-Induced ROS Production

ROS-mediated oxidative stress was assessed qualitatively and quantitatively through DCF-DA stain, as reported previously [41]. A total of 5×10^4 MCF-7 and MDA-MB-231 cells were initially allowed to adhere in each well of a 96-well plate under optimum culture conditions. Subsequently, the cells were exposed to varying concentrations of gedunin for

12 h and, after that, stained with DCFH-DA (10 µM) for 30 min at dark 37 °C. The cells were then washed cautiously using PBS, and finally, the cells were visualized through Carl Zeiss GmbH microscope (Model: LSM780NLO).

To quantify the generation of intracellular ROS, 1×10^4 cells were allowed to adhere in each 96-well black bottom plate well under optimum culture conditions. Cells were treated and incubated with gedunin for 12 h, as stated above. Eventually, the fluorescence of treated and untreated control MCF-7 cells was quantified in terms of fluorescence intensity percentage in comparison with untreated control at excitation: emission wavelength of 485:528 nm.

Effects of ROS Inhibitor

To ascertain the involvement of gedunin in augmenting ROS within human breast adenocarcinoma MCF-7 cells, a potent ROS inhibitor, N-acetyl cysteine (NAC), was used. Briefly, post-adherence 5×10^4 MCF-7 and MDA-MB-231 cells in each well of a 96-well plate were pretreated with NAC (10 mM) and incubated under standard conditions for 2 h. Subsequently, the cells were re-exposed to the above-stated concentrations of gedunin and incubated for 12 h. This was followed by treated and untreated control treatment with DCFH-DA (10 µM; 37 °C for 30 min) in the dark as described previously [42]. Finally, the fluorescence intensity of different treated and untreated cells was quantified, as stated above in evaluation of Gedunin-induced ROS production.

Assessment of Caspase-3 Activation

Caspase-3 activation in gedunin-treated human breast adenocarcinoma MCF-7 and triple negative MDA-MB-231 cells was assessed colorimetrically using a commercially available kit (BioVision). Around 3×10^6 gedunin-treated and/or untreated cells were lysed using lysis buffer (50 µL). The lysate was centrifuged at $10,000 \times g$, and the resulting supernatant was collected and immediately transferred on ice. The lysate belonging to various treated and control group (50 µL) was aliquot in each well of the 96-well plate and mixed with reaction buffer (50 µL; 10 mM DTT). Subsequently, DEVD-pNA substrate was also supplemented in each well at a volume of 50 µL for one h** at 37 °C. Finally, the absorbance of each well was recorded at 405 nm. Compared with the untreated control, the observations were interpolated as caspase-3 activity percentage (%).

Effects of Caspase-3 Inhibitor

To further characterize the cytotoxic effects of gedunin, MCF-7 and MDA-MB-231 cells with pretreated for 2 h with caspase-3 specific inhibitor and subsequently were re-exposed to varying concentrations of gedunin as stated above for 24 h. Finally, the cell viability of cells belonging to different groups was estimated through MTT assay, as stated above in Cytotoxic Effects of Gedunin against Breast Cancer.

Quantitative Real-Time PCR (qRT-PCR)

A total of 1×10^6 MCF-7 and MDA-MB-231 cells, after adherence, were subjected to varying stated concentrations of gedunin for 24 h. Subsequently, the mRNA content of both treated and untreated control cells was isolated and **two µg of this was used for cDNA synthesis using commercially available cDNA synthesis kits. The primers involved in the present investigation were synthesized using the NCBI pick primer designing tool, which is mentioned in Table 2. GAPDH was used as a housekeeping gene for normalization. The results were interpolated by the $2^{\Delta\Delta}$CT method [42].

Table 2. List of the primer sequences used in the study.

Genes	Forward Primer	Reverse Primer	NCBI Gene Number
GAPDH	GTCTCCTCTGACTTCAACAGCG	ACCACCCTGTTGCTGTAGCCAA	2597
Bcl2	ATCGCCCTGTGGATGACTGAGT	GCCAGGAGAAATCAAACAGAGGC	596
Bcl$_{XL}$	GCCACTTACCTGAATGACCACC	AACCAGCGGTTGAAGCGTTCCT	598
Bax	TCAGGATGCGTCCACCAAGAAG	TGTGTCCACGGCGGCAATCATC	581
Cyclin D1	TGAACTACCTGGACCGCT	GCCTCTGGCATTTTGGAG	595
c-myc	AGCGACTCTGAGGAGGAACAAG	GTGGCACCTCTTGAGGACCA	26,292
p21^{Cip1}	AGGTGGACCTGGAGACTCTCAG	TCCTCTTGGAGAAGATCAGCCG	5058
p53	CCTCAGCATCTTATCCGAGTGG	TGGATGGTGGTACAGTCAGAGC	7157
JAK1	GAGACAGGTCTCCCACAAACAC	GTGGTAAGGACATCGCTTTTCCG	3716
STAT3	CTTTGAGACCGAGGTGTATCACC	GGTCAGCATGTTGTACCACAGG	6774

4.4. Statistical Inferences

Data of the present investigation are the average + SEM of discrete experiments performed thrice at least in triplicate. Differences in comparison with control and different groups were considered statistically significant in the case of $p < 0.05$ and were analyzed using one-way ANOVA followed by Dunnett's post hoc and Student t-test using GraphPad Prism Ver. 5 software as per their applicability. * $p < 0.05$, ** $p < 0.01$, and *** $p < 0.001$.

5. Conclusions

Conclusively, these findings demonstrated the anticancer efficacy of gedunin against MCF-7 and MDA-MB-231 breast cancer cells by inhibiting the JAK1/STAT3 signaling pathway. Gedunin competently instigated apoptotic cell death by altering the expression of BcL-2, Bcl$_{XL}$, and Bax genes involved in apoptosis. Significantly, the other target genes of the JAK1/STAT3 pathway, such as c-Myc, cyclin D1, and p21^{Cip1}, were modulated upon treatment with gedunin. Therefore, it may be affirmed that gedunin could be a plausible therapeutic against breast cancer, owing to its capability of regulating the JAK1/STAT3 pathway, which warrants a further detailed mechanistic study of gedunin in preclinical disease models.

Author Contributions: Conceptualization, T.H. and S.M.D.R.; Formal analysis, M.A., J.A. and A.M.A.; Funding acquisition, T.H. and A.O.E.; Investigation, A.M.A. and S.M.D.R.; Methodology, M.A., J.A. and T.N.A.; Project administration, T.H. and A.O.E.; Resources, S.S.; Software, M.M.A. and S.S.; Supervision, A.O.E. and S.M.D.R.; Validation, M.A., J.A., A.U. and T.N.A.; Visualization, A.M.A., M.M.A. and S.S.; Writing—original draft, A.U., T.N.A. and M.M.A.; Writing—review & editing, A.U. All authors have read and agreed to the published version of the manuscript.

Funding: This work was funded by the Research Deanship, University of Hai'l, Hai'l, Kingdom of Saudi Arabia, under Project grant no. RG-20159.

Institutional Review Board Statement: Not applicable.

Informed Consent Statement: Not applicable.

Data Availability Statement: Data are contained within the article.

Conflicts of Interest: The authors declare no conflict of interest.

References

1. Global Cancer Observatory Factsheet on Cancers. Last Updated: December 2020. Available online: https://gco.iarc.fr/today/data/factsheets/cancers/20-Breast-fact-sheet.pdf (accessed on 8 August 2022).
2. Waks, A.G.; Winer, E.P. Breast Cancer Treatment: A Review. *JAMA* **2019**, *321*, 288–300. [CrossRef] [PubMed]
3. Pistilli, B.; Lohrisch, C.; Sheade, J.; Fleming, G.F. Personalizing Adjuvant Endocrine Therapy for Early-Stage Hormone Receptor-Positive Breast Cancer. *Am. Soc. Clin. Oncol. Educ. Book* **2022**, *42*, 60–72. [CrossRef] [PubMed]
4. Shyam, M.M.; Moin, A.; Medishetti, R.; Rajendra, K.M.; Raichur, A.; Prashantha, K.B.R. Dual drug conjugate loaded nanoparticles for the treatment of cancer. *Curr. Drug Deliv.* **2015**, *12*, 782–794. [CrossRef]

5. Baudino, T.A. Targeted Cancer Therapy: The Next Generation of Cancer Treatment. *Curr. Drug Discov. Technol.* **2015**, *12*, 3–20. [CrossRef]
6. Ibraheem, A.; Stankowski-Drengler, T.J.; Gbolahan, O.B.; Engel, J.M.; Onitilo, A.A. Chemotherapy-induced cardiotoxicity in breast cancer patients. *Breast Cancer Manag.* **2016**, *5*, 31–41. [CrossRef]
7. Kooti, W.; Servatyari, K.; Behzadifar, M.; Asadi-Samani, M.; Sadeghi, F.; Nouri, B.; Zare Marzouni, H. Effective Medicinal Plant in Cancer Treatment, Part 2: Review Study. *J. Evid. Based Complement. Altern. Med.* **2017**, *22*, 982–995. [CrossRef]
8. Jeon, H.J.; Kim, K.; Kim, C.; Kim, M.J.; Kim, T.O.; Lee, S.E. Molecular mechanisms of anti-melanogenic gedunin derived from neem tree (*Azadirachta indica*) using B16F10 mouse melanoma cells and early-stage zebrafish. *Plants* **2021**, *10*, 330. [CrossRef]
9. Braga, T.M.; Rocha, L.; Chung, T.Y.; Oliveira, R.F.; Pinho, C.; Oliveira, A.I.; Morgado, J.; Cruz, A. Biological Activities of Gedunin-A Limonoid from the Meliaceae Family. *Molecules* **2020**, *25*, 493. [CrossRef]
10. Kapinova, A.; Kubatka, P.; Golubnitschaja, O.; Kello, M.; Zubor, P.; Solar, P.; Pec, M. Dietary phytochemicals in breast cancer research: Anticancer effects and potential utility for effective chemoprevention. *Environ. Health Prev. Med.* **2018**, *23*, 36. [CrossRef]
11. Moin, A.; Wani, S.U.D.; Osmani, R.A.; Abu Lila, A.S.; Khafagy, E.S.; Arab, H.H.; Gangadharappa, H.V.; Allam, A.N. Formulation, characterization, and cellular toxicity assessment of tamoxifen-loaded silk fibroin nanoparticles in breast cancer. *Drug Deliv.* **2021**, *28*, 1626–1636. [CrossRef]
12. Wylie, M.R.; Merrell, D.S. The Antimicrobial Potential of the Neem Tree *Azadirachta indica*. *Front. Pharmacol.* **2022**, *13*, 1535. [CrossRef] [PubMed]
13. Aarthy, T.; Mulani, F.A.; Pandreka, A.; Kumar, V.; Nandikol, S.S.; Haldar, S.; Thulasiram, H.V. Tracing the biosynthetic origin of limonoids and their functional groups through stable isotope labeling and inhibition in neem tree (*Azadirachta indica*) cell suspension. *BMC Plant Biol.* **2018**, *18*, 230. [CrossRef] [PubMed]
14. Gupta, A.; Ansari, S.; Gupta, S.; Narwani, M.; Gupta, M.; Singh, M. Therapeutics role of neem and its bioactive constituents in disease prevention and treatment. *J. Pharmacogn. Phytochem.* **2019**, *8*, 680–691.
15. Tan, Q.G.; Luo, X.D. Meliaceous limonoids: Chemistry and biological activities. *Chem. Rev.* **2011**, *111*, 7437–7522. [CrossRef]
16. Patwardhan, C.A.; Fauq, A.; Peterson, L.B.; Miller, C.; Blagg, B.S.; Chadli, A. Gedunin inactivates the co-chaperone p23 protein causing cancer cell death by apoptosis. *J. Biol. Chem.* **2013**, *288*, 7313–7325. [CrossRef]
17. Wehde, B.L.; Rädler, P.D.; Shrestha, H.; Johnson, S.J.; Triplett, A.A.; Wagner, K.U. Janus Kinase 1 Plays a Critical Role in Mammary Cancer Progression. *Cell Rep.* **2018**, *25*, 2192–2207.e5. [CrossRef]
18. Ma, J.H.; Qin, L.; Li, X. Role of STAT3 signaling pathway in breast cancer. *Cell Commun. Signal.* **2020**, *18*, 33. [CrossRef]
19. Aggarwal, V.; Tuli, H.S.; Varol, A.; Thakral, F.; Yerer, M.B.; Sak, K.; Varol, M.; Jain, A.; Khan, M.A.; Sethi, G. Role of Reactive Oxygen Species in Cancer Progression: Molecular Mechanisms and Recent Advancements. *Biomolecules* **2019**, *9*, 735. [CrossRef]
20. Bao, L.; Zhang, H.; Chan, L.S. The involvement of the JAK-STAT signaling pathway in chronic inflammatory skin disease atopic dermatitis. *JAK-STAT* **2013**, *2*, e24137. [CrossRef]
21. Yu, H.; Lee, H.; Herrmann, A.; Buettner, R.; Jove, R. Revisiting STAT3 signalling in cancer: New and unexpected biological functions. Nature reviews. *Cancer* **2014**, *14*, 736–746. [CrossRef]
22. Ioannidou, E.; Moschetta, M.; Shah, S.; Parker, J.S.; Ozturk, M.A.; Pappas-Gogos, G.; Sheriff, M.; Rassy, E.; Boussios, S. Angiogenesis and Anti-Angiogenic Treatment in Prostate Cancer: Mechanisms of Action and Molecular Targets. *Int. J. Mol. Sci.* **2021**, *22*, 9926. [CrossRef] [PubMed]
23. Thomas, S.J.; Snowden, J.A.; Zeidler, M.P.; Danson, S.J. The role of JAK/STAT signalling in the pathogenesis, prognosis and treatment of solid tumours. *Br. J. Cancer* **2015**, *113*, 365–371. [CrossRef]
24. Verma, N.K.; Davies, A.M.; Long, A.; Kelleher, D.; Volkov, Y. STAT3 knockdown by siRNA induces apoptosis in human cutaneous T-cell lymphoma line Hut78 via downregulation of Bcl-xL. *Cell Mol. Biol. Lett.* **2010**, *15*, 342–355. [CrossRef] [PubMed]
25. Brooks, A.J.; Putoczki, T. JAK-STAT Signalling Pathway in Cancer. *Cancers* **2020**, *12*, 1971. [CrossRef] [PubMed]
26. Hussain, T.; Bajpai, S.; Saeed, M.; Moin, A.; Alafnan, A.; Khan, M.; Kamal, M.A.; Ganash, M.; Ashraf, G.M. Potentiating effect of ethnomedicinal plants against proliferation on different cancer cell lines. *Curr. Drug Metab.* **2018**, *19*, 584–795. [CrossRef]
27. Teiten, M.H.; Gaascht, F.; Dicato, M.; Diederich, M. Anticancer bioactivity of compounds from medicinal plants used in European medieval traditions. *Biochem. Pharm.* **2013**, *86*, 1239–1247. [CrossRef]
28. Razak, N.A.; Abu, N.; Ho, W.Y.; Zamberi, N.R.; Tan, S.W.; Alitheen, N.B.; Long, K.; Yeap, S.K. Cytotoxicity of eupatorin in MCF-7 and MDA-MB-231 human breast cancer cells via cell cycle arrest, anti-angiogenesis and induction of apoptosis. *Sci. Rep.* **2019**, *9*, 1514. [CrossRef]
29. Brentnall, M.; Rodriguez-Menocal, L.; De Guevara, R.L.; Cepero, E.; Boise, L.H. Caspase-9, caspase-3 and caspase-7 have distinct roles during intrinsic apoptosis. *BMC Cell Biol.* **2013**, *14*, 32. [CrossRef]
30. Rah, B.; Rather, R.A.; Bhat, G.R.; Baba, A.B.; Mushtaq, I.; Farooq, M.; Yousuf, T.; Dar, S.B.; Parveen, S.; Hassan, R.; et al. JAK/STAT Signaling: Molecular Targets, Therapeutic Opportunities, and Limitations of Targeted Inhibitions in Solid Malignancies. *Front. Pharmacol.* **2022**, *13*, 821344. [CrossRef]
31. Lall, R.K.; Syed, D.N.; Adhami, V.M.; Khan, M.I.; Mukhtar, H. Dietary polyphenols in prevention and treatment of prostate cancer. *Int. J. Mol. Sci.* **2015**, *16*, 3350–3376. [CrossRef]
32. Bolomsky, A.; Vogler, M.; Köse, M.C.; Heckman, C.A.; Ehx, G.; Ludwig, H.; Caers, J. MCL-1 inhibitors, fast-lane development of a new class of anti-cancer agents. *J. Hematol. Oncol.* **2020**, *13*, 173. [CrossRef] [PubMed]

33. Rana, M.S.; Ediriweera, M.K.; Rajagopalan, U.; Karunaratne, D.N.; Tennekoon, K.H.; Samarakoon, S.R. A new liposomal nanocarrier for co-delivery of gedunin and p-glycoprotein siRNA to target breast cancer stem cells. *Nat. Prod. Res.* **2022**, *36*, 6389–6392. [CrossRef] [PubMed]
34. Khan, M.K.; Ansari, I.A.; Khan, M.S.; Arif, J.M. Dietary phytochemicals as potent chemotherapeutic agents against breast cancer: Inhibition of NF-κB pathway via molecular interactions in rel homology domain of its precursor protein p105. *Pharmacogn. Mag.* **2013**, *9*, 51–57. [CrossRef] [PubMed]
35. Trott, O.; Olson, A.J. AutoDock Vina: Improving the speed and accuracy of docking with a new scoring function, efficient optimization, and multithreading. *J. Comput. Chem.* **2010**, *31*, 455–461. [CrossRef]
36. Zev, S.; Raz, K.; Schwartz, R.; Tarabeh, R.; Gupta, P.K.; Major, D.T. Benchmarking the Ability of Common Docking Programs to Correctly Reproduce and Score Binding Modes in SARS-CoV-2 Protease Mpro. *J. Chem. Inf. Model.* **2021**, *61*, 2957–2966. [CrossRef]
37. Lill, M.A.; Danielson, M.L. Computer-aided drug design platform using PyMOL. *J. Comput. Aided Mol. Des.* **2011**, *25*, 13–19. [CrossRef]
38. Alafnan, A.; Alamri, A.; Alanazi, J.; Hussain, T. Farnesiferol C Exerts Antiproliferative Effects on Hepatocellular Carcinoma HepG2 Cells by Instigating ROS-Dependent Apoptotic Pathway. *Pharmaceuticals* **2022**, *15*, 1070. [CrossRef]
39. Husain, I.; Bala, K.; Wani, A.; Makhdoomi, U.; Malik, F.; Sharma, A. Arginase purified from endophytic Pseudomonas aeruginosa IH2: Induce apoptosis through both cell cycle arrest and MMP loss in human leukemic HL-60 cells. *Chem.-Biol. Interact.* **2017**, *274*, 35–49. [CrossRef]
40. Husain, I.; Sharma, A.; Kumar, S.; Malik, F. Purification and Characterization of Glutaminase Free Asparaginase from Enterobacter cloacae: In-Vitro Evaluation of Cytotoxic Potential against Human Myeloid Leukemia HL-60 Cells. *PLoS ONE* **2016**, *11*, e0148877. [CrossRef]
41. Ahmad, A.; Tiwari, R.K.; Almeleebia, T.M.; Al Fayi, M.S.; Alshahrani, M.Y.; Ahmad, I.; Abohassan, M.S.; Saeed, M.; Ansari, I.A. Swertia chirayita suppresses the growth of non-small cell lung cancer A549 cells and concomitantly induces apoptosis via downregulation of JAK1/STAT3 pathway. *Saudi J. Biol. Sci.* **2021**, *28*, 6279–6288. [CrossRef]
42. Ahmad, A.; Ansari, I.A. Carvacrol Exhibits Chemopreventive Potential against Cervical Cancer Cells via Caspase-Dependent Apoptosis and Abrogation of Cell Cycle Progression. *Anti-Cancer Agents Med. Chem.* **2021**, *21*, 2224–2235. [CrossRef] [PubMed]

Disclaimer/Publisher's Note: The statements, opinions and data contained in all publications are solely those of the individual author(s) and contributor(s) and not of MDPI and/or the editor(s). MDPI and/or the editor(s) disclaim responsibility for any injury to people or property resulting from any ideas, methods, instructions or products referred to in the content.

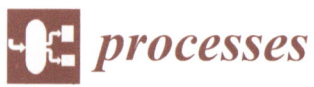

Article

STITCH, Physicochemical, ADMET, and In Silico Analysis of Selected *Mikania* Constituents as Anti-Inflammatory Agents

Narayanaswamy Radhakrishnan [1,*], Vasantha-Srinivasan Prabhakaran [2], Mohammad Ahmad Wadaan [3], Almohannad Baabbad [3], Ramachandran Vinayagam [4,*] and Sang Gu Kang [4,*]

[1] Department of Biochemistry, Saveetha Medical College and Hospital, Saveetha Institute of Medical and Technical Sciences (Deemed to be University), Chennai 602105, India
[2] Department of Bio-Informatics, Saveetha School of Engineering, Saveetha Institute of Medical and Technical Sciences (Deemed to be University), Chennai 602105, India; vasanthasrinivasanp.sse@saveetha.com
[3] Department of Zoology, College of Science, King Saud University, P.O. Box 2455, Riyadh 11451, Saudi Arabia; wadaan@ksu.edu.sa (M.A.W.); almbaabbad@ksu.edu.sa (A.B.)
[4] Department of Biotechnology, Institute of Biotechnology, College of Life and Applied Sciences, Yeungnam University, 280 Daehak-Ro, Gyeongsan 38541, Gyeongbuk, Republic of Korea
* Correspondence: nrkishnan@gmail.com (N.R.); rambio85@gmail.com (R.V.); kangsg@ynu.ac.kr (S.G.K.)

Citation: Radhakrishnan, N.; Prabhakaran, V.-S.; Wadaan, M.A.; Baabbad, A.; Vinayagam, R.; Kang, S.G. STITCH, Physicochemical, ADMET, and In Silico Analysis of Selected *Mikania* Constituents as Anti-Inflammatory Agents. *Processes* **2023**, *11*, 1722. https://doi.org/10.3390/pr11061722

Academic Editors: Alina Bora and Luminita Crisan

Received: 5 May 2023
Revised: 21 May 2023
Accepted: 23 May 2023
Published: 5 June 2023

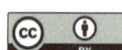

Copyright: © 2023 by the authors. Licensee MDPI, Basel, Switzerland. This article is an open access article distributed under the terms and conditions of the Creative Commons Attribution (CC BY) license (https://creativecommons.org/licenses/by/4.0/).

Abstract: The *Mikania* genus has been known to possess numerous pharmacological activities. In the present study, we aimed to evaluate the interaction of 26 selected constituents of *Mikania* species with (i) cyclooxygenase 2 (COX 2), (ii) human neutrophil elastase (HNE), (iii) lipoxygenase (LOX), matrix metalloproteinase ((iv) MMP 2 and (v) MMP 9), and (vi) microsomal prostaglandin E synthase 2 (mPGES 2) inhibitors using an in silico approach. The 26 selected constituents of *Mikania* species, namely mikamicranolide, kaurenoic acid, stigmasterol, grandifloric acid, kaurenol, spathulenol, caryophyllene oxide, syringaldehyde, dihydrocoumarin, o-coumaric acid, taraxerol, melilotoside, patuletin, methyl-3,5-di-*O*-caffeoyl quinate, 3,3′,5-trihydroxy-4′,6,7-trimethoxyflavone, psoralen, curcumene, herniarin, 2,6-dimethoxy quinone, bicyclogermacrene, α-bisabolol, γ-elemene, provincialin, dehydrocostus lactone, mikanin-3-*O*-sulfate, and nepetin, were assessed based on the docking action with COX 2, HNE, LOX, MMP 2, MMP 9, and mPGES 2 using Discovery Studio (in the case of LOX, the Autodock method was utilized). Moreover, STITCH (Search Tool for Interacting Chemicals), physicochemical, drug-likeness, and ADMET (Absorption, Distribution, Metabolism, Excretion, and Toxicity) analyses were conducted utilizing the STITCH web server, the Mol-inspiration web server, and Discovery Studio, respectively. In the present study, STITCH analysis revealed only six ligands (dihydrocoumarin, patuletin, kaurenol, psoralen, curcumene, and nepetin) that showed interactions with human proteins. Physicochemical analysis showed that seventeen ligands complied well with Lipinski's rule. ADMET analysis showed eleven ligands to possess hepatotoxic effects. Significantly, the binding free energy estimation displayed that the ligand methyl-3, 5-di-*O*-caffeoyl quinate revealed the highest binding energy for all the target enzymes, excluding LOX, suggesting that this may have efficacy as a non-steroidal anti-inflammatory drug (NSAID). The current study presents a better understanding of how *Mikania* is used as a traditional medicinal plant. Specifically, the 26 ligands of the *Mikania* plant are potential inhibitor against COX 2, HNE, LOX, MMP 2, MMP 9, and mPGES 2 for treatments for acute and/or chronic inflammatory diseases.

Keywords: STITCH; ADMET; docking; *Mikania*; methyl-3,5-di-*O*-caffeoyl quinate; cyclooxygenase; human neutrophil elastase; lipoxygenase

1. Introduction

The *Mikania* genus belongs to the Asteraceae (Daisy) family and it is reported to have around 450 subspecies in the Central America and Asia–Pacific regions [1]. Traditionally, the decoction of *M. micrantha* leaves has been used indigenously to treat tumors by the ethnic people of Assam, India [2,3]. Moreover, the Mizoram tribes in India have traditionally used *M. micrantha* juice to treat cuts and open wounds [4]. *M. cordata* has been used indigenously in Bangladesh to treat various ailments, such as bronchitis, cough, diabetes, fever, influenza, jaundice, muscle spasms, septic sores, and snake bites [5]. Da Silva et al. [6] have reviewed the pharmacological properties of the *Mikania* genus and reported that it possesses antibacterial, antidiarrheal, antifungal, anti-inflammatory, antinociceptive, antiophidian, antiparasitic, antiprotozoal, antispasmodic, antiulcerogenic, antiviral, bronchodilating, cytotoxic, mutagenic, and vasodilating properties. Recently, Radhakrishnan et al. [7] have reported the mosquitocidal activity of *M. scandens*.

Our research team identified 26 ligands of the phytoconstituents of *Mikania* species during the development of mosquito repellents [7]. The present study focuses on *Mikania* species to demonstrate the relationships among their pharmacological actions and the phytochemicals. Recently, species of *Mikania* have attracted the interest of researchers due to their numerous pharmacological actions [6]. In this work, therefore, we conducted a docking study with the phytoconstituents of *Mikania* species, viz., mikamicranolide (sesquiterpene dilactone), kaurenoic acid (diterpenoid), stigmasterol (phytosterol), grandifloric acid (diterpenoid), kaurenol (diterpenoid), spathulenol (sesquiterpenoid), caryophyllene oxide (sesquiterpenoid oxide), syringaldehyde (hydroxybenzaldehyde), dihydrocoumarin (benzopyrone), o-coumaric acid (hydroxycinnamic acid), taraxerol (triterpenoid), melilotoside (phenylpropanoid), patuletin (flavonol), methyl-3,5-di-*O*-caffeoyl quinate (cyclitol derivative), 3,3′,5-trihydroxy-4′,6,7-trimethoxyflavone (flavonol), psoralen (furanocoumarin), curcumene (sesquiterpenoid), herniarin (coumarin), 2,6-dimethoxyquinone (quinone derivative), bicyclogermacrene (sesquiterpenoid), α-bisabolol (monocyclic sesquiterpene), γ-elemene (triterpenoid), provincialin (sesquiterpene lactone), dehydrocostus lactone (sesquiterpene lactone), mikanin-3-*O*-sulfate (flavonoid sulfate), and nepetin (flavonoid). The above-mentioned phytoconstituents of *Mikania* species were investigated for docking with (i) cyclooxygenase 2 (COX 2), (ii) human neutrophil elastase (HNE) (iii) lipoxygenase (LOX), matrix metalloproteinase ((iv) MMP 2 and (v) MMP 9), and (vi) microsomal prostaglandin E synthase 2 (mPGES 2), with an examination of the enzymes' apparent binding sites using Discovery Studio (in the case of LOX, the Autodock method was applied). Furthermore, STITCH (Search Tool for Interacting Chemicals), physicochemical, drug-likeness, and ADMET analyses were conducted utilizing the STITCH web server, the Mol-inspiration web server, and Discovery Studio, respectively.

2. Results and Discussion

Computational approaches have been emerging as a new tool for evaluating the therapeutic potential of medicinal plants. In particular, molecular docking is used to select protein (enzymes/biomarkers) targets of interest and to identify the docking behavior of particular phytoconstituents on these targets [8]. Computational approaches have great potential for drug repositioning, target identification, ligand profiling, and receptor deorphanization [9].

Da Silva et al. [6] have demonstrated the anti-inflammatory activity of the *Mikania* genus and they further reported that *Mikania scandens* (leaf extract) possesses stronger anti-inflammatory activity than *M. scandens* (stem extract). Suyenaga et al. [10] have shown the anti-inflammatory activity of *Mikania laevigata* (leaf decoction) under an in vivo (animal model) approach. Perez-Amador et al. [11] have described the anti-inflammatory activity of *Mikania micrantha* ethyl acetate (EA) extract in a TPA (12-O-tetradecanoylphorbol-13-acetate)-induced animal model in an in vivo experiment. Della Pasqua et al. [12] have demonstrated that *M. laevigata* (leaf aqueous extract) possesses superior anti-inflammatory activity compared to *M. glomerata* (leaf aqueous extract). Thus, the above-summarized anti-inflammatory studies were evaluated to perform the present study.

The search tool for interacting chemicals (STITCH) free web server provides comprehensive particulars regarding: (i) metabolic pathways of interactions, (ii) crystal structure information, (iii) binding investigations, and (iv) target–drug correlations [13]. In the present study, the STITCH analysis revealed that only six ligands, namely (a) dihydrocoumarin, (b) patuletin, (c) kaurenol, (d) psoralen, (e) curcumene, and (f) nepetin (eupafolin), showed interactions with human proteins (Figure 1). Interestingly, patuletin interacted with the human lipooxygenase (LOX, inflammatory) protein, as presented in Figure 1b.

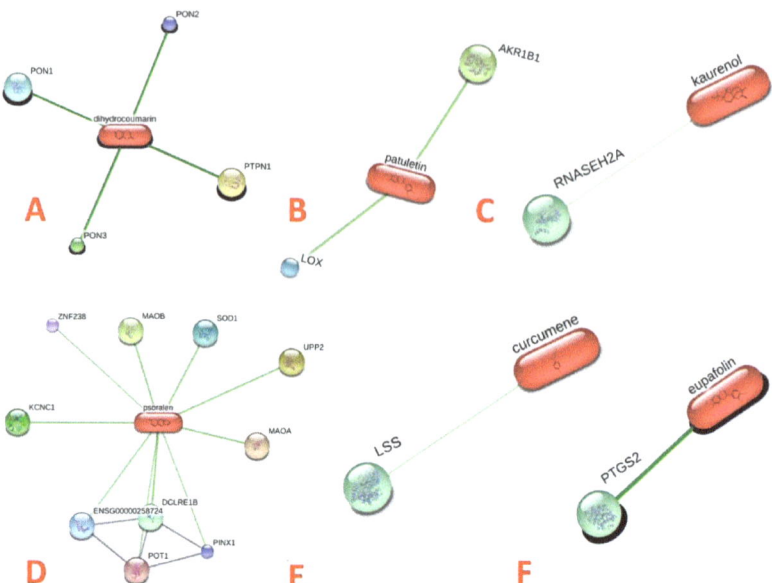

Figure 1. Representation of the protein network analysis (selected ligands of *Mikania* with human enzymes). (**A**) Dihydrocoumarin, (**B**) patuletin, (**C**) kaurenol, (**D**) psoralen, (**E**) curcumene, and (**F**) nepetin (eupafolin).

Prior to the docking experiments, it is vital to understand the (i) physicochemical, (ii) drug- likeness/bioactivity score, (iii) ADME, and finally, (iv) the toxicity of the 26 chosen phytoconstituents of the *Mikania* species. These analyses have been shown to help in the computer-aided drug development (CADD) process [14]. Regarding the physicochemical properties, six ligands (stigmasterol, taraxerol, curcumene, bicyclogermacrene, γ-elemene, and provincialin) showed one violation, while only one ligand (3,5-methyl-di-O-caffeoyl quinate) displayed three violations for the rule of five (Table 1). Similarly, with reference to supporting the drug-likeness or the score of the bioactivity analysis, only one ligand (mikamicranolide) revealed a bioactivity score of >0 towards the six descriptors; on the other hand, the other ligands showed a bioactivity score range of active to moderate. Moreover, the other 26 selected ligands showed an inactive score (<−5.0) (Table 2).

Table 1. The physicochemical analysis of 26 (*Mikania*) ligands using the Mol-inspiration free web server.

Ligand	Log A ◊	Natoms ■	MW ■	noN ••	nOH NH ◊◊	Nviolations *	Nrotb **
Mikamicranolide	−2.14	22	308.3	7	1	0	0
Kaurenoic acid	4.67	22	302.5	2	1	0	1
Stigmasterol	7.87	30	412.7	1	1	1	5
Grandifloric acid	3.75	23	318.5	3	2	0	1
Kaurenol	4.79	21	288.5	1	1	0	1
Spathulenol	3.91	16	220.4	1	1	0	0
Caryophyllene oxide	4.14	16	220.4	1	0	0	0
Syringaldehyde	1.08	13	182.2	4	1	0	3
Dihydrocoumarin	1.79	11	148.2	2	0	0	0

Table 1. Cont.

Ligand	Log A ◊	Natoms ■	MW ■	noN ••	nOH NH ◊◊	Nviolations *	Nrotb **
o-Coumaric acid	1.67	12	164.2	3	2	0	2
Taraxerol	8.02	31	426.7	1	1	1	0
Melilotoside	−0.58	23	326.3	8	5	0	5
Patuletin	1.70	24	332.3	8	5	0	2
Methyl-3,5-di-O-caffeoyl quinate	2.04	38	530.5	12	6	3	10
3,3′,5-Trihydroxy-4′,6,7-trimethoxyflavone	2.31	26	360.3	8	3	0	4
Psoralen	2.29	14	186.2	3	0	0	0
Curcumene	5.82	15	202.3	0	0	1	4
Herniarin	2.05	13	176.2	3	0	0	1
2,6-Dimethoxyquinone	0.53	12	168.2	4	0	0	2
Bicyclogermacrene	5.29	15	204.4	0	0	1	0
α-Bisabolol	4.68	16	222.4	1	1	0	4
γ-Elemene	5.42	15	204.4	0	0	1	2
Provincialin	1.91	37	518.6	10	2	1	11
Dehydrocostus lactone	2.29	17	230.3	2	0	0	0
Mikanin-3-O-sulfate	0.36	29	424.4	10	2	0	6
Nepetin	1.99	23	316.3	7	4	0	2

Note: ◊-Octanol–Water (O/W) partition coefficient; ■-molecular weight; ■-number of non-hydrogen atoms; ◊◊- number of hydrogen bond donors [OH and NH groups]; •• number of hydrogen bond acceptors [O and N atoms]; *- no. of rule of five violations, and ** no. of rotatable bonds (Nrotb).

Table 2. The drug-likeness or bioactivity analysis of 26 (*Mikania*) ligands utilized the Mol-inspiration free web server.

Ligand	GPCR ■ Ligand	Ion-Channel Modulator	Kinase Inhibitor	Nuclear Receptor Ligand	Protease Inhibitor	Enzyme Inhibitor
Mikamicranolide	0.28	0.03	0.01	0.66	0.07	0.56
Kaurenoic acid	0.29	0.15	−0.39	0.75	0.06	0.46
Stigmasterol	0.12	−0.08	−0.49	0.74	−0.02	0.53
Grandifloric acid	0.21	0.12	−0.47	0.78	0.10	0.43
Kaurenol	0.21	0.10	−0.21	0.67	−0.02	0.44
Spathulenol	−0.42	−0.28	−0.68	0.28	−0.36	0.05
Caryophyllene oxide	−0.08	0.14	−0.86	0.62	0.00	0.57
Syringaldehyde	−0.95	−0.36	−0.80	−0.69	−1.27	−0.39
Dihydrocoumarin	−0.90	−0.48	−1.25	−0.75	−1.13	−0.47
o-Coumaric acid	−0.64	−0.37	−0.98	−0.25	−0.90	−0.21
Taraxerol	0.21	0.02	−0.20	0.54	0.00	0.49
Melilotoside	0.17	−0.03	−0.13	0.27	0.04	0.40
Patuletin	−0.14	−0.34	0.22	0.13	−0.35	0.17
3,5-Methyl-di-O-caffeoyl quinate	0.11	−0.07	−0.06	0.34	0.07	0.25
3,3′,5-Trihydroxy−4′,6,7-trimethoxyflavone	−0.14	−0.33	0.20	0.09	−0.34	0.14
Psoralen	−0.89	−0.38	−1.11	−1.13	−1.19	−0.37
Curcumene	−0.47	−0.12	−0.80	−0.24	−0.72	−0.14
Herniarin	−1.23	−0.84	−1.28	−1.06	−1.28	−0.47
2,6-Dimethoxyquinone	−1.48	−0.69	−0.78	−1.50	−1.36	−0.42
Bicyclogermacrene	−0.75	−0.69	−1.11	−0.65	−0.88	−0.16
α-Bisabolol	−0.06	0.26	−0.78	0.37	−0.38	0.43
γ-Elemene	−0.46	0.02	−1.01	0.51	−0.71	0.24
Provincialin	0.32	0.23	−0.15	0.95	0.07	0.82
Dehydrocostus lactone	−0.04	−0.02	−0.56	1.00	−0.22	0.66
Mikanin-3-O-sulfate	0.08	−0.30	0.02	0.01	0.06	0.45
Nepetin	−0.08	−0.23	0.22	0.17	−0.31	0.16

Note: ■- G Protein-coupled receptors (GPCR).

Before docking, it is vital to know a compound's/ligand's properties, such as (i) physicochemical, (ii) drug-likeness or score of bioactivity, and (iii) ADMET, along with its (iv) toxicity. Moreover, standardized rule (Lipinski's rule of five) and ADMET are available for determining such properties [15]. Concerning ADMET analysis, eleven ligands (mikamicranolide, spathulenol, caryophyllene oxide, patuletin, 3,3′,5-trihydroxy-4′,6,7-trimethoxyflavone, psoralen, herniarin, 2,6-dimethoxyquinone, dehydrocostus lactone, mikanin-3-O-sulfate, and nepetin) have hepatotoxic properties, as displayed in Table 3.

Table 3. ADMET analysis of 26 (*Mikania*) ligands using Discovery Studio.

Ligand	HIA ◇	AS ■	BBB [a]	PPB **	CYP2D6 ◊◊	HT [b]
	L *	L **	L ***	Predication		
Mikamicranolide	0	4	3	F	F	T
Kaurenoic acid	0	2	0	T	F	F
Stigmasterol	3	1	4	T	F	F
Grandifloric acid	0	2	1	T	F	F
Kaurenol	0	2	0	T	F	F
Spathulenol	0	3	1	T	F	T
Caryophyllene oxide	0	2	0	T	F	T
Syringaldehyde	0	4	3	T	F	F
Dihydrocoumarin	0	3	1	T	F	F
o-Coumaric acid	0	4	3	F	F	F
Taraxerol	3#	0	4	T	F	F
Melilotoside	1#	4	4	F	F	F
Patuletin	1	3	4	F	F	T
3,5-Methyl-di-O-caffeoyl quinate	3#	3	4	F	F	F
3,3′,5-Trihydroxy-4′,6,7-trimethoxyflavone	0	3	4	T	F	T
Psoralen	0	3	2	F	F	T
Curcumene	1	2	0	T	F	F
Herniarin	0	3	2	T	F	T
2,6-Dimethoxyquinone	0	4	3	F	F	T
Bicyclogermacrene	1	2	0	T	F	F
α-Bisabolol	0	2	0	T	F	F
γ-Elemene	1	2	0	T	F	F
Provincialin	2	3	4	F	F	F
Dehydrocostus lactone	0	2	1	T	F	T
Mikanin-3-O-sulfate	1	3	4	T	F	T
Nepetin	0	3	4	T	T	T

Note: (■ AS—Aqueous solubility; ◇ HIA—Human intestinal absorption; ** PPB—Plasma protein binding; [a] BBB—Blood–brain barrier; [b] HT—Hepatotoxicity; ◊◊ CYP2D6—Cytochrome P450 2D6; T—True, F—False, and L—Level). * [0—Strong. 1—Medium. 2—Weak, and 3—Very weak]; ** [0—Extremely weak, 1—Very weak, 2—Weak, 3—Strong, 4—Optimal, 5—Soluble, and 6—Warning]; *** [0—Very strong penetration, 1—Strong, 2—Moderate, 3—Low, and 4—Undefined].

Regarding the toxicological screening of 26 ligands, as illustrated in Table 4, 5 ligands (dihydrocoumarin, patuletin, 3,3′,5-trihydroxy-4′,6, 7-trimethoxyflavone, 3-O-mikanin-sulfate along with nepetin) are non-degradable in terms of aerobic biodegradability nature. Two ligands (patuletin and 3, 3′, 5-trihydroxy-4′, 6, 7-trimethoxyflavone) are predicated as mutagens.

The C-docking study and free energy binding analysis (Table 5) showed that 3,5-methyl-di-O-caffeoyl quinate possesses the maximum energy interaction (−42.51 kcal/mol) with the COX 2 enzyme (as presented in Figure 2a). In contrast, psoralen revealed the least interaction energy (−15.57 kcal/mol). Moreover, eight ligands (grandifloric acid, kaurenol, o-coumaric acid, melilotoside, patuletin, 3,5-methyl-di-O-caffeoylquinate, mikanin-3-O-sulfate, and nepetin) showed interaction with the Glu539 residues of the COX 2 enzyme, as displayed in Table 5. The present results were in good conformity with our previous findings where 4-hydroxyisoleucine (4-HIL) and phytic acid (PA) showed interaction with

(i) Glu539; (ii) Glu350; (iii) Asn546; and (iv) Trp531 amino acid (AA) residues of the COX 2 enzyme [16].

Table 4. The toxicological screening of 26 (*Mikania*) ligands using Discovery Studio.

Ligands	AB ■	AM ◊	OI •	SI ◊◊	Oral Toxicity *
Mikamicranolide	D	NM	I	I	1.02
Kaurenoic acid	D	NM	I	I	1.53
Stigmasterol	D	NM	I	I	1.18
Grandifloric acid	D	NM	I	I	1.44
Kaurenol	D	NM	I	I	1.85
Spathulenol	D	NM	I	I	0.75
Caryophyllene oxide	D	NM	I	I	1.13
Syringaldehyde	D	NM	I	I	1.26
Dihydrocoumarin	ND	NM	I	I	0.74
o-Coumaric acid	D	NM	I	NI	1.59
Taraxerol	D	NM	I	I	0.93
Melilotoside	D	NM	I	NI	1.32
Patuletin	ND	M	I	NI	1.08
Methyl-3,5-di-*O*-caffeoyl quinate	D	NM	I	NI	2.37
3,3′,5-Trihydroxy-4′,6,7-trimethoxyflavone	ND	M	I	NI	0.93
Psoralen	D	NM	I	I	0.30
Curcumene	D	NM	NI	I	2.47
Herniarin	D	NM	NI	I	0.68
2,6-Dimethoxyquinone	D	NM	I	I	0.63
Bicyclogermacrene	D	NM	I	I	0.48
α-Bisabolol	D	NM	I	I	1.65
γ-Elemene	D	NM	I	I	2.00
Provincialin	D	NM	I	I	3.11
Dehydrocostus lactone	D	NM	I	I	1.45
Mikanin-3-*O*-sulfate	ND	NM	I	NI	NA **
Nepetin	ND	NM	I	NI	0.68

Note: (AM ◊—Ames mutagenicity, AB ■—Aerobic biodegradability, SI ◊◊—Skin irritancy, I •—Ocular irritancy, and Oral toxicity *—Oral toxicity in rat [LD_{50} in g/Kg]; D—Degradable, ND—Non-degradable, M—Mutagen, NM—Non-mutagen, I—Irritant, NI—Non-irritant, and NA **—Not analyzed).

Stigmasterol has been described to inhibit thromboxane B_2 (TXB_2) production, which afterwards leads to inhibition of cyclooxygenase 1 (COX 1) activity [17]. However, no reports are available for stigmasterol's cyclooxygenase 2 (COX 2) inhibition activity. Additionally, caryophyllene has been reported to exhibit cyclooxygenase-2 (COX-2) inhibition activity in THP-1 (human monocytic) cells [18]. Psoralen, spathulenol, syringaldehyde, and taraxerol acetate have been found to exhibit cyclooxygenase-2 (COX-2) inhibition activity [19–23]. All the above findings were in agreement with our results on cyclooxygenase 2 (COX 2) inhibition activity.

The HNE is an additional targeted enzyme whose docking analysis and free energy binding analysis showed that 3,5-methyl-di-*O*-caffeoyl quinate displayed the maximum energy of interactions (−54.66 kcal/mol), as presented in Figure 2b. Thirteen ligands (kaurenol, syringaldehyde, o-coumaric acid, melilotoside, patuletin, 3,5-methyl-di-*O*-caffeoyl quinate, trihydroxy-3,3′,5-trimethoxy-4′,6,7-flavone, psoralen, herniarin, 2,6-dimethoxyquinone, provincialin, mikanin-3-*O*-sulfate, and nepetin) exhibited interaction with Ser195 amino acid residue of HNE, as shown in Table 6. The present finding was in good agreement with our previous study, where phytic acid (PA) and 4-hydroxyisoleucine (4-HIL) demonstrated interaction with (i) Ser195; (ii) Arg147; (iii) Cys191; (iv) Phe192; (v) Gly193; (vi) Asp194; and (vii) Ser214 amino acid (AA) residues of the HNE enzyme [16].

Five sesquiterpene lactones, namely (15- (3′-Hydroxy)-methacryloyloxy-micrantholide, isobutyryloxy-15-(2′,3′-Epoxy)-micrantholide, isobutyryloxy-15-(2′-Hydroxy)-micrantholide, 4α hydroxy-1β-Acetoxy-15- eudesma-isobutyryloxy-12-8β-olide11-13-en from *M. cordifolia*, and Scandenolide from *M. micrantha* have been reported to exhibit human neutrophil elastase (HNE) inhibition activity [24]. Similarly, p-coumaric acid and di-O-caffeoyl-3,5-quinic acid, two phytochemicals, were described as possessing human neutrophil elastase (HNE) inhibition activity [25]. Both reports were in close agreement with the present findings on the human neutrophil elastase (HNE) inhibition activity.

Table 5. Energy interaction analysis of twenty-six (*Mikania*) ligands along with cyclooxygenase 2 (COX 2) utilizing Discovery Studio.

Ligands	c-Docker Energy Interaction (-kcal/mol)	Amino Acid Interaction Residue (AA)	Bond Distance (Å)
Mikamicranolide	22.37	Asn546	1.1
Kaurenoic acid	F *	-	-
Stigmasterol	34.51	Lys346	2.5
		Asp348	1.2
Grandifloric acid	24.17	Glu539	0.91
		Asn546	1.5 and 1.7
Kaurenol	21.75	Glu539	0.55
Spathulenol	18.08	No interaction	-
Caryophyllene oxide	17.20	No interaction	-
Syringaldehyde	21.57	Asn546	1.5
Dihydrocoumarin	16.97	No interaction	-
o-Coumaric acid	18.23	Glu539	2.0
		Asn546	1.5
		Lys543 ♦	6.5
Taraxerol	29.03	Glu350	0.96
		Lys346	2.2
		Asp348	1.9
Melilotoside	32.06	Glu539	1.7
		Asn546	1.7
		Lys328 ♦	6.3
Patuletin	28.65	Asp348	0.53
		Glu350	2.2
		Trp531	1.4
		Glu539	2.3
		Lys346	2.4
Methyl-3,5-di-O-caffeoyl quinate	42.51	Asp348	0.96
		Glu350	1.8
		Glu539	2.4
		Asn546	2.2 and 2.3
3,3′,5-Trihydroxy-4′,6,7-trimethoxyflavone	28.20	Asn546	2.4
Psoralen	15.57	Asn546	0.8 and 2.2
		Lys543 ♦	5.1 and 5.8
Curcumene	19.47	No interaction	-
Herniarin	17.10	Asn546	2.4
2,6-Dimethoxyquinone	18.20	Asn546	1.3
Bicyclogermacrene	17.12	No interaction	-
α-Bisabolol	23.26	Asn546	2.2
γ-Elemene	17.41	No interaction	-
Provincialin	37.74	Lys346	1.8
Dehydrocostus lactone	19.95	No interaction	-
Mikanin-3-O-sulfate	29.99	Glu539	2.1
		Asn546	2.2 and 2.5
		Lys328 ♦	6.6
Nepetin	32.50	Asp348	0.31
		Glu350	2.2
		Trp531	1.7
		Glu539	2.1

Note: [F *—Failed to dock; ♦—+-π interaction].

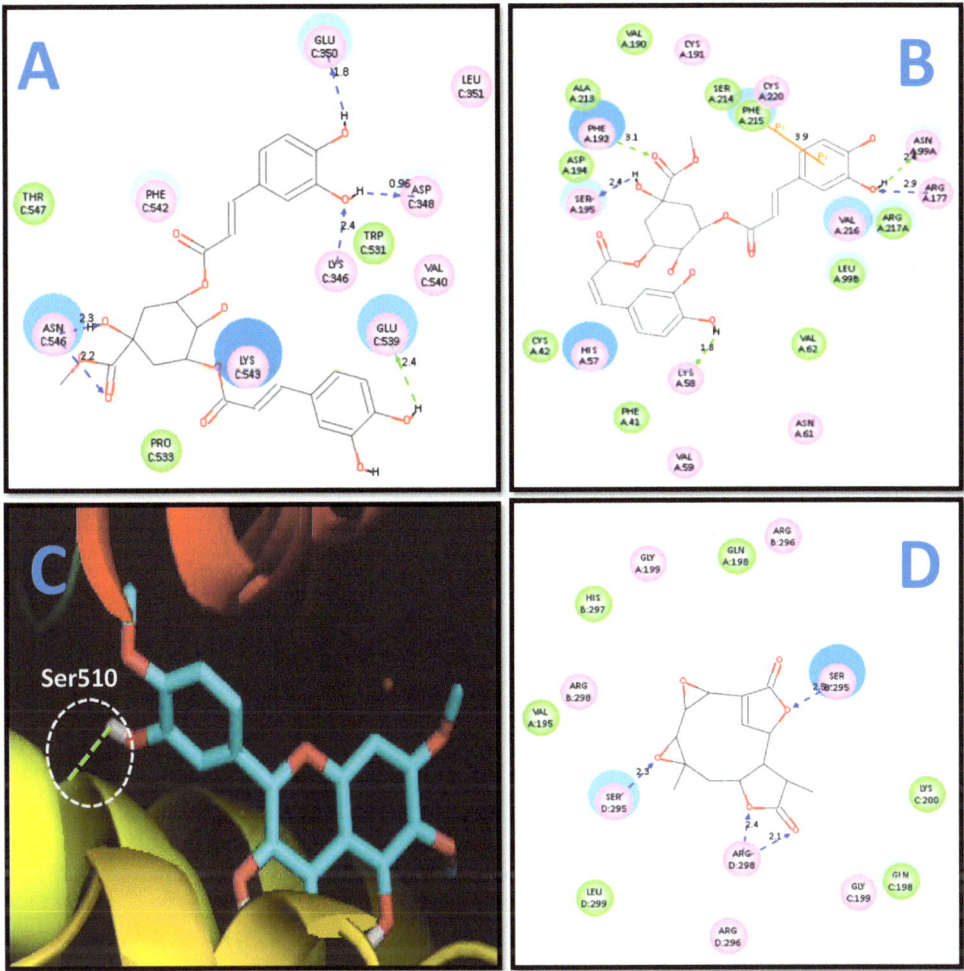

Figure 2. The two-dimensional (2D) structure of methyl-3,5-di-O-caffeoyl quinate with (**A**) COX 2 and (**B**) HNE; hydrogen atoms have been excluded in two-dimensional (2D) images for good explanation and bond distances are expressed in (Å) angstroms; (**C**) three-dimensional (3D) structure of 3,3′,5-trihydroxy-4′,6,7-trimethoxyflavone with LOX (docked using Autodock and analyzed using pyMOL method) and (**D**) two-dimensional (2D) structure of provincialin with mPGES 2.

The docking study and free binding energy analysis showed that 3,3′,5-trihydroxy-4′,6,7-trimethoxyflavone (Figure 2c) had the least binding energy (−9.71 kcal/mol) (Table 7). Moreover, five ligands (mikamicranolide, syringaldehyde, patuletin, 2,6-dimethoxyquinone, and mikanin-3-O-sulfate) exhibited interactions with the His518 amino acid residue of LOX. The current finding was in good accord with our previous study, where the compound-3e (Geranylacetophenone derivative) showed interaction with His518 amino acid residue of the LOX enzyme [26]. Similarly, our earlier study also displayed that 4-hydroxyisoleucine (4-HIL) showed interaction with (i) Ser510; (ii) His513; and (iii) Gln716 amino acid (AA) residues of the LOX enzyme [16].

Table 6. Energy interaction analysis of 26 ligands (*Mikania*) along with HNE using Discovery Studio.

Ligands	Energy Interaction of c-Docker (-kcal/mol)	Amino Acid Interaction Residue (AA)	Bond Distance (Å)
Mikamicranolide	31.32	No interaction	-
Kaurenoic acid	F *	-	-
Stigmasterol	34.31	No interaction	-
Grandifloric acid	26.95	Gly219	2.8
Kaurenol	28.05	Ser195	2.3
Spathulenol	23.55	No interaction	-
Caryophyllene oxide	23.54	No interaction	-
Syringaldehyde	30.11	Cys191	1.8
		Gly193	2.6
		Asp194	2.8
		Ser195	2.8
		Val216	3.1
Dihydrocoumarin	20.95	Arg147	2.2
		Phe192	2.8
o-Coumaric acid	22.74	Cys191	2.0
		Gly193	2.8
		Asp194	3.1
		Ser195	1.9, 2.6 and 2.9
		Ser214	2.1
Taraxerol	28.96	No interaction	-
Melilotoside	37.79	Arg147	2.4
		Phe192	1.9 and 2.9
		Gly193	3.0
		Ser195	3.1
		Gly219	2.5
Patuletin	35.32	Cys191	2.0
		Gly193	2.8
		Asp194	3.1
		Ser195	2.8
		Ser214	2.1
		Gly218	3.0
		Gly219	2.8
3,5-Methyl-di-O-caffeoyl quinate	54.66	Cys58	1.8
		Asn99A	2.4
		Arg177	2.9
		Phe192	3.1
		Ser195	2.4
		Phe215◊	3.9
4′,6,7-trimethoxy-3,3′,5-Trihydroxyflavone	34.66	Gly193	3.0
		Ser195	3.1 and 3.1
		Gly219	2.9
Psoralen	19.74	Phe192	3.2
		Ser195	2.1
Curcumene	24.66	No interaction	-
Herniarin	24.89	Arg147	2.9
		Phe192	2.8
		Ser195	2.1
2,6-Dimethoxyquinone	22.60	Gly193	2.7
		Ser195	2.9 and 3.0
Bicyclogermacrene	23.35	No interaction	-
α-Bisabolol	25.75	No interaction	-
γ-Elemene	18.53	No interaction	-
Provincialin	49.20	Gly193	2.9
		Ser195	2.7 and 3.1
		Gly219	2.6
		Val216	3.1
Dehydrocostus lactone	25.02	No interaction	-

Table 6. Cont.

Ligands	Energy Interaction of c-Docker (-kcal/mol)	Amino Acid Interaction Residue (AA)	Bond Distance (Å)
Mikanin-3-O-sulfate	40.31	Cys191	1.8
		Phe192	2.6
		Gly193	3.0
		Ser195	2.8 and 3.1
		Ser214	3.2
		Val216	1.7 and 2.7
Nepetin	31.90	Cys191	2.1
		Gly193	2.9
		Ser195	3.0
		Gly218	2.8
		Gly219	2.6

Note: [F *—Failed to dock].

Table 7. Energy interaction analysis of twenty-six (*Mikania*) ligands along with LOX utilizing Autodock.

Ligands	Minimal Binding Energy (-kcal/mol)	Amino Acid Interaction Residue (AA)	Bond Distance (Å)
Mikamicranolide	8.21	His518	2.2
		Trp519	3.2
Kaurenoic acid	6.50	His513	3.3
		Gln716	2.0 and 3.2
Stigmasterol	7.03	Ile557	2.6
Grandifloric acid	4.82	No interaction	-
Kaurenol	8.37	No interaction	-
Spathulenol	7.43	No interaction	-
Caryophyllene oxide	8.00	No interaction	-
Syringaldehyde	5.33	Gln514	2.0
		His518	2.7
Dihydrocoumarin	5.74	His523	3.6
		Ile557	3.2
o-Coumaric acid	4.44	Ser510	2.1
		Gln514	2.1
Taraxerol	+11.79	ND *	ND *
Melilotoside	6.79	Ser510	1.8 and 3.4
		Gln514	2.3
		His513	1.9 and 3.4
Patuletin	9.32	Gln514	2.7
		His518	3.2
		Arg726	2.1
3,5-Methyl-di-O-caffeoyl quinate	+30.23	ND *	ND *
4′,6,7-3,3′,5-Trihydroxy-trimethoxyflavone	9.71	Ser510	2.1
Psoralen	6.51	No interaction	-
Curcumene	7.73	No interaction	-
Herniarin	5.79	No interaction	-
2,6-Dimethoxyquinone	4.93	His518	3.1
Bicyclogermacrene	7.94	No interaction	-
α-Bisabolol	8.11	Gln716	1.9 and 3.2
γ-Elemene	7.54	No interaction	-
Provincialin	+46.86	ND *	ND *
Dehydrocostus lactone	8.26	His523	2.7
		Ser510	1.7
Mikanin-3-O-sulfate	4.88	His513	3.2
		Gln514	1.8 and 2.4
		His518	3.5
Nepetin	9.21	Arg726	2.1 and 3.4

Note: [+—Positive sign represents the (weak) binding energy, which may be due to an improper binding feature as demonstrated by Castro et al. [27]; ND *—Not determined].

Mikania micrantha (leaves and stems—ethyl acetate extract) [11], *Mikania lindleyana* (aerial parts of the plant—methanolic extract), and *Mikania cordata* (root—methanolic extract) have been described to have anti-inflammatory properties [28,29], whereas three other *Mikania* species (*M. glomerata*, *M. hirsutissima*, and *M. laevigata*) have been reported to inhibit 5- lipoxygenase (5-LOX) activity in a dose-dependent manner [30,31]. Jyothi Lakshmi [32] reported the cyclooxygenase (COX), lipoxygenase (LOX), and nitric oxide synthase (iNOS) inhibition activities of *Mikania micrantha* (leaf and flower extract). Similarly, (i) 6,7-dihydroxy coumarin, (ii) β- caryophyllene, and (iii) β- caryophyllene oxide have been reported to inhibit 5- lipoxygenase (5-LOX) activity [33], whereas stigmasterol has been described to inhibit 15- lipoxygenase (15-LOX) activity [34]. Kaurenoic acid has been reported to have weak lipoxygenase (LOX) inhibition activity [35]. All the above-mentioned studies are in good correlation with the current results on lipoxygenase (LOX) inhibition activity.

The docking study and binding free energy analysis with MMP 2 showed that 3,5-methyl-di-O-caffeoylquinate possessed the maximum interaction energy (-83.34 kcal/mol), and five ligands (syringaldehyde, o-coumaric acid, 3,5-methyl-di-O-caffeoylquinate, 3-O-mikanin-sulfate, and nepetin) showed interaction with the MMP2 amino acid residue Glu-202 (Table 8). This observation was in agreement with previous findings, where 4-hydroxyisoleucine (4-HIL) has shown interaction with the (i) Glu202; (ii) Ala165; and (iii) His201 amino acid (AA) residues of the MMP 2 enzyme [16].

Table 8. Energy interaction analysis of twenty-six ligands of (*Mikania*) MMP 2 utilizing Discovery Studio.

Ligands	Minimal Binding Energy (-kcal/mol)	Amino Acid Interaction Residue (AA)	Bond Distance (Å)
Mikamicranolide	F *	-	-
Kaurenoic acid	F *	-	-
Stigmasterol	F *	-	-
Grandifloric acid	F *	-	-
Kaurenol	F *	-	-
Spathulenol	F *	-	-
Caryophyllene oxide	F *	-	-
Syringaldehyde	33.92	Ala167	2.5
		Glu202	2.0
Dihydrocoumarin	31.67	No interaction	-
o-Coumaric acid	38.99	Glu202	1.7
Taraxerol	F *	-	-
Melilotoside	F *	-	-
Patuletin	47.85	Gly162	2.5
		Leu164	2.0
		Ala167	1.2 and 1.7
		Zn501 ♦	3.6
		His201 ◊	4.7
3,5-Methyl-di-O-caffeoylquinate	83.34	Glu202	1.3
		Glu210	1.9
		His166	2.0
4′,6,7-trimethoxyflavone-3,3′,5-Trihydroxy	48.36	Ala167	2.3
		Pro221	2.4
Psoralen	34.40	No interaction	-
Curcumene	34.54	Zn501 ♦	3.4
Herniarin	36.51	No interaction	-
2,6-Dimethoxyquinone	33.27	Leu164	2.0
		Ala165	1.6
Bicyclogermacrene	19.70	No interaction	-
α-Bisabolol	39.85	His201	2.5
γ-Elemene	F *	-	-
Provincialin	F *	-	-
Dehydrocostus lactone	F *	-	-
Mikanin-3-O-sulfate	52.36	Leu163 ■	2.2
		His166	2.3
		Ala167	1.7
		Glu202	1.9
		Pro221	1.8
Nepetin	46.27	Gly162	2.4
		Ala167	2.1
		Glu202	1.5

Note: [F *—Failed to dock; ♦ —+–π interaction; ◊ — π–π interaction; ■—Sigma–π interaction].

Similarly, in the C-docking study and binding energy analysis with MMP 9, 3,5-methyl-di-O-caffeoyl quinate exhibited the maximum binding energy (−81.65 kcal/mol), and three ligands (3,5-methyl-di-O-caffeoylquinate, curcumene, and 2,6-dimethoxyquinone) displayed an interaction with His226 amino acid (AA) residue of MMP 9 (Table 9). The current result was in good correlation with our preceding study, where 3-phenyllactic acid (3-PLA) showed interaction with His226 amino acid (AA) residues of the MMP 9 enzyme [36]. Stigmasterol has been reported to reduce matrix metalloproteinase 3 (MMP 3) mRNA expression in humans and mouses, MMP 3 protein in mice, and matrix metalloproteinase 13 (MMP 13) mRNA expression in humans and mice [37]. However, in the present study, stigmasterol failed to dock with both enzymes (MMP 2 and 9).

Table 9. Energy interaction analyzes of twenty-six ligands (*Mikania*) MMP 9 utilizing Discovery Studio.

Ligands	Energy Interaction of c-Docker (-kcal/mol)	Amino Acid Interaction Residue (AA)	Bond Distance (Å)
Mikamicranolide	F *	-	-
Kaurenoic acid	F *	-	-
Stigmasterol	F *	-	-
Grandifloric acid	F *	-	-
Kaurenol	F *	-	-
Spathulenol	F *	-	-
Caryophyllene oxide	F *	-	-
Syringaldehyde	36.26	Tyr248	3.2 and 3.2
Dihydrocoumarin	33.03	No interaction	-
o-Coumaric acid	40.73	Ala189	2.0
Taraxerol	F *	-	-
Melilotoside	F *	-	-
Patuletin	43.96	Leu188	2.3
Methyl-3,5-di-O-caffeoyl quinate	81.65	His226 ■	5.1
		Gln227	1.7
3,3′,5-Trihydroxy-4′,6,7-trimethoxyflavone	45.60	Pro180	2.4
		His190	2.7
Psoralen	33.72	No interaction	-
Curcumene	32.74	His226 ■	3.7
Herniarin	35.71	Tyr248	2.8
		Leu188	2.9
2,6-Dimethoxyquinone	31.79	Ala189	2.7
		His226	3.2
Bicyclogermacrene	F *	-	-
α-Bisabolol	42.26	No interaction	-
γ-Elemene	F *	-	-
Provincialin	F *	-	-
Dehydrocostus lactone	F *	-	-
Mikanin-3-O-sulfate	48.76	Gln227	3.0
Nepetin	44.73	Pro180	2.3 and 2.5
		His190	2.7

Note: [F *—Failed to dock, ■—π–π interaction].

Docking and energy binding analysis (Table 10) shows that the provincialin had maximum energy binding (−54.18 kcal/mol) with the mPGES 2 enzyme (as illustrated in Figure 2d) and twelve ligands (syringaldehyde, o-coumaric acid, melilotoside, patuletin, 3,5-methyl-di-O-caffeoylquinate, 4′,6,7-trimethoxyflavone-3,3′,5-trihydroxy, psoralen, herniarin, provincialin, dehydrocostus lactone, mikanin-3-O-sulfate, and nepetin) had interaction with Arg298 amino acid (AA) residue of mPGES 2. Interestingly, in the present study, all 25 ligands (except for 2,6-dimethoxyquinone) showed docking and binding affinities with microsomal prostaglandin E synthase 2 (mPGES 2). Maione et al. [38] have reported that the amino acids (i) Cys110, (ii) His241, (iii) His244, (iv) Ser247, (v) Arg292, and (vi) Arg296 are the key binding residues for mPGES 2. However, there are no reports on their mPGES 2 inhibition activity.

Table 10. Energy interaction analyzes of twenty-six ligands (*Mikania*) of mPGES 2 utilizing Discovery Studio.

Ligands	Energy Interaction of c-Docker (-kcal/mol)	Amino Acid Interaction Residue (AA)	Bond Distance (Å)
Mikamicranolide	26.05	SerB295	2.3 and 2.5
		SerD295	1.9
		ArgD292	2.1
Kaurenoic acid	22.92	SerD295	1.9
		ArgD296	2.3
Stigmasterol	32.09	Lys200	2.0
Grandifloric acid	23.59	SerD295	1.9
Kaurenol	22.25	No interaction	-
Spathulenol	24.46	SerD295	1.3 and 1.4
Caryophyllene oxide	19.57	No interaction	-
Syringaldehyde	28.24	SerD295	1.8, 1.8 and 2.4
		ArgD298	1.7
Dihydrocoumarin	23.83	No interaction	-
o-Coumaric acid	26.40	SerD295	1.5
		ArgB298	1.7
Taraxerol	29.16	SerB295	1.7 and 2.3
		GlnA198	1.6 and 2.2
Melilotoside	42.13	SerB295	1.3 and 2.2
		ArgB298	1.7
		GlnA198	1.6
		GlyA199	0.96
Patuletin	39.66	GlyC199	1.6
		ArgB298	1.7 and 1.8
		ArgD298	1.7
		GlnA198	1.8
		GlnC198	1.9
		GlyC199	2.3
3,5-Methyl-di-O-caffeoyl quinate	52.22	SerB295	1.9, 2.4 and 2.5
		ArgD296	1.5 and 1.8
		ArgD296 ■	2.8
		ArgD298	1.8
		GlyA199	1.3
6,7-Trimethoxyflavone-3,3',5-Trihydroxy-4'	39.70	GlyC199	1.8
		ArgB298	2.0 and 2.5
		ArgD298	1.3
Psoralen	26.93	ArgB298	1.5 and 1.9
Curcumene	26.84	No interaction	-
Herniarin	25.62	SerD295	2.3
		ArgD298	1.8
2,6-Dimethoxyquinone	F *	-	-
Bicyclogermacrene	22.19	No interaction	-
α-Bisabolol	28.37	SerB295	1.1 and 2.7
γ-Elemene	20.98	No interaction	-
		ArgB292	2.2
		ArgD292	2.3
		SerB295	2.0 and 2.4
Provincialin	54.18	ArgB296	2.4
		ArgB298	1.6
		ArgD298	1.7
Dehydrocostus lactone	21.58	SerB295	1.8
		ArgD298	2.2
Mikanin-3-O-sulfate	42.38	SerD295	2.5
		ArgB298	1.5
		GlyA199	1.4
Nepetin	39.41	GlyC199	1.9
		SerD295	1.4
		ArgB298	1.4 and 1.7

Note: [F *—docking failed, ■—π–sigma interaction].

3. Materials and Methods

3.1. Ligand (Small Molecule of Interest) Preparation

The simplified molecular input line entry specification (SMILES) of the 26 selected ligands: (i) mikamicranolide (Chemspider ID 10189069); (ii) kaurenoic acid (CID 73062); (iii) stigmasterol (CID 5280794); (iv) grandifloric acid (CID 159930); (v) kaurenol (CID 443465); (vi) spathulenol (CID 522266); (vii) caryophyllene oxide (CID 14350); (viii) syringaldehyde (CID 8655); (ix) dihydrocoumarin (CID 660); (x) o-coumaric acid (Chemspider ID 553146); (xi) taraxerol (CID 92097); (xii) melilotoside (CID 5280759); (xiii) patuletin (CID 5281678); (xiv) methyl-3,5-di-O-caffeoyl quinate (ChEBI ID 66708); (xv) 3,3',5-trihydroxy-4',6,7-trimethoxyflavone (Chemspider ID 4476175); (xvi) psoralen (CID 6199); (xvii) curcumene (CID 92139); (xviii) herniarin (Chemspider ID 10295); (xix) 2,6-dimethoxyquinone; (xx) bicyclogermacrene (CID 5315347); (xxi) α-bisabolol (CID 442343); (xxii) γ-elemene (CID 6432312); (xxiii) provincialin (ChEBI ID 8599); (xxiv) dehydrocostus lactone (CID 73174); (xxv) mikanin-3-O-sulfate (CID 14630674); and (xxvi) nepetin (Chemspider ID 4476172) were obtained from (i) Chemspider, (ii) PubMed, and (iii) Chemical Entities of Biological Interest. A three-dimensional structure of 2, 6-dimethoxy quinone was generated using ChemBioDraw Ultra 12.0. All the 26 ligands [above-mentioned] were sketched using Ultra 12.0 ChemBioDraw software and further MM2—molecular mechanics ligand minimization—was performed using Ultra 12.0 ChemBio3D software. Thus, these minimized energy ligands [3D images] were engaged for Autodock and in the C-docker case, and the ligand in-build preparation procedure (Accelrys, San Diego, CA, USA) was applied [16].

3.2. Protein Network Interaction Analysis

The search tool for interacting chemicals [STITCH] free web server [39] was employed to identify the interaction between ligands (26 selected phyto-constituents of *Mikania* species) and human proteins.

3.3. Selection of Target Protein (Enzyme) and Preparation

The 3D enzymes of (i) COX 2 (3LN1), with a resolution of 2.40 Å; (ii) HNE (1H1B [PDB number], with a resolution of 2.00 Å; (iii) LOX (1JNQ [PDB number], with a resolution of 2.10 Å; (iv) MMP 2 (1QIB [PDB number], with 2.80 angstrom (Å) resolution; (v) MMP9 (4H1Q) with 1.59 Å resolution; and (vi) mPGES 2 (1Z9I1), with 2.60 Å resolution. were retrieved from the RCSB Protein Data Bank. In COX2, the C chain was processed, and mPGES 2, all chains were processed individually by eliminating the B, C, and D ligands along with the crystallographically detected water (H_2O) particles. The enzymes mentioned above were primed using Chimera UCSF software for Autodocking and C-docker in-built protein preparation procedure (Accelrys, San Diego, CA, USA) was applied [16].

3.4. Physicochemical and Drug-Likeness or Bioactivity Score Analyses

The physicochemical and drug-likeness or biological activity score analyses were conducted for the selected twenty-six selected (*Mikania*) ligands utilizing the Mol-inspiration-free web server [16].

3.5. ADMET and TOPKAT Analyses

The ADMET and TOPKAT analyses were performed using Discovery Studio (Accelrys, San Diego, CA, USA) for the 26 selected (*Mikania*) ligands [16].

3.6. Docking Analysis

The docking analysis was performed for twenty-six screened compounds extracted from *Mikania* utilizing C-docker. The 3D structures of COX 2; MMP 2; HNE; MMP 9; and mPGES 2 were recovered from the Protein Data Bank and further processed with the C-docker procedure [40] along the protein–ligand interaction section using 3.1. Discovery Studio® (Accelrys, San Diego, CA, USA) was utilized. A model of Autodock 4.2 was used for LOX alone, where all rotatable bonds [rotb] along the twenty-six Mikania ligands were withheld for the flexible docking approach. The grid size was fixed (60 × 60 × 60) with a space of 0.375 Å between the grid points. Lamarckian Genetic Algorithm (LGA) was used to choose the good conformers. Similarly, a genetic algorithm was used to produce 100 individual docking runs for each selected *Mikania* ligand. In summary, the standardized Autodock step-wise docking protocol was used for the current study [16].

4. Conclusions

The present study found that 3,5-methyl-di-*O*-caffeoylquinate was efficient in binding with five target enzymes, whereas kaurenoic acid did not bind with the selected four targeted proteins. These two phytochemicals showed good efficacy as potential anti-inflammatory drugs of non-steroid [NSAIDs] nature. Interestingly, all 26 selected ligands (except 2, 6-dimethoxy quinone) from *Mikania* species showed good docking and binding to mPGES 2. Thus, the findings of this study indicate that it is possible to suppress COX 2, HNE, LOX, MMP 2 and 9, and mPGES 2 in the treatment of acute and chronic inflammatory diseases using these ligands of *Mikania* species.

Author Contributions: Conceptualization, software and methodology, N.R.; formal analysis and validation, V.-S.P.; data manager, M.A.W.; report documentation—initial manuscript draft preparation, N.R.; report documentation—reviewing and redrafting, S.G.K., R.V. and A.B.; supervision, R.V.; funding acquisition, A.B. All authors have read and agreed to the published version of the manuscript.

Funding: The authors express their sincere appreciation to the Researchers Supporting Project Number (RSP2023R466), King Saud University, Riyadh, Saudi Arabia.

Institutional Review Board Statement: Not applicable.

Informed Consent Statement: Not applicable.

Data Availability Statement: All of the study data details are readily available from the corresponding authors and are available upon request.

Conflicts of Interest: The authors declare no conflict of interest.

References

1. Ismail, B.S.; Mah, L.S. Effects of *Mikania micrantha* HBK on germination and growth of weed species. *Plant Soil* **1993**, *157*, 107–113.
2. Bora, A.R.; Deka, J.; Barua, I.C.; Barman, B. Intensity of *Mikania micrantha* in coffee and other plantations of Karbi Anglong district, Assam. *Indian J. Weed Sci.* **2019**, *51*, 95–97. [CrossRef]
3. Debaprotim, D.; Suvakanta, D.; Jashabir, C. Evaluation of anticancer activity of *Mikania micrantha* Kunth (Asteraceae) against ehrlich ascites carcinoma in swiss albino mice. *Int. J. Pharm. Res. Allied Sci.* **2014**, *3*, 9–18.
4. Zohmachhuana, A.; Tlaisun, M.; Mathipi, V.; Khawlhring, L.; Priya, J.S. Suppression of the RAGE gene expression in RAW 264.7 murine leukemia cell line by ethyl acetate extract of *Mikania micrantha* (L.) Kunth. *J. Appl. Biol. Biotechnol.* **2022**, *10*, 107–114. [CrossRef]
5. Rahman, M.M.; Kabir, M.M.; Noman, M.A.A.; Islam, M.R.; Dash, B.K.; Akhter, S.; Uddin, M.J.; Rahman, A. *Mikania cordata* leaves extract promotes activity against pathogenic bacteria and anticancer activity in EAC cell-bearing swiss albino mice. *J. Appl. Pharm. Sci.* **2020**, *10*, 112–122.
6. Da Silva, A.B.; Owiti, A.; Barbosa, W. Pharmacology of *Mikania* genus: A systematic review. *Pharmacogn. Rev.* **2018**, *12*, 230–237.
7. Radhakrishnan, N.; Karthi, S.; Raghuraman, P.; Ganesan, R.; Srinivasan, K.; Edwin, E.S.; Ganesh-Kumar, S.; Mohd Esa, N.; Senthil-Nathan, S.; Vasantha-Srinivasan, P.; et al. Chemical screening and mosquitocidal activity of essential oil derived from *Mikania scandens* (L.) Willd. against Anopheles gambiae Giles and their non-toxicity on mosquito predators. *All Life* **2023**, *16*, 2169959. [CrossRef]
8. Barlow, D.J.; Buriani, A.; Ehrman, T.; Bosisio, E.; Eberini, I.; Hylands, P.J. In-silico studies in Chinese herbal medicines' research: Evaluation of in-silico methodologies and phytochemical data sources, and a review of research to date. *J. Ethnopharmacol.* **2012**, *140*, 526–534. [CrossRef]
9. Prachayasittikul, V.; Worachartcheewan, A.; Shoombuatong, W.; Songtawee, N.; Simeon, S.; Prachayasittikul, V.; Nantasenamat, C. Computer-aided drug design of bioactive natural products. *Curr. Top. Med. Chem.* **2015**, *15*, 1780–1800. [CrossRef]
10. Suyenaga, E.S.; Reche, E.; Farias, F.M.; Schapoval, E.E.S.; Chaves, C.G.M.; Henriques, A.T. Antiinflammatory investigation of some species of Mikania. *Phytother. Res.* **2002**, *16*, 519–523. [CrossRef]
11. Perez-Amador, M.C.; Munoz Ocotero, V.; Ibarra Balcazar, R.; Garcia Jimenez, F. Phytochemical and pharmacological studies on *Mikania micrantha* HBK (Asteraceae). *Phyton* **2010**, *79*, 77–80.

12. Della Pasqua, C.S.P.; Iwamoto, R.D.; Antunes, E.; Borghi, A.A.; Sawaya, A.C.H.F.; Landucci, E.C.T. Pharmacological study of anti-inflammatory activity of aqueous extracts of *Mikania glomerata* (Spreng.) and *Mikania laevigata* (Sch. Bip. ex Baker). *J. Ethnopharmacol.* **2019**, *231*, 50–56. [CrossRef] [PubMed]
13. Kuhn, M.; von Mering, C.; Campillos, M.; Jensen, L.J.; Bork, P. STITCH: Interaction networks of chemicals and proteins. *Nucleic Acids Res.* **2007**, *36*, D684–D688. [CrossRef] [PubMed]
14. Kumaraswamy, S.; Arumugam, G.; Pandurangan, A.K.; Prabhakaran, V.S.; Narayanaswamy, R. Molecular docking analysis of organic acids (OA) from honey as modulators of human ferritin, transferrin, and hepcidin. *J. Microbiol. Biotechnol. Food Sci.* **2023**, *12*, 5743. [CrossRef]
15. Lipinski, C.A.; Lombardo, F.; Dominy, B.W.; Feeney, P.J. Experimental and computational approaches to estimate solubility and permeability in drug discovery and development settings. *Adv. Drug Deliv. Rev.* **2001**, *46*, 03–26. [CrossRef]
16. Narayanaswamy, R.; Wai, L.K.; Esa, N.M. Molecular docking analysis of phytic acid and 4-hydroxyisoleucine as cyclooxygenase-2, microsomal prostaglandin E synthase-2, tyrosinase, human neutrophil elastase, matrix metalloproteinase-2 and-9, xanthine oxidase, squalene synthase, nitric oxide synthase, human aldose reductase, and lipoxygenase inhibitors. *Pharmacogn. Mag.* **2017**, *13*, S512–S518.
17. Saadawi, S.; Jalil, J.; Jasamai, M.; Jantan, I. Inhibitory effects of acetylmelodorinol, chrysin and polycarpol from *Mitrella kentii* on prostaglandin E2 and thromboxane B2 production and platelet activating factor receptor binding. *Molecules* **2012**, *17*, 4824–4835. [CrossRef]
18. Park, K.R.; Nam, D.; Yun, H.M.; Lee, S.G.; Jang, H.J.; Sethi, G.; Cho, S.K.; Ahn, K.S. β-Caryophyllene oxide inhibits growth and induces apoptosis through the suppression of PI3K/AKT/mTOR/S6K1 pathways and ROS-mediated MAPKs activation. *Cancer Lett.* **2011**, *312*, 178–188. [CrossRef]
19. Lomarat, P.; Sripha, K.; Phanthong, P.; Kitphati, W.; Thirapanmethee, K.; Bunyapraphatsara, N. In vitro biological activities of black pepper essential oil and its major components relevant to the prevention of Alzheimer's disease. *Thai J. Pharm. Sci.* **2015**, *39*, 94–101.
20. Zheng, M.; Jin, W.; Son, K.H.; Chang, H.W.; Kim, H.P.; Bae, K.; Kang, S.S. The constituents isolated from *Peucedanum japonicum* Thunb. and their cyclooxygenase (COX) inhibitory activity. *Korean J. Med. Crop Sci.* **2005**, *13*, 75–79.
21. Jayaprakasam, B.; Alexander-Lindo, R.L.; DeWitt, D.L.; Nair, M.G. Terpenoids from Stinking toe (*Hymneae courbaril*) fruits with cyclooxygenase and lipid peroxidation inhibitory activities. *Food Chem.* **2007**, *105*, 485–490. [CrossRef]
22. Stanikunaite, R.; Khan, S.I.; Trappe, J.M.; Ross, S.A. Cyclooxygenase-2 inhibitory and antioxidant compounds from the truffle *Elaphomyces granulatus*. *Phytother. Res.* **2009**, *23*, 575–578. [CrossRef]
23. Rehman, U.U.; Shah, J.; Khan, M.A.; Shah, M.R.; Khan, I. Molecular docking of taraxerol acetate as a new COX inhibitor. *Bangladesh J. Pharmacol.* **2013**, *8*, 194–197. [CrossRef]
24. Siedle, B.; Cisielski, S.; Murillo, R.; Löser, B.; Castro, V.; Klaas, C.A.; Hucke, O.; Labahn, A.; Melzig, M.F.; Merfort, I. Sesquiterpene lactones as inhibitors of human neutrophil elastase. *Bioorg. Med. Chem.* **2002**, *10*, 2855–2861. [CrossRef]
25. Siedle, B.; Hrenn, A.; Merfort, I. Natural compounds as inhibitors of human neutrophil elastase. *Planta Med.* **2007**, *73*, 401–420. [CrossRef] [PubMed]
26. Ng, C.H.; Rullah, K.; Aluwi, M.F.F.M.; Abas, F.; Lam, K.W.; Ismail, I.S.; Narayanaswamy, R.; Jamaludin, F.; Shaari, K. Synthesis and docking studies of 2, 4, 6-trihydroxy-3-geranylacetophenone analogs as potential lipoxygenase inhibitor. *Molecules* **2014**, *19*, 11645–11659. [CrossRef]
27. Castro, J.S.; Trzaskowski, B.; Deymier, P.A.; Bucay, J.; Adamowicz, L.; Hoying, J.B. Binding affinity of fluorochromes and fluorescent proteins to Taxol™ crystals. *Mater. Sci. Eng. C* **2009**, *29*, 1609–1615. [CrossRef]
28. Ríos, E.V.; León, A.; Chávez, M.I.; Torres, Y.; Ramírez-Apan, M.T.; Toscano, R.A.; Bravo-Monzón, Á.E.; Espinosa-García, F.J.; Delgado, G. Sesquiterpene lactones from Mikania micrantha and Mikania cordifolia and their cytotoxic and anti-inflammatory evaluation. *Fitoterapia* **2014**, *94*, 155–163. [CrossRef]
29. Vanderlinde, F.A.; Rocha, F.F.; Malvar, D.C.; Ferreira, R.T.; Costa, E.A.; Florentino, I.F.; Guilhon, G.; Lima, T. Anti-inflammatory and opioid-like activities in methanol extract of *Mikania lindleyana*, sucuriju. *Rev. Bras. Farmacogn.* **2012**, *22*, 150–156. [CrossRef]
30. Kumar, S.; Bajwa, B.S.; Singh, K.; Kalia, A.N. Anti-inflammatory activity of herbal plants: A review. *Int. J. Adv. Pharm. Biol. Chem.* **2013**, *2*, 272–281.
31. Chagas-Paula, D.A.; Oliveira, T.B.; Faleiro, D.P.; Oliveira, R.B.; Da Costa, F.B. Outstanding anti-inflammatory potential of selected Asteraceae species through the potent dual inhibition of cyclooxygenase-1 and 5-lipoxygenase. *Planta Med.* **2015**, *81*, 1296–1307. [CrossRef] [PubMed]
32. Jyothilakshmi, M.; Jyothis, M.; Latha, M.S. Cyclooxygenase, Lipoxygenase, Nitric Oxide Synthase, Myeloperoxidase and Protease inhibiting activities of the leaves and flowers of *Mikania micrantha* Kunth. *J. Complement. Med. Res.* **2020**, *11*, 51. [CrossRef]
33. Werz, O. Inhibition of 5-lipoxygenase product synthesis by natural compounds of plant origin. *Planta Med.* **2007**, *73*, 1331–1357. [CrossRef] [PubMed]
34. El-Ahmady, S.H.; Ashour, M.L.; Wink, M. Chemical composition and anti-inflammatory activity of the essential oils of *Psidium guajava* fruits and leaves. *J. Essent. Oil Res.* **2013**, *25*, 475–481. [CrossRef]
35. de Vargas, F.S.; de Almeida, P.D.; Aranha, E.S.P.; de Boleti, A.P.A.; Newton, P.; de Vasconcellos, M.C.; Junior, V.F.V.; Lima, E.S. Biological activities and cytotoxicity of diterpenes from *Copaifera spp*. Oleoresins. *Molecules* **2015**, *20*, 6194–6210. [CrossRef]

36. Narayanaswamy, R.; Kok Wai, L.; Ismail, I.S. In silico analysis of selected honey constituents as human neutrophil elastase (HNE) and matrix metalloproteinases (MMP 2 and 9) inhibitors. *Int. J. Food Prop.* **2015**, *18*, 2155–2164. [CrossRef]
37. Gabay, O.; Sanchez, C.; Salvat, C.; Chevy, F.; Breton, M.; Nourissat, G.; Wolf, C.; Jacques, C.; Berenbaum, F. Stigmasterol: A phytosterol with potential anti-osteoarthritic properties. *Osteoarthr. Cartil.* **2010**, *18*, 106–116. [CrossRef]
38. Maione, F.; Minosi, P.; Di Giannuario, A.; Raucci, F.; Chini, M.G.; De Vita, S.; Bifulco, G.; Mascolo, N.; Pieretti, S. Long-lasting anti-inflammatory and antinociceptive effects of acute ammonium glycyrrhizinate administration: Pharmacological, biochemical, and docking studies. *Molecules* **2019**, *24*, 2453. [CrossRef]
39. Szklarczyk, D.; Santos, A.; Von Mering, C.; Jensen, L.J.; Bork, P.; Kuhn, M. STITCH 5: Augmenting protein–chemical interaction networks with tissue and affinity data. *Nucleic Acids Res.* **2016**, *44*, D380–D384. [CrossRef]
40. Wu, G.; Robertson, D.H.; Brooks, C.L.; Vieth, M. Detailed analysis of grid-based molecular docking: A case study of CDOCKER—A CHARMm-based MD docking algorithm. *J. Comput. Chem.* **2003**, *24*, 1549–1562. [CrossRef]

Disclaimer/Publisher's Note: The statements, opinions and data contained in all publications are solely those of the individual author(s) and contributor(s) and not of MDPI and/or the editor(s). MDPI and/or the editor(s) disclaim responsibility for any injury to people or property resulting from any ideas, methods, instructions or products referred to in the content.

Synthesis and Biological Evaluation of α-Tocopherol Derivatives as Potential Anticancer Agents

Aneta Baj [1,*], Lucie Rárová [2], Artur Ratkiewicz [3], Miroslav Strnad [4] and Stanislaw Witkowski [1]

1. Department of Organic Chemistry, Faculty of Chemistry, University of Bialystok, Ciołkowskiego 1K, 15-245 Białystok, Poland; wit@uwb.edu.pl
2. Department of Experimental Biology, Faculty of Science, Palacký University, Šlechtitelů 27, CZ-78371 Olomouc, Czech Republic; lucie.rarova@upol.cz
3. Department of Physical Chemistry, Faculty of Chemistry, University of Bialystok, Ciołkowskiego 1K, 15-245 Białystok, Poland; artrat@uwb.edu.pl
4. Laboratory of Growth Regulators, Institute of Experimental Botany of the Czech Academy of Sciences, Faculty of Science, Palacký University, Šlechtitelů 27, CZ-78371 Olomouc, Czech Republic; miroslav.strnad@upol.cz
* Correspondence: aneta.baj@uwb.edu.pl; Tel.: +48-85-738-80-41

Abstract: α-Tocopheryl succinate (α-TS) and α-tocopheryloxyacetic acid (α-TEA) are potent inducers of apoptosis in cancer cells and efficient suppressors of tumors in experimental model cancer cell lines. They exhibit selective cytotoxicity against tumor cells and very limited or no toxicity toward nonmalignant cells. In the present work, a series of new α-tocopherol derivatives were synthesized as analogs of α-TS and α-TEA. The cytotoxic activity of obtained compounds was tested using three human cancer cell lines, including chronic lymphoblastic leukemia (CEM), breast adenocarcinoma (MCF7), cervical adenocarcinoma (HeLa), and normal human fibroblasts (BJ). The introduction of an alkyl substituent into the ether-linked acetic acid moiety in α-TEA increased anticancer activity. α-Tocopheryloxy-2-methylpropanoic acid with two additional geminal methyl groups was more active against CEM cells compared to α-TEA and non-toxic to normal cells. In order to acquire a deeper understanding of the biological activity of synthesized compounds, a molecular docking study was also conducted. Our research confirmed that vitamin E derivatives are interesting and valuable compounds in terms of their potential therapeutic use as anticancer agents.

Keywords: vitamin E derivatives; α-tocopheryloxyacetic acid (α-TEA); α-tocopheryl succinate (α-TS); cancer; mitocans; apoptosis

1. Introduction

Treatment of cancer to date remains a significant challenge, mainly due to continuous mutations, which make the tumor cells resistant to established chemotherapeutics [1]. Mitochondria provide a novel targeting site that can selectively kill cancer cells without affecting normal cells [2]. Mitocans (mitochondria-targeted drugs) act by destabilizing mitochondria in cancer cells, causing them to unleash their pro-apoptotic potential, ultimately leading to reduced growth or death of tumor cells [3–5]. To this group belong redox-silent vitamin E analogs (Figure 1), represented by α-tocopheryl succinate (α-TS), which is mainly nontoxic to normal cells and tissues. Its pro-apoptotic activity was detected in various epithelial cancer cell types, particularly in breast, colon, and prostate cancers [6–9]. Significant anticancer activity show TS nanovesicles, both in vitro and in vivo [10]. However, α-TS is effective only by intraperitoneal injection, not by oral administration, since it is hydrolyzed by nonspecific esterases in the intestinal tract and in normal cells [11]. α-Tocopheryl malonate (TM) and α-tocopheryl oxalate (TO) show higher in vitro activity than α-TS. They are strong apoptogens in vitro but often show non-selective toxicity [12,13]. α-Tocopheryl phosphate (α-TP), a water-soluble form of α-T, has been detected in low amounts in human and animal tissues and plasma. Since the hydroxyl group is phosphorylated, α-T gains a redox-silent character and reveals new activities [14,15]. According to some authors, α-TP is a potentially stronger anti-proliferative agent than α-T [16,17]. Due to its potent biological activity, α-TP is still the subject of numerous investigations [18–20].

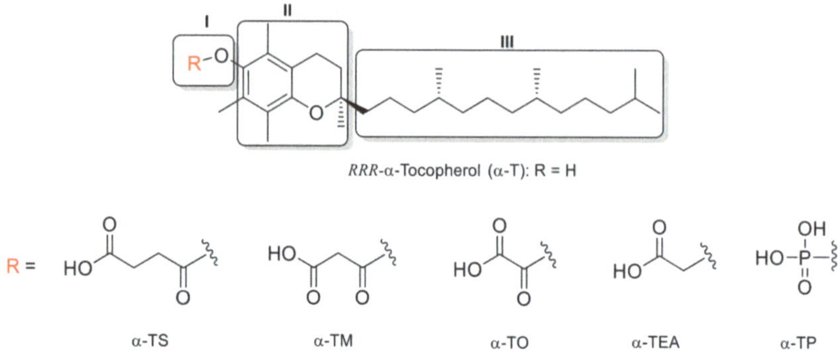

Figure 1. Chemical structure of α-tocopherol (α-T), α-tocopheryl succinate (α-TS), α-tocopheryl malonate (α-TM), α-tocopheryl oxalate (α-TO), α-tocopheryloxyacetic acid (α-TEA), and α-tocopheryl phosphate (α-TP) (Domains in vitamin E molecule and its analogs: I—functional, II—signaling, III—hydrophobic).

α-TS is unstable under physiological conditions because of cellular esterases' activity. To overcome this problem, the succinic moiety was substituted by an acetic acid part linked to the phenolic oxygen by ether linkage to give α-tocopheryloxyacetic acid (α-TEA) with a stable, non-hydrolysable entity [21–26]. This α-tocopherol derivative can be administered orally with high antitumor efficacy [26,27]. Studies in the past decade have shown that α-TEA is a potent inducer of apoptosis in various types of cancer epithelial cells [28] in tests both in vitro and in vivo [29]. α-TEA induces autophagy in lung and mammary tumor cells. The autophagy-mediated cell death is partially responsible for the cytotoxic properties of α-TEA [30]. Tests in vivo showed an even stronger antitumor effect than α-TS [21]. Similarly to α-TS, α-TEA is a potent inducer of apoptosis in human endometrial, breast, ovarian, lung, colon, prostate, and lymphoid cells [31]. It induces apoptosis through an increase in death-promoting factors and a decrease in survival-promoting factors in human prostate cancer cells [32]. It was demonstrated that α-TEA inhibits proliferation, migration, and invasion in colon cancer cells [25,33]. On the other hand, α-TEA does not induce apoptosis in normal human mammary epithelial cells, normal PrEC human prostate cells, and healthy tissues. Several chemical modifications of the α-TEA as a leading structure have been reported. They primarily concerned alterations in the ethereal moiety or in the ending of the acidic fragment. In α-tocopheryloxybutyric acid, the butyric acid residue is linked by the ethereal bond to the α-tocopheryloxyl part [34]. In another modification, the ending carboxylic group was replaced with sulphonic or phosphonic groups linked to three or four carbon-containing linkers [35]. Previous investigations have shown that α-TEA and α-TS can be effective adjuvants in chemoprevention and cancer treatment, enhancing the antitumor effect of drug substances [25,33,36]. They were tested in combination with known anticancer drugs: celecoxib [37] and cisplatin [38–40].

Three domains are distinguished in the structure of α-T and its derivatives (Figure 1). Domain I as the functional domain, is essential for the antioxidant or pro-apoptotic action of vitamin E. Acylation at the C-6 position with succinic anhydride makes α-tocopheryl succinate (α-TS) a dormant antioxidant with strong pro-apoptotic properties. Domain II consists of the chroman ring and is responsible for the signaling function affecting, among others, the activity of PP2A phosphatase and protein kinase C (PKC). Domain III includes the lipophilic side chain, which is responsible for docking tocopherol molecules in cell membranes and plasma lipoproteins [6,41,42].

The aim of the present study was to obtain some new α-tocopherol derivatives with higher anticancer activity than α-TS and α-TEA. For this purpose, we planned to modify the substituent at the C-6 position of tocopheroxyl moiety, which can modulate the original pro-apoptotic activity. We decided to introduce an additional group (carboxyl or alkyl) in the α-position relative to the terminal carboxyl group.

2. Results and Discussion

The synthesis of target vitamin E derivatives **3–10** was performed according to the synthetic route, as shown in Scheme 1. *RRR*-α-tocopherol (α-T) was the substrate in the described reactions. In the first variant, an additional carboxyl group was introduced into the α-position to the carboxyl group in the α-TS molecule. For this purpose, dibenzyl malonate was alkylated with α-tocopheryl chloroacetate (**1**), followed by hydrogenolysis of dibenzyl ester **2** to give compound **3**. In another experiment, α-T was alkylated with diethyl bromomalonate followed by alkaline hydrolysis to give tocopheryloxymalonic acid (**4**). The analogs of α-TEA (**5–10**) with additional alkyl substituents in ether-linked acetic acid moiety were obtained by alkylation of α-T with corresponding α-bromoacid ethyl esters (i.e., 2-bromopropionate, 2-bromobutyrate, α-bromoisobutyrate, 2-bromovalerate, 2-bromo-3-methylbutyrate, 2-bromocaprylate, respectively). All reactions were carried out in mild conditions to give very good yields. The synthesized compounds were characterized by NMR, FT-IR, and HRMS analysis, and the obtained data were consistent with the desired structures.

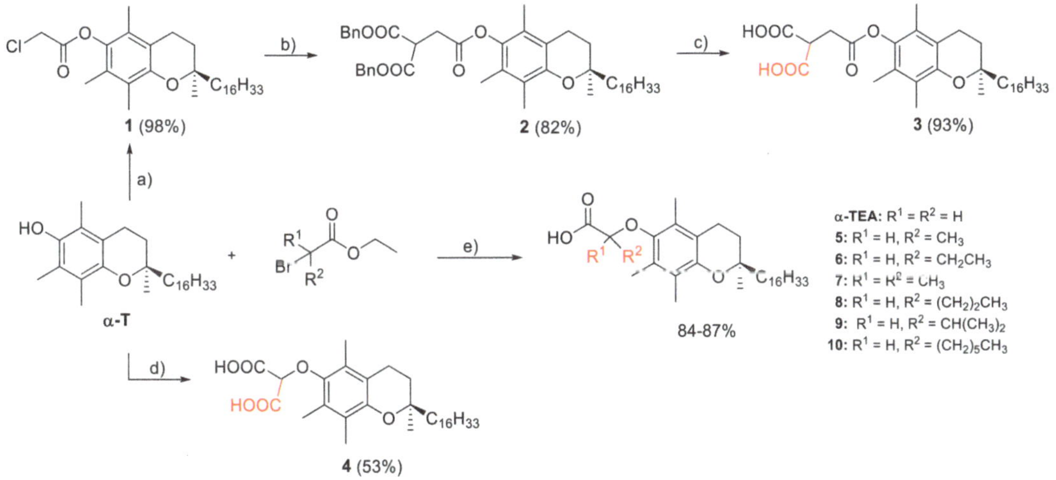

Scheme 1. Synthesis of vitamin E derivatives (**2–10**) from *RRR*-α-tocopherol (α-T). Reagents and conditions: (**a**) chloroacetyl chloride, pyridine, toluene, rt; (**b**) $CH_2(COOBn)_2$, *t*-BuOK, THF, rt; (**c**) H_2 (1 atm), Pd/C, ethyl acetate; (**d**) 1. diethyl bromomalonate, K_2CO_3, acetone, reflux, 2. KOH_{aq}, THF, rt; (**e**) NaOH, DMF, rt.

To determine the cytotoxic activity, the synthesized compounds **3–10** were screened for their in vitro antiproliferative action against a panel of three different human cancer cell lines, namely human chronic lymphoblastic leukemia (CEM), human breast adenocarcinoma (MCF7), human cervical adenocarcinoma (HeLa), and normal human fibroblasts (BJ). For a better comparison, known compounds, namely α-TEA, α-TS, α-TM, α-TO, and α-TP, were also tested in our laboratory conditions. Furthermore, we used Doxorubicin (Dox), a known, anti-cancer drug, as a reference in cytotoxic assay. The obtained results are listed in Table 1.

Table 1. IC$_{50}$ (µM) on three cancer cell lines (CEM, MCF7, HeLa) and normal human fibroblasts (BJ) after 72 h of incubation with the tested compounds. The data are means ± standard deviation (SD) obtained from at least three independent experiments performed in triplicate.

Compound	R	CEM	MCF7	HeLa	BJ	Complex II Affinity (kcal/mol)
α-TS		33.8 ± 0.0	48.6 ± 2.1	45.8 ± 0.8	43.3 ± 2.3	−7.4
α-TO		24.6 ± 3.6	31.0 ± 7.4	28.1 ± 0.3	45.1 ± 2.4	−6.9
α-TM		17.8 ± 1.2	41.1 ± 6.3	26.9 ± 7.4	45.0 ± 0.8	−7.4
α-TEA		32.0 ± 1.2	48.2 ± 1.1	40.9 ± 3.9	40.4 ± 6.6	−7.2
α-TP		>50	>50	>50	>50	−7.5
3		>50	>50	>50	>50	−7.1
4		>50	>50	35.3 ± 0.8	>50	−7.0
5		24.5 ± 2.1	47.3 ± 0.1	17.2 ± 3.4	43.6 ± 2.2	−7.4
6		24.5 ± 6.3	46.6 ± 0.4	13.1 ± 0.1	41.8 ± 1.7	−7.3
7		14.1 ± 0.8	>50	>50	>50	−7.5
8		31.5 ± 3.7	26.9 ± 4.5	31.5 ± 3.6	>50	−7.3
9		28.7 ± 1.0	21.6 ± 1.0	29.9 ± 2.0	35.5 ± 3.7	−7.4
10		>50	>50	>50	>50	−7.4
Dox	–	0.255 ± 0.022	0.273 ± 0.019	0.868 ± 0.054	0.278 ± 0.036	–

As expected, Dox exhibited strong, non-selective cytotoxicity against all tested cell lines. α-T derivatives α-TEA, α-TS, α-MT, and α-TO showed moderate cytotoxicity against cancer cells and weak cytotoxicity toward normal human fibroblasts (BJ). This fact appears to be in accordance with the literature data, which reported a very limited or lack of toxicity toward non-malignant cells [13,42,43].

The selective toxicity of α-TS and α-TEA against malignant versus normal cells is probably related to the negative charge of the succinic or acetic part of the molecules at neutral pH [7,44]. This assumption was supported by an observation that pro-apoptotic action was increased in the acidic milieu [45]. The presence of a charged group appears to be essential for apoptosis induction. Methylation of the terminal carboxyl group deprives a compound of proapoptotic activity [46]. It was reported that pH of the interstitium of most tumors is 6.2–6.5, and for most normal tissues, it is in the range of 7.0–7.4 [47]. Thus, increasing the acidity in carboxylic moiety may result in higher apoptogenic activity. Such a tendency was observed for the α-tocopheryl dicarboxylic monoesters, increasing in the order: succinate < malonate < oxalate [12,13,48]. Following these observations, we decided to modify the acidic part in α-TS and α-TEA by introducing an additional carboxyl group into the α-position of the carboxyl group. Consequently, transformation into the malonic ending might result in stronger anticancer action due to increased acidity. Unexpectedly, the analog **3** (carboxylated α-TS) appeared inactive in the tests performed in three cancer cell lines. Similarly, α-tocopheryl phosphate (α-TP) was inactive against all investigated cancer cell lines. In turn, the compound **4** (carboxylated α-TEA) showed higher activity selectively against human cervical carcinoma cells (HeLa) compared to α-TEA. Particularly interesting anticancer profiles were obtained for the α-TEA analogs (**5–10**), in which alkyl substituents were introduced into the ether-linked acetic acid moiety. Only compound **10** containing the n-hexyl substituent in the α-position to the terminal carboxyl group was inactive against all tested cancer cell lines. 2-Tocopheryloxypropionic acid (**5**) showed higher cytotoxicity toward human chronic lymphoblastic leukemia CEM cells (24.5 ± 2.1) and much stronger action toward HeLa cells (17.2 ± 3.4) in comparison to the reference α-TEA. The replacing of methyl with ethyl group resulted in higher activity against HeLa (13.1 ± 0.1). Both compounds were also much less cytotoxic for normal fibroblasts (BJ). The most interesting results were obtained for compound **7** containing two geminal methyl groups (clofibric acid fragment), which revealed a considerable increase in activity against CEM cell line (14.1 ± 0.8). It also showed a relatively high therapeutic window because its cytotoxicity toward normal BJ cells was zero. Unexpectedly, it appeared inactive in assays in MCF7 and HeLa cell lines. Like most of the synthesized compounds, derivatives **8** and **9** showed moderate activity toward all cancer cell lines.

Based on the literature data, we have decided to determine the interaction of newly synthesized compounds with Complex II (CII), also known as succinate dehydrogenase (SDH), in silico via molecular docking simulation. Mitocans from the group of vitamin E derivatives interact with mitochondrial CII by interfering with ubiquinone (UbQ) functions, causing leakage of electrons and generation of reactive oxygen species (ROS), which induce selective apoptosis in cancer cells [3,49–51]. In the present work, the calculations were carried out in the Complex II active site for α-T derivatives **3–10** and, to compare, other species considered here, as detailed in the Section 3.3. The docking scores (affinities) of species tested here against their cytotoxicity are listed in Table 1. Additionally, for the sake of comparison, simulations were performed for α-T and ubiquinone-2 (UQ2) with affinities of −7.1 and −8.0 kcal/mol, respectively. Scores of newly synthesized species, changing in the range of −7.0 kcal/mol for **4** to −7.5 kcal/mol for **7**, are not particularly different from each other, making it difficult to decide explicitly which is the most active. Additionally, affinities for compounds already reported in the literature (α-TS, α-TO, α-TM, α-TEA, and α-TP) are within a similar scope. Interestingly, derivatives with higher anticancer activity (**5–8**) simultaneously possess affinities slightly higher than that for α-TEA. Although not large, the differences may, however, contribute to the observed increased cytotoxicity toward cancer cells. While the bonding score for the native ligand UQ2 of −8.0 kcal/mol is more favorable, the one for the α-T (−7.1 kcal/mol) is noticeably worse. This indicates that substitution has a beneficial effect on the molecule's ability to penetrate Complex II and thus confirms the consideration of α-T derivatives as new drug candidates. As shown below (Figure 2), ubiquinone-2 is bound to the active center of the protein via two hydrogen bonds to tryptophan (Trp164) from the subunit B of NEK1 and tyrosine (Tyr83, subunit C).

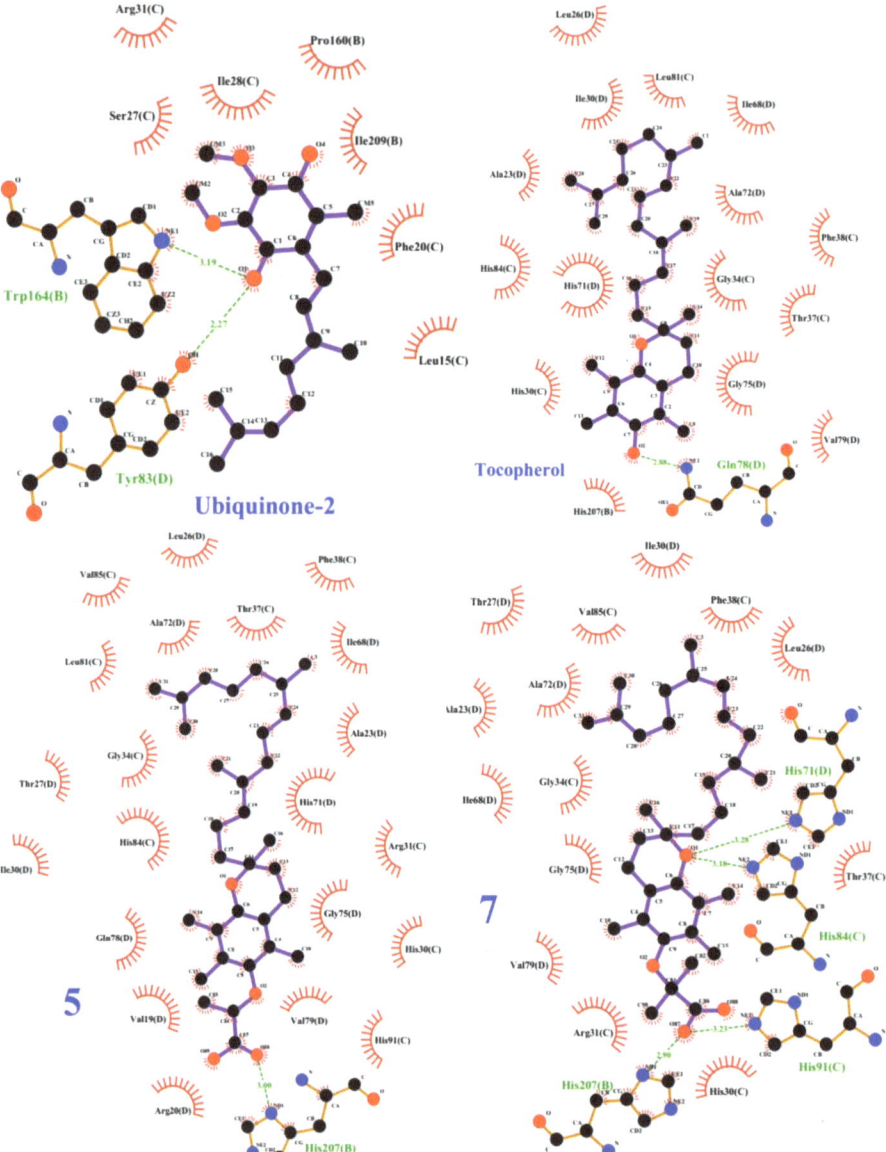

Figure 2. The pattern of hydrogen bonds for the best scored docking modes of ubiquinone-2, α-tocopherol (α-T), compound **5** and compound **7** to Complex II. Green dashed lines symbolize hydrogen bonds, whereas red half circles with outlines mean nonpolar interactions. Bond lengths are given in angstroms.

The key moieties involved in these interactions are N atoms from the pyrrole ring and the hydroxyl group from Tyr83 as hydrogen bond donors and ketone groups as acceptors, which further confirms the localization of ubiquinone-2 between three subunits of Complex 2 (B–D). As it is clearly seen in Figure 2, the arrangement of hydrogen bonds changes for α-T and its derivatives, replacing ubiquinone-2 in the protein. The peptide group from Gln78 is a H bond donor for α-T. In contrast, α-T derivatives interact with the N atoms from the aromatic rings of amino acids, as is the case for ubiquinone.

Figure 3 visualizes the exact spatial location of the best docking poses for the ligands in Figure 2. It is interesting to observe that the position of α-T differs significantly from that of the other three ligands. In fact, α-T seems to penetrate deeper into the structure of Complex II; in particular, it burrows more deeply into the D subunit. This could have significant consequences. Since it is reasonable to assume that the action of a ligand is most effective when it is located precisely in the active center of the enzyme itself, it can be inferred that the biological activity of α-T may be significantly less than that of its derivatives, which locate almost exactly at the site of ubiquinone-2 (UQ2), which is the native ligand. Indeed, similar conclusions also emerge from the experiments described in the previous section. As such, the in silico experiments also confirm the possible utility of the newly obtained compounds as drug candidates.

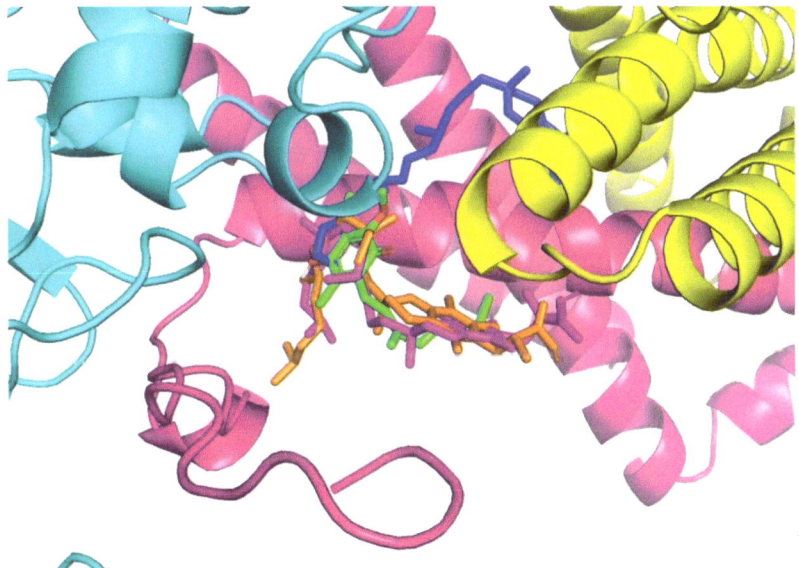

Figure 3. The best docking mods to the active center of Complex II for: ubiquinone-2 (UQ2, green color), α-tocopherol (blue color), compounds 5 (light brown color) and 7 (magenta). Subunits of Complex II are colored as follows: A—green, B—cyan, C—magenta, D—yellow.

3. Materials and Methods

3.1. Chemistry

3.1.1. General

All reagents were purchased from commercial sources and used without further purification. Anhydrous solvents (i.e., THF, DCM, DMF, toluene, acetone, pyridine) were dried by distillation over appropriate drying agents under an argon atmosphere. D-α-tocopherol (*RRR*-α-tocopherol, α-T), D-α-tocopheryl succinate (α-TS), and α-bromoacid ethyl esters (i.e., 2-bromopropionate, 2-bromobutyrate, α-bromoisobutyrate, 2-bromovalerate, 2-bromo-3-methylbutyrate, 2-bromocaprylate) were purchased from Merck Life Sciences Sigma-Aldrich (Darmstadt, Germany). α-Tocopheryl malonate (α-TM) and α-tocopheryl oxalate (α-TO) were synthesized according to procedures in the literature [48]. α-Tocopheryl phosphate (α-TP) was prepared using phase transfer catalyzed phosphorylation method of phenols in a two-phase system (see Supplementary Materials file) [52].

Thin layer chromatography (TLC) was performed using Merck silica gel plates (0.25 mm, 60F-254) and visualized with CAM stain (ceric-ammonium-molybdate solution containing H_2SO_4). Standard flash chromatography (FC) was accomplished using silica gel (230–400 mesh size, J. T. Baker). Solvents for FC were freshly distilled before use.

NMR spectra were recorded at room temperature on a Bruker Avance DPX 200 or Avance II 400 spectrometers operating at 200 and 400 MHz, respectively. The chemical shifts (δ) are given in parts per million (ppm) relative to tetramethylsilane (TMS) using a residual solvent signal as an internal standard: $CHCl_3$ = 7.26 ppm (^{1}H NMR) and $CDCl_3$ = 77.0 ppm (^{13}C NMR). The following abbreviations are used to describe peak patterns: s = singlet, br = broad signal, d = doublet, t = triplet, q = quartet, m = multiplet. Only selected signals in the ^{1}H NMR spectra are reported. The mean values of chemical shifts were given for signals for which the dynamic effects in ^{13}C NMR spectra were observed. The original ^{1}H and ^{13}C NMR spectra are contained in the Supplementary Materials. FT-IR spectra were recorded in the range between 4000 and 500 cm^{-1} on a Nicolet 6700 spectrometer. HRMS data were acquired on an Agilent Technologies 6530 Accurate-Mass Q-TOF LC/MS.

3.1.2. Steps for the Preparation of Compound 3

Synthesis of *RRR*-α-tocopheryl chloroacetate (**1**)

A solution of chloroacetyl chloride (0.24 mL, 3 mmol) in dry toluene (4 mL) was added to a stirred solution of *RRR*-α-T (861 mg, 2 mmol) in dry toluene (10 mL) and dry pyridine (0.5 mL, 6 mmol) at room temperature. After 30 min, the resulting precipitate was filtrated through a pad of Celite, and the filtrate was washed with brine (15 mL), dried over anhydrous Na_2SO_4, and concentrated under reduced pressure. The crude product was purified using FC (hexane/ethyl acetate, 98:2, v/v) to yield compound **1** as a light-yellow oil (995 mg, 98% yield). ^{1}H and ^{13}C NMR data were consistent with those available in the literature [53].

Synthesis of dibenzyl *RRR*-α-tocopheryloxy-2-oxoethylmalonate (**2**)

To a stirred solution of dibenzyl malonate (341 mg, 1.2 mmol) in dry THF (10 mL), *t*-BuOK (146 mg, 1.3 mmol) was added at room temperature. After 30 min, solution of chloroacetate **1** (510 mg, 1 mmol) in dry THF (2 mL) was added. The reaction mixture was stirred overnight (16 h), poured into saturated solution of NH_4Cl (20 mL), and extracted with diethyl ether (3 × 20 mL). The combined organic layers were washed with brine (20 mL), dried over anhydrous Na_2SO_4, and concentrated under vacuum. The crude product was purified using FC (hexane/ethyl acetate, 95:5, v/v) to yield compound **2** as a colorless oil (622 mg, 82% yield).

Compound **2**: ^{1}H NMR (200 MHz, $CDCl_3$) δ 7.38–7.31 (m, 10H, H-Ar), 5.23–5.16 (m, 4H, C$\underline{H}_2$Ph), 4.11 (t, *J* = 7.5 Hz, 1H, C$\underline{H}$COOBn), 3.30 (d, *J* = 7.5 Hz, 2H, C$\underline{H}_2$CHCOOBn), 2.59 (t, *J* = 6.6 Hz, 2H, H-4), 2.09, 1.99, 1.95 (3s, 9H, H-5a, H-7a, H-8b), 1.89–1.72 (m, 2H, H-3), 0.90–0.86 (m, 12H, H-4′a, H-8′a, H-12′a, H-13′); ^{13}C{^{1}H} NMR (100 MHz, $CDCl_3$) δ 169.5 (C), 168.0 (2 × C), 149.5 (C), 140.4 (C), 135.1 (2 x C), 128.9–128.1 (10 x CH), 126.6 (C), 124.9 (C), 123.0 (C), 117.4 (C), 75.05 (C), 67.6 (2 x CH_2), 47.9 (CH), 40.2 (CH_2), 39.4 (CH_2), 37.6, 37.5, 37.4, 37.3 (4 × CH_2), 32.8 (CH_2), 32.8 (CH), 32.7 (CH), 31.0 (CH_2), 28.0 (CH), 24.8 (CH_2), 24.4 (CH_2), 23.6 (CH_3), 22.7 (CH_3), 22.6 (CH_3), 21.0 (CH_2), 20.6 (CH_2), 19.73 (CH_3), 19.67 (CH_3), 12.9 (CH_3), 12.0 (CH_3), 11.8 (CH_3); IR (ATR) ν_{max} 2928, 1748, 1456, 1239, 1154 cm^{-1}.

Synthesis of *RRR*-α-tocopheryloxy-2-oxoethylmalonic acid (**3**)

The mixture of compound **2** (500 mg, 0.66 mmol) and 10% Pd/C (100 mg) in ethyl acetate (30 mL) was hydrogenated under atmospheric pressure at room temperature. After total conversion (4 h, TLC control), the reaction mixture was filtered through a pad of Celite, and the filtrate was evaporated under vacuum. The crude product was purified using flash chromatography (ethyl acetate) to yield compound **3** as a colorless oil (354 mg, 93% yield).

Compound **3**: ^{1}H NMR (400 MHz, CDCl$_3$): δ 9.41 (bs, 1H, COOH), 4.04 (t, J = 7.0 Hz, 1H, C$\underline{H}$COOH), 3.31 (d, J = 7.0 Hz, 2H, C$\underline{H_2}$CHCOOH), 2.58 (t, J = 6.6 Hz, 2H, H-4), 2.09, 2.01, 1.96 (3s, 9H, H-5a, H-7a, H-8b), 1.84–1.71 (m, 2H, H-3), 0.89–0.85 (m, 12H, H-4′a, H-8′a, H-12′a, H-13′); ^{13}C{^{1}H}NMR (100 MHz, CDCl$_3$) δ 173.0 (2 × C), 169.5 (C), 149.6 (C), 140.4 (C), 126.6 (C), 124.9 (C), 123.2 (C), 117.5 (C), 75.1 (C), 47.2 (CH), 40.4 (CH$_2$), 39.4 (CH$_2$), 37.6, 37.5, 37.4, 37.3 (4 × CH$_2$), 32.8 (CH), 32.7 (CH), 32.5 (CH$_2$), 31.0 (CH$_2$), 28.0 (CH), 24.8 (CH$_2$), 24.5 (CH$_2$), 23.8 (CH$_3$), 22.7 (CH$_3$), 22.6 (CH$_3$), 21.0 (CH$_2$), 20.6 (CH$_2$), 19.7 (CH$_3$), 19.6 (CH$_3$), 12.8 (CH$_3$), 12.0 (CH$_3$), 11.8 (CH$_3$); IR (ATR): 3448, 2927, 1752, 1735, 1655, 1459, 1261, 1156, 1107 cm^{-1}; HRMS m/z 575.3938 (calcd for C$_{34}$H$_{55}$O$_7$ t([M+H]$^+$ 575.3942).

3.1.3. Steps for the Preparation of Compound 4

Synthesis of ethyl *RRR*-α-tocopheryloxymalonate (**4-S**)

To a stirred solution of *RRR*-α-T (470 mg, 1.1 mmol) in dry acetone (20 mL), K$_2$CO$_3$ (1.2 g, 8.8 mmol) was added at room temperature. After 10 min, diethyl bromomalonate (981 mg, 4.1 mmol) was added to the reaction mixture. The resulting yellow suspension was refluxed for 18 h (TLC control). After cooling to room temperature, the inorganic material was filtered off, and the filtrate was concentrated under reduced pressure. The residue was dissolved in diethyl ether (20 mL), washed with brine (2 × 20 mL) and water (1 × 20 mL), dried over Na$_2$SO$_4$, and concentrated under vacuum. The crude product was purified by FC using hexane/ethyl acetate (gradient 50:1 → 10:1, v/v) as an eluent to give pure product as a colorless oil (530 mg, 87% yield).

Compound **4-S**: ^{1}H NMR (400 MHz, CDCl$_3$) δ 4.69 (s, 1H, OCH), 4.34–4.26 (m, 4H, C$\underline{H_2}$CH$_3$), 2.55 (t, J = 6.7 Hz, 2H, H-4), 2.15, 2.11, 2.06 (3s, 9H, H-5a, H-7a, H-8b), 1.80–1.76 (m, 2H, H-3), 0.88–0.84 (m, 12H, H-4′a, H-8′a, H-12′a, H-13′); ^{13}C{^{1}H} NMR (100 MHz, CDCl$_3$) δ 166.5 (2 × C), 148.3 (C), 148.0 (C), 127.3 (C), 125.6 (C), 123.1 (C), 117.6 (C), 81.4 (CH), 74.8 (C), 62.0 (2 × CH$_2$), 39.9 (CH$_2$), 39.3 (CH$_2$), 37.39–37.22 (4 × CH$_2$), 32.7 (CH), 32.6 (CH), 31.2 (CH$_2$), 27.9 (CH), 24.8 (CH$_2$), 24.4 (CH$_2$), 23.8 (CH$_3$), 22.7 (CH$_3$), 22.6 (CH$_3$), 21.0 (CH$_2$), 20.6 (CH$_2$), 19.7 (CH$_3$), 19.6 (CH$_3$), 14.0 (2 × CH$_3$), 13.2 (CH$_3$), 12.3 (CH$_3$), 11.8 (CH$_3$).

Synthesis of *RRR*-α-tocopheryloxymalonic acid (**4**)

A solution of KOH (190 mg, 3.39 mmol) in water (2.5 mL) was added to a solution of compound **4-S** (400 mg, 0.68 mmol) in THF (10 mL,) and the resulting mixture was stirred vigorously at room temperature. After 2 h, 6M HCl was added to reach pH 2 and extracted with ethyl acetate (3 × 50 mL). The combined organic extracts were washed with water (2 × 30 mL) and brine (2 × 30 mL), and dried over Na$_2$SO$_4$. The crude product was purified by FC using ethyl acetate as an eluent to yield compound **4** as a light-yellow oil (220 mg, 61% yield) and dried in vacuo for 48 h.

Compound **4**: ^{1}H NMR (400 MHz, CDCl$_3$): δ 7.27 (bs, 2H, COOH), 4.80 (s, 1H, OCH), 2.55 (t, J = 6.5 Hz, 2H, H-4), 2.15, 2.12, 2.07 (3s, 9H, H-5a, H-7a, H-8b), 1.83–1.72 (m, 2H, H-3), 0.88–0.84 (m, 12H, H-4′a, H-8′a, H-12′a, H-13′); ^{13}C{^{1}H} NMR (100 MHz, CDCl$_3$) δ: 169.8 (2 × C), 148.7 (C), 147.6 (C), 127.2 (C), 125.5 (C), 123.5 (C), 118.0 (C), 80.7 (CH), 75.1 (C), 40.2 (CH$_2$), 39.4 (CH$_2$), 37.6, 37.5, 37.4, 37.3 (4 × CH$_2$), 32.8 (CH), 32.7 (CH), 31.1 (CH$_2$), 28.0 (CH), 24.8 (CH$_2$), 24.4 (CH$_2$), 23.7 (CH$_3$), 22.7 (CH$_3$), 22.6 (CH$_3$), 21.0 (CH$_2$), 20.8 (CH$_2$), 19.7 (CH$_3$), 19.6 (CH$_3$), 13.3 (CH$_3$), 12.4 (CH$_3$), 11.8 (CH$_3$); IR (ATR): 3415, 2924 (broad), 2867, 1763, 1737, 1572, 1462, 1411, 1374, 1246, 1094 cm^{-1}; HRMS m/z 533.3863 (calcd for C$_{32}$H$_{53}$O$_6$ [M+H]$^+$ 533.3858).

3.1.4. General Procedure for the Synthesis of α-TEA and Compounds 5–10

A solution of respective α-bromoester (4.51 mmol, 8.5 eq) in dry DMF (2 mL) and powdered NaOH (635 mg, 15.9 mmol, 30 eq) were added to a solution of α-T (230 mg, 0.53 mmol, 1 eq) in dry DMF (8 mL). The resulting yellow suspension was stirred overnight (18–24 h) at room temperature. Then, the reaction mixture was poured into water, acidified with 6M HCl to pH 2 and extracted with diethyl ether (3 × 30 mL). The combined organic extracts were washed with water (2 × 30 mL) and brine (2 × 30 mL), dried over Na$_2$SO$_4$, and concentrated under reduced pressure. The crude product was purified using flash column chromatography (gradient 60–100% ethyl acetate in hexane). The pure product was dried in vacuo for 48 h.

α-TEA (RRR-α-tocopheryloxyacetic acid): yellowish waxy solid; yield: 87%; ^{1}H NMR (400 MHz, CDCl$_3$) δ 4.25 (brs, 2H, OCH$_2$), 2.56 (t, J = 6.6 Hz, 2H, H-4), 2.14, 2.10, 2.08 (3s, 9H, H-5a, H-7a, H-8b), 1.81–1.75 (m, 2H, H-3), 0.88–0.84 (m, 12H, H-4′a, H-8′a, H-12′a, H-13′); ^{13}C{^{1}H} NMR (100 MHz, CDCl$_3$) δ 173.9 (C), 148.5 (C), 146.7 (C), 127.3 (C), 125.4 (C), 123.2 (C), 117.7 (C), 75.0 (C), 69.4 (OCH$_2$), 40.1 (CH$_2$), 39.3 (CH$_2$), 37.43–37.26 (4 × CH$_2$), 32.8 (CH), 32.7 (CH), 31.1 (CH$_2$), 28.0 (CH), 24.8 (CH$_2$), 24.4 (CH$_2$), 23.8 (2 × CH$_3$), 22.7 (CH$_3$), 22.6 (CH$_3$), 21.0 (CH$_2$) 20.6 (CH$_2$), 19.7 (CH$_3$), 19.6 (CH$_3$), 12.7 (CH$_3$), 11.8 (2 × CH$_3$); IR (ATR) ν_{max} 2927 (broad), 1724, 1446, 1410, 1248, 1093, 1060 cm^{-1}; HRMS m/z 487.3795 (calcd for C$_{31}$H$_{51}$O$_4$ [M–H]$^-$ 487.3793).

Compound 5 (2-(RRR-α-tocopheryloxy)propanoic acid): yellowish waxy solid; yield: 85%; ^{1}H NMR (400 MHz, CDCl$_3$) δ 4.44 (q, 1H, J = 6.8 Hz, OCH), 2.56 (t, J = 6.4 Hz, 2H, H-4), 2.16, 2.12, 2.10 (3s, 9H, H-5a, H-7a, H-8b), 1.83–1.79 (m, 2H, H-3), 0.88–0.84 (m, 12H, H-4′a, H-8′a, H-12′a, H-13′); ^{13}C{^{1}H} NMR (100 MHz, CDCl$_3$) δ 148.4 (C), 145.4 (C), 127.7 (C), 125.9 (C), 123.4 (C), 117.9 (C), 77.0 (OCH), 75.0 (C), 40.0 (CH$_2$), 39.4 (CH$_2$), 37.54–37.23 (4 × CH$_2$), 32.8 (CH), 32.7 (CH), 31.2 (CH$_2$), 28.0 (CH), 24.8 (CH$_2$), 24.4 (CH$_2$), 23.8 (CH$_3$), 22.7 (CH$_3$), 22.6 (CH$_3$), 21.0 (CH$_2$), 20.7 (CH$_2$), 19.7 (CH$_3$), 19.6 (CH$_3$), 17.4 (CH$_3$), 13.8 (CH$_3$), 12.9 (CH$_3$), 11.9 (CH$_3$); IR (ATR) ν_{max} 2923 (broad), 2867, 1715, 1460, 1409, 1375, 1249, 1094 cm^{-1}; HRMS m/z 501.3953 (calcd for C$_{32}$H$_{53}$O$_4$ [M–H]$^-$ 501.3949).

Compound 6 (2-(RRR-α-tocopheryloxy)butanoic acid): white waxy solid; yield: 84%; ^{1}H NMR (400 MHz, CDCl$_3$) δ 4.28 (t, J = 5.7 Hz, 1H, OCH), 2.57 (t, J = 6.6 Hz, 2H, H-4), 2.17, 2.14, 2.09 (3s, 9H, H-5a, H-7a, H-8b), 1.95–1.92 (m, 2H), 1.80–1.78 (m, 2H), 0.89–0.85 (m, 12H, H-4′a, H-8′a, H-12′a, H-13′); ^{13}C{^{1}H} NMR (100 MHz, CDCl$_3$): δ 175.0 (C), 148.2 (C), 146.8 (C), 127.6 (C), 125.7 (C), 123.3 (C), 117.8 (C), 82.5 (OCH), 74.9 (C), 40.0 (CH$_2$), 39.4 (CH$_2$), 37.54–37.27 (4 × CH$_2$), 32.8 (CH), 32.7 (CH), 31.2 (CH$_2$), 28.0 (CH), 24.9 (CH$_2$), 24.8 (CH$_2$), 24.4 (CH$_2$), 23.8 (CH$_3$), 22.7 (CH$_3$), 22.6 (CH$_3$), 21.0 (CH$_2$), 20.8 (CH$_2$), 19.7 (CH$_3$), 19.6 (CH$_3$), 13.7 (CH$_3$), 12.9 (CH$_3$), 11.9 (CH$_3$), 8.9 (CH$_3$); IR (ATR) ν_{max} 2924 (broad), 2867, 1722, 1459, 1407, 1374, 1248, 1085 cm^{-1}; HRMS m/z 517.4248 (calcd for C$_{33}$H$_{57}$O$_4$ [M+H]$^+$ 517.4251).

Compound 7 (2-(RRR-α-tocopheryloxy)-2-methylpropanoic acid): white waxy solid; yield: 86%; ^{1}H NMR (400 MHz, CDCl$_3$) δ 6.58 (bs, 1H, COOH), 2.57 (t, J = 6.4 Hz, 2H, H-4), 2.14, 2.10, 2.09 (3s, 9H, H-5a, H-7a, H-8b), 1.85–1.76 (m, 2H), 0.89–0.85 (m, 12H, H-4′a, H-8′a, H-12′a, H-13′); ^{13}C{^{1}H} NMR (100 MHz, CDCl$_3$) δ 177.5 (C), 148.2 (C), 143.9 (C), 129.6 (C), 127.7 (C), 122.9 (C), 117.5 (C), 81.8 (O-C), 74.9 (C), 39.9 (CH$_2$), 39.3 (CH$_2$), 37.54–37.27 (4 × CH$_2$), 32.8 (CH), 32.6 (CH), 31.3 (CH$_2$), 28.0 (CH), 24.9 (2 × CH$_3$), 24.8 (CH$_2$), 24.4 (CH$_2$), 23.7 (CH$_3$), 22.7 (CH$_3$), 22.6 (CH$_3$), 21.0 (CH$_2$), 20.8 (CH$_2$), 19.7 (CH$_3$), 19.6 (CH$_3$), 14.9 (CH$_3$), 14.0 (CH$_3$), 11.9 (CH$_3$); IR (ATR) ν_{max} 2924 (broad), 1708, 1569, 1461, 1405, 1249, 1148, 1083 cm^{-1}; HRMS m/z 515.4109 (calcd for C$_{33}$H$_{55}$O$_4$ [M–H] 515.4106).

Compound 8 (2-(RRR-α-tocopheryloxy)-pentanoic acid): yellowish waxy solid; yield: 85%; ^{1}H NMR (400 MHz, CDCl$_3$) δ 9.63 (bs, 1H, COOH), 4.32 (t, J = 5.8 Hz, 1H, CH-O), 2.57 (t, J = 6.7 Hz, 2H, H-4), 2.17, 2.16, 2.09 (3s, 9H, H-5a, H-7a, H-8b), 1.88–1.73 (m, 2H), 2.96 (t, J = 7.3 Hz, 3H, CH$_2$CH$_3$), 0.89–0.85 (m, 12H, H-4′a, H-8′a, H-12′a, H-13′); ^{13}C{^{1}H} NMR (100 MHz, CDCl$_3$) δ 175.2 (C), 148.2 (C), 146.9 (C), 127.5 (C), 125.7 (C), 123.3 (C), 117.8 (C), 81.4 (OCH), 74.9 (C), 40.0 (CH$_2$), 39.4 (CH$_2$), 37.45–37.28 (4 x CH$_2$), 34.0 (CH$_2$), 32.8 (CH), 32.7 (CH), 31.2 (CH$_2$), 28.0 (CH), 24.8 (CH$_2$), 24.4 (CH$_2$), 23.8 (CH$_3$), 22.7 (CH$_3$), 22.6 (CH$_3$), 21.0 (CH$_2$), 20.7 (CH$_2$), 19.7 (CH$_3$), 19.6 (CH$_3$), 17.9 (CH$_2$), 14.0 (CH$_3$), 13.7 (CH$_3$), 12.8 (CH$_3$), 11.9 (CH$_3$); IR (ATR) ν_{max} 2927 (broad), 1708, 1572, 1466, 1409, 1086 cm^{-1}; HRMS m/z 529.4267 (calcd for C$_{34}$H$_{57}$O$_4$ [M–H]$^-$ 529.4262).

Compound 9 (2-(RRR-α-tocopheryloxy)-3-methylbutanoic acid): yellowish waxy solid; yield: 86%; ^{1}H NMR (400 MHz, CDCl$_3$) δ 8.90 (bs, 1H, COOH), 4.21 (d, J = 4.7 Hz, 1H, CH-O), 2.58 (t, J = 6.7 Hz, 2H, H-4), 2.19, 2.15, 2.10 (3s, 9H, H-5a, H-7a, H-8b), 1.84–1.75 (m, 2H), 0.90–0.86 (m, 12H, H-4′a, H-8′a, H-12′a, H-13′); ^{13}C NMR{^{1}H} (100 MHz, CDCl$_3$)

δ 175.3 (C), 147.9 (C), 147.2 (C), 127.5 (C), 125.6 (C), 123.2 (C), 117.7 (C), 85.9 (OCH), 74.8 (C), 40.0 (CH$_2$), 39.4 (CH$_2$), 37.44–37.27 (4 × CH$_2$), 32.8 (CH), 32.7 (CH), 31.3 (CH$_2$), 31.1 (CH), 28.0 (CH), 24.8 (CH$_2$), 24.4 (CH$_2$), 23.8 (CH$_3$), 22.7 (CH$_3$), 22.6 (CH$_3$), 21.0 (CH$_2$), 20.7 (CH$_2$), 19.7 (CH$_3$), 19.6 (CH$_3$), 18.6 (CH$_3$), 17.3 (CH$_3$), 13.9 (CH$_3$), 13.0 (CH$_3$), 11.9 (CH$_3$); IR (ATR) ν_{max} 2927 (broad), 1709, 1573, 1467, 1409, 1085 cm^{-1}; HRMS m/z 529.4269 (calcd for C$_{34}$H$_{57}$O$_4$ [M–H]$^-$ 529.4262).

Compound **10** (2-(*RRR*-α-tocopheryloxy)-octanoic acid): yellowish waxy solid; yield: 84%; ^{1}H NMR (400 MHz, CDCl$_3$) δ 10.09 (bs, 1H, COOH), 4.31 (t, *J* = 5.8 Hz, 1H, CH-O), 2.57 (t, *J* = 6.4 Hz, 2H, H-4), 2.17, 2.13, 2.09 (3s, 9H, H-5a, H-7a, H-8b), 0.89–0.85 (m, 15H, H-4′a, H-8′a, H-12′a, H-13′, CH$_2$C$\underline{\text{H}}$$_3$); ^{13}C{^{1}H} NMR (100 MHz, CDCl$_3$) δ 175.3 (C), 148.1 (C), 147.0 (C), 127.5 (C), 125.7 (C), 123.2 (C), 117.8 (C), 81.5 (OCH), 74.9 (C), 40.0 (CH$_2$), 39.4 (CH$_2$), 37.44–37.27 (4 × CH$_2$), 32.8 (CH), 32.7 (CH), 32.0 (CH$_2$), 31.6 (CH$_2$), 31.2 (CH$_2$), 29.2 (CH$_2$), 28.0 (CH), 24.8 (CH$_2$), 24.4 (CH$_2$), 23.8 (CH$_3$), 22.7 (CH$_3$), 22.6 (CH$_3$), 22.5 (CH$_2$), 21.0 (CH$_2$), 20.7 (CH$_2$), 19.7 (CH$_3$), 19.6 (CH$_3$), 14.0 (CH$_3$), 13.7 (CH$_3$), 12.8 (CH$_3$), 11.9 (CH$_3$) ppm; IR (ATR): 2929 (broad), 1710, 1572, 1467, 1411, 1087 cm^{-1}; HRMS m/z 571.4738 (calcd for C$_{37}$H$_{59}$O$_4$ [M–H]$^-$ 571.4732).

The NMR spectra of compounds **3-10**, α-TEA, and α-TP are presented in the Supplementary Materials file (Figures S3–S24 from Supplementary Materials).

3.2. Cytotoxicity Test Assay

T-lymphoblastic leukemia CEM, cervix epithelioid carcinoma HeLa, and breast carcinoma MCF7 cell lines, all of which were obtained from the European Collection of Authenticated Cell Cultures (ECACC, London, UK) were used for screening. Human foreskin fibroblasts (BJ) were purchased from the American Type Culture Collection (Manassas, VA, USA). The cytotoxicity of tested compounds in the described cell lines and normal cells was determined using resazurin assay following the manufacturer's protocol (Sigma Aldrich, St. Louis, MO, USA).

Stock solutions of compounds were prepared in DMSO at 7.5 mM and the highest tested concentration in cultivation medium in well was 50 μM. The concentration of DMSO in well never exceeded 0.6%. Briefly, 5.0 × 10^4 cells·mL^{-1} cells were seeded into 96-well plates (TPP, Trasadingen, Switzerland) and incubated for 24 h. Then, compounds solved in DMSO were added into cultivation medium and incubated further for 72 h. Cell viability was determined using resazurin. The procedure has been reported [54].

3.3. Molecular Docking

In order to acquire a deeper understanding of the biological activity of α-tocopherol derivatives, a molecular docking study was conducted with the AutoDock Vina (version 1.1.3) [55] program, provided by Scripps Research Institute. The visualization was carried out in Pymol [56] and LigPlus [57] programs. The crystal structure of Complex II (succinate dehydrogenase, SDH) from *Escherichia Coli* was obtained from the Protein Data Bank (PDB:1NEK) [58]. The enzyme was prepared for docking by cleansing its structure of water molecules and other co-crystallized species. Additionally, polar hydrogens and Kollman charges [59] were added. The search box was set to cover the co-crystallized ubiquinone-2 molecule (PDb:UQ2), which is located on the edge of the subunit D of 1NEK. A cubical (20 × 0 × 20 Å) grid box was utilized during the simulations. For the sake of validation, a redocking procedure for the ubiquinone-2 (a native ligand) was conducted. To improve docking accuracy, the EXHAUSTIVENESS parameter had been set to 100 (default = 8), ensuring the best performance [60] in treating large ligands with long phytyl chains. Additionally, for the same purpose, the SPACING parameter was set to 0.15, which is far below its default value of 0.375. The best (in the sense of docking score) pose was compared to UQ2 from the crystal structure, obtained with the resolution of 2.6 Å. Both conformations were found to be in satisfactory agreement, with RMSD = 1.313Å. The aligned structures are pictured in Figure 4.

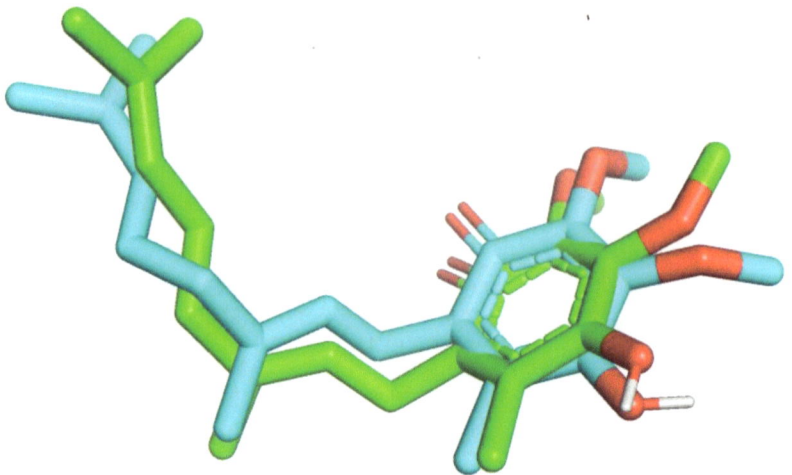

Figure 4. The alignment of the native UQ2 ligand (green scaffold) compared to the best pose from the redocking procedure (cyan scaffold).

4. Conclusions

In this project, a series of α-TS and α-TEA analogs have been synthesized by modification of the substituent in the C-6 position of the α-T molecule. All compounds possess the structural requirements described for their proapoptotic activity of α-tocopherol esters, i.e., the combination of three structural domains: functional, signaling, and hydrophobic. All compounds were examined for their in vitro cytotoxic activity against three human cancer cell lines (CEM, MCF7, HeLa), and normal human fibroblasts (BJ). Our results showed a relationship between anticancer properties and the structure of the substituent located at the C-6 position in the α-T molecule. Surprisingly, the analogs of α-TEA and α-TS (**3** and **4**, respectively) in which the acidic parts (acetic or succinic, respectively) contained an additional carboxyl group proved to be inactive. On the other hand, the introduction of an alkyl substituent (e.g., methyl or ethyl) into the ether-linked acetic acid moiety in α-TEA increases cytotoxic activity. Promising drug candidates seem to be compounds **5–8**. They all had moderate activity toward tested cancer cell lines and relatively high therapeutic window as their cytotoxicity toward normal fibroblasts was very low or zero. Molecular docking to Complex II has shown that the affinities of newly synthesized compounds as ligands are approximately on the same level, and there is no easy way to indicate which one is potentially most useful. However, the differences between α-T and its derivatives clearly indicate that, while behaving similarly in affinity to the native ligand (UQ2), they differ significantly from α-T in terms of the localization and interaction with the receptor. Combined with better affinities, this may explain their significantly higher anticancer activity and confirm their suitability as drug candidates. Our results demonstrate that it is possible to achieve good selectivity and higher proapoptotic activity with the introduction of larger substituents into the acidic ethereal part in the α-TEA molecule. However, it should be taken into account that the results of enzymatic assays may differ from cytotoxic ones and may shed new light on the mechanism of action of the tested compounds. Further investigations are in progress.

Supplementary Materials: The following supporting information can be downloaded at: https://www.mdpi.com/article/10.3390/pr11061860/s1. S2, Experimental procedures for the preparation of α-tocopheryl phosphate (α-TP); S3–S24, ^{1}H and ^{13}C NMR spectra of the synthesized compounds.

Author Contributions: Conceptualization, A.B. and S.W.; methodology, A.B., L.R. and S.W.; formal analysis, A.B., L.R. and A.R.; investigation, A.B., L.R. and A.R.; visualization, A.B. and A.R.; writing—original draft preparation, A.B.; writing—review and editing, A.B., L.R., A.R., M.S. and S.W.; supervision, S.W. and M.S. All authors have read and agreed to the published version of the manuscript.

Funding: This work was carried out as part of the project "Synthesis of vitamin E derivatives with potential anticancer activity" (Research of Young Scientists, 2019–2020, Faculty of Chemistry, University of Bialystok) financed by the Ministry of Science and Higher Education, Poland (MNiSW).

Institutional Review Board Statement: Not applicable.

Informed Consent Statement: Not applicable.

Data Availability Statement: All relevant data that support the findings of this study are included in this article.

Acknowledgments: Authors are grateful to Leszek Siergiejczyk for recording the NMR spectra (Faculty of Chemistry, University of Bialystok) and Aneta M. Tomkiel (Faculty of Chemistry, University of Bialystok) for HRMS measurements. The authors would like to thank the Computational Center of the University of Bialystok (Grant GO-008) for providing access to the supercomputer resources and the AutoDock VINA program.

Conflicts of Interest: The authors declare no conflict of interest.

References

1. Chorawala, M.R.; Oza, P.M.; Shah, G.B. Mechanism of Anticancer Drugs Resistance: An Overview. *Int. J. Pharm. Sci. Drug Res.* **2012**, *4*, 1–9.
2. Panda, V.; Khambat, P.; Patil, S. Mitocans as Novel Agents for Anticancer Therapy: An Overview. *Int. J. Clin. Med.* **2011**, *2*, 515–529. [CrossRef]
3. Dong, L.-F.; Jameson, V.J.A.; Tilly, D.; Cerny, J.; Mahdavian, E.; Marín-Hernández, A.; Hernández-Esquivel, L.; Rodríguez-Enríquez, S.; Stursa, J.; Witting, P.K.; et al. Mitochondrial Targeting of Vitamin E Succinate Enhances Its Pro-Apoptotic and Anti-Cancer Activity via Mitochondrial Complex II. *J. Biol. Chem.* **2011**, *286*, 3717–3728. [CrossRef]
4. Neuzil, J.; Dyason, J.C.; Freeman, R.; Dong, L.-F.; Prochazka, L.; Wang, X.-F.; Scheffler, I.; Ralph, S.J. Mitocans as Anti-Cancer Agents Targeting Mitochondria: Lessons from Studies with Vitamin E Analogues, Inhibitors of Complex II. *J. Bioenerg. Biomembr.* **2007**, *39*, 65–72. [CrossRef] [PubMed]
5. Dong, L.; Gopalan, V.; Holland, O.; Neuzil, J. Mitocans Revisited: Mitochondrial Targeting as Efficient Anti-Cancer Therapy. *Int. J. Mol. Sci.* **2020**, *21*, 7941. [CrossRef]
6. Neuzil, J.; Tomasetti, M.; Mellick, A.; Alleva, R.; Salvatore, B.; Birringer, M.; Fariss, M. Vitamin E Analogues: A New Class of Inducers of Apoptosis with Selective Anti-Cancer Effects. *CCDT* **2004**, *4*, 355–372. [CrossRef] [PubMed]
7. Neuzil, J.; Weber, T.; Schröder, A.; Lu, M.; Ostermann, G.; Gellert, N.; Mayne, G.C.; Olejnicka, B.; Nègre-Salvayre, A.; Stícha, M.; et al. Induction of Cancer Cell Apoptosis by α-Tocopheryl Succinate: Molecular Pathways and Structural Requirements. *FASEB J.* **2001**, *15*, 403–415. [CrossRef] [PubMed]
8. Weber, T.; Lu, M.; Andera, L.; Lahm, H.; Gellert, N.; Fariss, M.W.; Korinek, V.; Sattler, W.; Ucker, D.S.; Terman, A.; et al. Vitamin E Succinate Is a Potent Novel Antineoplastic Agent with High Selectivity and Cooperativity with Tumor Necrosis Factor-Related Apoptosis-Inducing Ligand (Apo2 Ligand) In Vivo. *Clin. Cancer Res.* **2002**, *8*, 863.
9. Yu, Z.-Q.; Wang, L.-M.; Yang, W.-X. How Vitamin E and Its Derivatives Regulate Tumour Cells via the MAPK Signalling Pathway? *Gene* **2022**, *808*, 145998. [CrossRef]
10. Majima, D.; Mitsuhashi, R.; Fukuta, T.; Tanaka, T.; Kogure, K. Biological Functions of α-Tocopheryl Succinate. *J. Nutr. Sci. Vitaminol.* **2019**, *65*, S104–S108. [CrossRef]
11. Wang, X.-F.; Dong, L.; Zhao, Y.; Tomasetti, M.; Wu, K.; Neuzil, J. Vitamin E Analogues as Anticancer Agents: Lessons from Studies with α-Tocopheryl Succinate. *Mol. Nutr. Food Res.* **2006**, *50*, 675–685. [CrossRef] [PubMed]
12. Kogure, K.; Manabe, S.; Suzuki, I.; Tokumura, A.; Fukuzawa, K. Cytotoxicity of Alpha-Tocopheryl Succinate, Malonate and Oxalate in Normal and Cancer Cells in vitro and Their Anti-Cancer Effects on Mouse Melanoma in vivo. *J. Nutr. Sci. Vitaminol.* **2005**, *51*, 392–397. [CrossRef] [PubMed]
13. Zhao, Y.; Neuzil, J.; Wu, K. Vitamin E Analogues as Mitochondria-Targeting Compounds: From the Bench to the Bedside? *Mol. Nutr. Food Res.* **2009**, *53*, 129–139. [CrossRef] [PubMed]
14. Goh, S.H.; Hew, N.F.; Ong, A.S.H.; Choo, Y.M.; Brumby, S. Tocotrienols from Palm Oil: Electron Spin Resonance Spectra of Tocotrienoxyl Radicals. *J. Am. Oil Chem. Soc.* **1990**, *67*, 250–254. [CrossRef]
15. Ghayour-Mobarhan, M.; Saghiri, Z.; Ferns, G.; Sahebkar, A. α-Tocopheryl Phosphate as a Bioactive Derivative of Vitamin E: A Review of the Literature. *J. Diet. Suppl.* **2015**, *12*, 359–372. [CrossRef] [PubMed]

16. Ju, J.; Picinich, S.C.; Yang, Z.; Zhao, Y.; Suh, N.; Kong, A.-N.; Yang, C.S. Cancer-Preventive Activities of Tocopherols and Tocotrienols. *Carcinogenesis* **2010**, *31*, 533–542. [CrossRef]
17. Rezk, B.M. Alpha-Tocopheryl Phosphate Is a Novel Apoptotic Agent. *Front. Biosci.* **2007**, *12*, 2013. [CrossRef]
18. Bidossi, A.; Bortolin, M.; Toscano, M.; De Vecchi, E.; Romanò, C.L.; Mattina, R.; Drago, L. In Vitro Comparison between α-Tocopheryl Acetate and α-Tocopheryl Phosphate against Bacteria Responsible of Prosthetic and Joint Infections. *PLoS ONE* **2017**, *12*, e0182323. [CrossRef]
19. Harper, R.A.; Saleh, M.M.; Carpenter, G.; Abbate, V.; Proctor, G.; Harvey, R.D.; Gambogi, R.J.; Geonnotti, A.; Hider, R.; Jones, S.A. Soft, Adhesive (+) Alpha Tocopherol Phosphate Planar Bilayers That Control Oral Biofilm Growth through a Substantive Antimicrobial Effect. *Nanomed. Nanotechnol. Biol. Med.* **2018**, *14*, 2307–2316. [CrossRef]
20. Hama, S.; Kirimura, N.; Obara, A.; Takatsu, H.; Kogure, K. Tocopheryl Phosphate Inhibits Rheumatoid Arthritis-Related Gene Expression In Vitro and Ameliorates Arthritic Symptoms in Mice. *Molecules* **2022**, *27*, 1425. [CrossRef]
21. Dong, L.-F.; Grant, G.; Massa, H.; Zobalova, R.; Akporiaye, E.; Neuzil, J. α-Tocopheryloxyacetic Acid Is Superior to α-Tocopheryl Succinate in Suppressing HER2-High Breast Carcinomas Due to Its Higher Stability. *Int. J. Cancer* **2012**, *131*, 1052–1058. [CrossRef] [PubMed]
22. Lawson, K.A.; Anderson, K.; Menchaca, M.; Atkinson, J.; Sun, L.; Knight, V.; Gilbert, B.E.; Conti, C.; Sanders, B.G.; Kline, K. Novel Vitamin E Analogue Decreases Syngeneic Mouse Mammary Tumor Burden and Reduces Lung Metastasis. *Mol. Cancer Ther.* **2003**, *2*, 437. [PubMed]
23. Lawson, K.A.; Anderson, K.; Simmons-Menchaca, M.; Atkinson, J.; Sun, L.; Sanders, B.G.; Kline, K. Comparison of Vitamin E Derivatives α-TEA and VES in Reduction of Mouse Mammary Tumor Burden and Metastasis. *Exp. Biol. Med.* **2004**, *229*, 954–963. [CrossRef] [PubMed]
24. Hahn, T.; Akporiaye, E.T. α-TEA as a Stimulator of Tumor Autophagy and Enhancer of Antigen Cross-Presentation. *Autophagy* **2013**, *9*, 429–431. [CrossRef] [PubMed]
25. Hahn, T.; Bradley-Dunlop, D.J.; Hurley, L.H.; Von-Hoff, D.; Gately, S.; Mary, D.L.; Lu, H.; Penichet, M.L.; Besselsen, D.G.; Cole, B.B.; et al. The Vitamin E Analog, Alpha-Tocopheryloxyacetic Acid Enhances the Anti-Tumor Activity of Trastuzumab against HER2/Neu-Expressing Breast Cancer. *BMC Cancer* **2011**, *11*, 471. [CrossRef]
26. Kawamura, K.; Kume, A.; Umemiya-Shirafuji, R.; Kasai, S.; Suzuki, H. Effect of α-Tocopheryloxy Acetic Acid, a Vitamin E Derivative Mitocan, on the Experimental Infection of Mice with Plasmodium Yoelii. *Malar. J.* **2021**, *20*, 280. [CrossRef]
27. Hahn, T.; Szabo, L.; Gold, M.; Ramanathapuram, L.; Hurley, L.H.; Akporiaye, E.T. Dietary Administration of the Proapoptotic Vitamin E Analogue Alpha-Tocopheryloxyacetic Acid Inhibits Metastatic Murine Breast Cancer. *Cancer Res.* **2006**, *66*, 9374–9378. [CrossRef]
28. Kline, K.; Yu, W.; Sanders, B.G. Vitamin E and Breast Cancer. *J. Nutr.* **2004**, *134*, 3458S–3462S. [CrossRef]
29. Tiwary, R.; Yu, W.; Sanders, B.G.; Kline, K. α-TEA Cooperates with Chemotherapeutic Agents to Induce Apoptosis of P53 Mutant, Triple-Negative Human Breast Cancer Cells via Activating P73. *Breast Cancer Res.* **2011**, *13*, R1. [CrossRef]
30. Li, Y.; Hahn, T.; Garrison, K.; Cui, Z.-H.; Thorburn, A.; Thorburn, J.; Hu, H.-M.; Akporiaye, E.T. The Vitamin E Analogue α-TEA Stimulates Tumor Autophagy and Enhances Antigen Cross-Presentation. *Cancer Res.* **2012**, *72*, 3535–3545. [CrossRef]
31. Neuzil, J.; Kågedal, K.; Andera, L.; Weber, C.; Brunk, U.T. Vitamin E Analogs: A New Class of Multiple Action Agents with Anti-Neoplastic and Anti-Atherogenic Activity. *Apoptosis* **2002**, *7*, 179–187. [CrossRef]
32. Jia, L.; Yu, W.; Wang, P.; Sanders, B.G.; Kline, K. In Vivo and in vitro Studies of Anticancer Actions of α-TEA for Human Prostate Cancer Cells. *Prostate* **2008**, *68*, 849–860. [CrossRef]
33. Yao, J.; Gao, P.; Xu, Y.; Li, Z. α-TEA Inhibits the Growth and Motility of Human Colon Cancer Cells via Targeting RhoA/ROCK Signaling. *Mol. Med. Rep.* **2016**, *14*, 2534–2540. [CrossRef]
34. Wu, Y.; Zu, K.; Ni, J.; Yeh, S.; Kasi, D.; James, N.S.; Chemler, S.; Ip, C. Cellular and Molecular Effects of Alpha-Tocopheryloxybutyrate: Lessons for the Design of Vitamin E Analog for Cancer Prevention. *Anticancer Res.* **2004**, *24*, 3795–3802.
35. Ni, J.; Mai, T.; Pang, S.-T.; Haque, I.; Huang, K.; DiMaggio, M.A.; Xie, S.; James, N.S.; Kasi, D.; Chemler, S.R.; et al. In Vitro and In Vivo Anticancer Effects of the Novel Vitamin E Ether Analogue RRR-Tocopheryloxybutyl Sulfonic Acid in Prostate Cancer. *Clin. Cancer Res.* **2009**, *15*, 898–906. [CrossRef] [PubMed]
36. Khallouki, F.; Hajji, L.; Saber, S.; Bouddine, T.; Edderkaoui, M.; Bourhia, M.; Mir, N.; Lim, A.; El Midaoui, A.; Giesy, J.P.; et al. An Update on Tamoxifen and the Chemo-Preventive Potential of Vitamin E in Breast Cancer Management. *JPM* **2023**, *13*, 754. [CrossRef]
37. Zhang, S.; Lawson, K.A.; Simmons-Menchaca, M.; Sun, L.; Sanders, B.G.; Kline, K. Vitamin E Analog α-TEA and Celecoxib Alone and Together Reduce Human MDA-MB-435-FL-GFP Breast Cancer Burden and Metastasis in Nude Mice. *Breast Cancer Res. Treat.* **2004**, *87*, 111–121. [CrossRef]
38. Anderson, K.; Lawson, K.A.; Simmons-Menchaca, M.; Sun, L.; Sanders, B.G.; Kline, K. Alpha-TEA plus Cisplatin Reduces Human Cisplatin-Resistant Ovarian Cancer Cell Tumor Burden and Metastasis. *Exp. Biol. Med.* **2004**, *229*, 1169–1176. [CrossRef]
39. Yu, W.; Shun, M.; Anderson, K.; Chen, H.; Sanders, B.G.; Kline, K. α-TEA Inhibits Survival and Enhances Death Pathways in Cisplatin Sensitive and Resistant Human Ovarian Cancer Cells. *Apoptosis* **2006**, *11*, 1813–1823. [CrossRef] [PubMed]
40. Suntharalingam, K.; Song, Y.; Lippard, S.J. Conjugation of Vitamin E Analog α-TOS to Pt(Iv) Complexes for Dual-Targeting Anticancer Therapy. *Chem. Commun.* **2014**, *50*, 2465. [CrossRef] [PubMed]

41. Neuzil, J. α-Tocopheryl Succinate Epitomizes a Compound with a Shift in Biological Activity Due to pro-Vitamin-to-Vitamin Conversion. *Biochem. Biophys. Res. Commun.* **2002**, *293*, 1309–1313. [CrossRef] [PubMed]
42. Birringer, M.; EyTina, J.H.; Salvatore, B.A.; Neuzil, J. Vitamin E Analogues as Inducers of Apoptosis: Structure–Function Relation. *Br. J. Cancer* **2003**, *88*, 1948–1955. [CrossRef] [PubMed]
43. Neuzil, J.; Tomasetti, M.; Zhao, Y.; Dong, L.-F.; Birringer, M.; Wang, X.-F.; Low, P.; Wu, K.; Salvatore, B.A.; Ralph, S.J. Vitamin E Analogs, a Novel Group of "Mitocans", as Anticancer Agents: The Importance of Being Redox-Silent. *Mol. Pharmacol.* **2007**, *71*, 1185–1199. [CrossRef] [PubMed]
44. Neuzil, J.; Weber, T.; Gellert, N.; Weber, C. Selective Cancer Cell Killing by Alpha-Tocopheryl Succinate. *Br. J. Cancer* **2001**, *84*, 87–89. [CrossRef]
45. Neuzil, J.; Zhao, M.; Ostermann, G.; Sticha, M.; Gellert, N.; Weber, C.; Eaton, J.W.; Brunk, U.T. α-Tocopheryl Succinate, an Agent with in vivo Anti-Tumour Activity, Induces Apoptosis by Causing Lysosomal Instability. *Biochem. J.* **2002**, *362*, 709–715. [CrossRef] [PubMed]
46. Mazzini, F.; Betti, M.; Canonico, B.; Netscher, T.; Luchetti, F.; Papa, S.; Galli, F. Anticancer Activity of Vitamin E-Derived Compounds in Murine C6 Glioma Cells. *ChemMedChem* **2010**, *5*, 540–543. [CrossRef]
47. Gerweck, L.E.; Seetharaman, K. Cellular PH Gradient in Tumor versus Normal Tissue: Potential Exploitation for the Treatment of Cancer. *Cancer Res.* **1996**, *56*, 1194–1198.
48. Kogure, K.; Hama, S.; Kisaki, M.; Takemasa, H.; Tokumura, A.; Suzuki, I.; Fukuzawa, K. Structural Characteristic of Terminal Dicarboxylic Moiety Required for Apoptogenic Activity of α-Tocopheryl Esters. *Biochim. Biophys. Acta (BBA) Gen. Subj.* **2004**, *1672*, 93–99. [CrossRef]
49. Yan, B.; Stantic, M.; Zobalova, R.; Bezawork-Geleta, A.; Stapelberg, M.; Stursa, J.; Prokopova, K.; Dong, L.; Neuzil, J. Mitochondrially Targeted Vitamin E Succinate Efficiently Kills Breast Tumour-Initiating Cells in a Complex II-Dependent Manner. *BMC Cancer* **2015**, *15*, 401. [CrossRef]
50. Dong, L.-F.; Low, P.; Dyason, J.C.; Wang, X.-F.; Prochazka, L.; Witting, P.K.; Freeman, R.; Swettenham, E.; Valis, K.; Liu, J.; et al. α-Tocopheryl Succinate Induces Apoptosis by Targeting Ubiquinone-Binding Sites in Mitochondrial Respiratory Complex II. *Oncogene* **2008**, *27*, 4324–4335. [CrossRef]
51. Neuzil, J.; Cerny, J.; Dyason, J.C.; Dong, L.-F.; Ralph, S.J. Affinity of Vitamin E Analogues for the Ubiquinone Complex II Site Correlates with Their Toxicity to Cancer Cells. *Mol. Nutr. Food Res.* **2011**, *55*, 1543–1551. [CrossRef]
52. Zwierzak, A. Phase-Transfer-Catalysed Phosphorylation of Alcohols in a Two-Phase System. *Synthesis* **1976**, *1976*, 305–306. [CrossRef]
53. López, G.V.; Batthyány, C.; Blanco, F.; Botti, H.; Trostchansky, A.; Migliaro, E.; Radi, R.; González, M.; Cerecetto, H.; Rubbo, H. Design, Synthesis, and Biological Characterization of Potential Antiatherogenic Nitric Oxide Releasing Tocopherol Analogs. *Bioorg. Med. Chem.* **2005**, *13*, 5787–5796. [CrossRef]
54. Rárová, L.; Steigerová, J.; Kvasnica, M.; Bartůněk, P.; Křížová, K.; Chodounská, H.; Kolář, Z.; Sedlák, D.; Oklestkova, J.; Strnad, M. Structure Activity Relationship Studies on Cytotoxicity and the Effects on Steroid Receptors of AB-Functionalized Cholestanes. *J. Steroid Biochem. Mol. Biol.* **2016**, *159*, 154–169. [CrossRef]
55. Trott, O.; Olson, A.J. AutoDock Vina: Improving the Speed and Accuracy of Docking with a New Scoring Function, Efficient Optimization, and Multithreading. *J. Comput. Chem.* **2009**, *31*, 455–461. [CrossRef] [PubMed]
56. Schrödinger, L.; DeLano, W. The PyMOL Molecular Graphics System, Version 1.3r1. PyMOL. Available online: http://www.pymol.org/pymol (accessed on 26 May 2023).
57. Wallace, A.C.; Laskowski, R.A.; Thornton, J.M. LIGPLOT: A Program to Generate Schematic Diagrams of Protein-Ligand Interactions. *Protein Eng. Des. Sel.* **1995**, *8*, 127–134. [CrossRef] [PubMed]
58. Yankovskaya, V.; Horsefield, R.; Törnroth, S.; Luna-Chavez, C.; Miyoshi, H.; Léger, C.; Byrne, B.; Cecchini, G.; Iwata, S. Architecture of Succinate Dehydrogenase and Reactive Oxygen Species Generation. *Science* **2003**, *299*, 700–704. [CrossRef] [PubMed]
59. Singh, U.C.; Kollman, P.A. An Approach to Computing Electrostatic Charges for Molecules. *J. Comput. Chem.* **1984**, *5*, 129–145. [CrossRef]
60. Agarwal, R.; Smith, J.C. Speed vs Accuracy: Effect on Ligand Pose Accuracy of Varying Box Size and Exhaustiveness in AutoDock Vina. *Mol. Inform.* **2023**, *42*, 2200188. [CrossRef]

Disclaimer/Publisher's Note: The statements, opinions and data contained in all publications are solely those of the individual author(s) and contributor(s) and not of MDPI and/or the editor(s). MDPI and/or the editor(s) disclaim responsibility for any injury to people or property resulting from any ideas, methods, instructions or products referred to in the content.

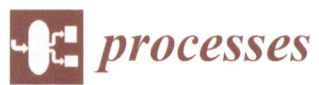

Article

Anticancer Activity of Anti-Tubercular Compound(s) Designed on Pyrrolyl Benzohydrazine Scaffolds: A Repurposing Study

Turki Al Hagbani [1], Afrasim Moin [1], Talib Hussain [2], N. Vishal Gupta [3], Farhan Alshammari [1], Syed Mohd Danish Rizvi [1,*] and Sheshagiri Dixit [4,*]

[1] Department of Pharmaceutics, College of Pharmacy, University of Ha'il, Ha'il 81442, Saudi Arabia; t.alhagbani@uoh.edu.sa (T.A.H.); a.moinuddin@uoh.edu.sa (A.M.); frh.alshammari@uoh.edu.sa (F.A.)
[2] Department of Pharmacology and Toxicology, College of Pharmacy, University of Ha'il, Ha'il 81442, Saudi Arabia; md.talib@uoh.edu.sa
[3] Department of Pharmaceutics, JSS College of Pharmacy, JSS Academy of Higher Education and Research, Mysore 570015, India; vishalkumargupta@jssuni.edu.in
[4] Department of Pharmaceutical Chemistry, JSS College of Pharmacy, JSS Academy of Higher Education and Research, Mysore 570015, India
* Correspondence: sm.danish@uoh.edu.sa (S.M.D.R.); sheshagiridixit@jssuni.edu.in (S.D.)

Abstract: The present study explored anti-tubercular pyrrole derivatives against cancer targets using different in silico and in vitro approaches. Initially, nineteen anti-tubercular pyrrolyl benzohydrazide derivatives were screened against a potent cancer target PLK1 using an AutoDock Vina approach. Out of the nineteen derivatives, the two most potent derivatives **C8** [N′-(4-(1H-pyrrol-1-yl) benzoyl)-3-chlorobenzohydrazide] and **C18** [N′-(4-(1H-pyrrol-1-yl) benzoyl)-4-nitrobenzohydrazide], were subjected to molecular simulation analysis for a 100 ns trajectory. Further, these two derivatives were tested against A549, MCF-7, and HepG2 cell lines using an MTT proliferation assay. Apoptotic cell cycle and DAPI assays were also performed for **C8** on A549 cell lines. Molecular dynamic analysis revealed that the stability of the **C8**–PLK1 protein complex during the 100 ns trajectory run was better than that of the **C18**–PLK1 protein complex. In addition, **C8** showed lower IC_{50} values against the tested cell lines, in comparison to **C18**. Thus, **C8** was selected for cell cycle, apoptosis, and DAPI analysis. Interestingly, **C8** resulted in the significant cell cycle arrest of A549 cells at the G2/M phase, and annexin V-FITC/PI showed a significant increase (from 6.27% to 60.52%) in the percentage of apoptotic A549 cells. The present findings suggest that the anti-tubercular compound (**C8**) could be translated into a potent repurposed candidate against lung cancer. Nevertheless, in vivo assessment is necessary to further confirm the outcome and its clinical translation.

Keywords: anti-tubercular; anti-cancer; drug repurposing; PLK1; pyrrolyl benzohydrazide derivative

Citation: Hagbani, T.A.; Moin, A.; Hussain, T.; Gupta, N.V.; Alshammari, F.; Rizvi, S.M.D.; Dixit, S. Anticancer Activity of Anti-Tubercular Compound(s) Designed on Pyrrolyl Benzohydrazine Scaffolds: A Repurposing Study. *Processes* 2023, 11, 1889. https://doi.org/10.3390/pr11071889

Academic Editors: Alina Bora and Luminita Crisan

Received: 24 April 2023
Revised: 1 June 2023
Accepted: 19 June 2023
Published: 23 June 2023

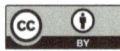

Copyright: © 2023 by the authors. Licensee MDPI, Basel, Switzerland. This article is an open access article distributed under the terms and conditions of the Creative Commons Attribution (CC BY) license (https://creativecommons.org/licenses/by/4.0/).

1. Introduction

Onco-therapy is a major concern for the scientific community due to the multifactorial features of cancer disease. According to a report, every year, 50 billion dollars are spent on cancer research and development to develop new onco-drug candidates [1], but the WHO reported 10 million cancer-associated deaths worldwide in the year 2020 [2]. In addition, the cancer-linked deaths are increasing at an alarming rate with time [3]. Thus, solutions are urgently warranted to cope with the current grave situation. However, drug repurposing has opened a new avenue for effective cancer treatment [4,5]. Repurposing can reduce the developmental cost, timeline, processing, and approval requirements. In other words, repurposing can overcome the bottlenecks associated with cancer drug development. Several reports have suggested that anti-tubercular agents could be repurposed for cancer therapy [6–11]. Bedaquiline, isoniazid, ethionamide, prothionamide, and thioacetazone are some examples of anti-tubercular drugs/agents that were successfully repurposed for cancer treatment. These findings prompted us to explore anti-tubercular pyrrolyl benzohydrazide derivatives as anti-cancer agents.

Earlier, in the year 2017, several pyrrolyl benzohydrazide derivatives were synthesized and tested for anti-tubercular potential [12]. In the present study, the same pyrrolyl benzohydrazide derivatives [12] were used, to obtain deeper insight into their anticancer potential, with the reason being the well-reported potent anticancer activity of pyrrole analogs and benzohydrazide derivatives [13,14]. The pyrrole scaffold has its due relevance while designing important medicinal drugs. Pyrrole has a typical aromatic nitrogen-containing heterocycle, and the existence of nitrogen atom significantly improves the polarity of the pyrrole analogs [15]. In addition, the pyrrole ring is an important component of plant chlorophyll and animal vitamin B12, hemin, and myoglobin [14]. Moreover, their derivatives have shown a valuable pharmacological profile and potent anticancer activities in different investigations [14–19]. In fact, some of marketed drugs already have pyrrole moieties in them to enhance their potency [14,15]. On the other hand, there are a plethora of reports suggesting the potent anticancer activities of benzohydrazide derivatives [13,20–25]. Benzohydrazide derivatives might follow different mechanisms of action against different cancer cells; they could act as inhibitors of VEGFR-2 [21], lysine-specific histone demethylase 1A [22], tubulin polymerization [23], Bcl-2/Bcl-xL [24], and CD44 [25]. However, reports [13,20–25] clearly suggest that benzohydrazide derivatives could be applied for a variety of cancer cells. Taking into consideration the pharmacological and anticancer activities of benzohydrazide and pyrrole derivatives, the compounds derived from them via a hybridization approach [12] were used in the present study to assess their anticancer potential.

Prior to wet lab investigations, nineteen anti-tubercular pyrrolyl benzohydrazide derivatives were screened through computational analysis to select the best compounds out of them. This computational study was performed using molecular docking interaction analysis and molecular dynamics. Further, the selected compounds (**C8** [N′-(4-(1H-pyrrol-1-yl) benzoyl)-3-chlorobenzohydrazide] and **C18** [N′-(4-(1H-pyrrol-1-yl) benzoyl)-4-nitrobenzohydrazide]) were investigated using different cell lines i.e., A549, MCF-7, and HepG2. Moreover, compound **C8** was further subjected to cell cycle, apoptosis, and DAPI analysis using A549 cells. The repurposing of anti-tubercular compounds into anticancer drugs, as well as against lung cancer, seems to be an appealing approach. It is like hitting two birds with one stone, as tuberculosis is one of the strong risk factors of lung cancer.

2. Materials and Methods

2.1. Synthesis of Pyrrolyl Benzohydrazide Derivatives

Nineteen pyrrolyl benzohydrazide derivatives were selected from the prior study [12] conducted for anti-tuberculosis potential. In the study [12], the Pall–Knorr pyrrole synthesis approach, as shown in Scheme 1, was used to synthesize the derivatives. The most active compound, **C8** [N′-(4-(1H-pyrrol-1-yl) benzoyl)-3-chlorobenzohydrazide], was synthesized by using ethyl 4-amino benzoate as a starting material, which was refluxed with 2,5-dimethoxy tetrahydrofuran at 150–160 °C for 45 min. The formed pyrrolyl ester was hydrazide by using hydrazine hydrate, and the formed hydrazide was stirred at room temperature for 24–30 h with 3-chlorobenzaldehyde with the help of HBTU [2-(1H-benzotriazole-1-yl)-1,1,3,3-tetramethyl uronium hexa fluorophosphate] and DIEA (diisopropyl ethylamine), a coupling agent and a catalyst to form **C8**.

2.2. Dry Lab Investigations

2.2.1. Ligand Preparation for Molecular Docking

Three dimensional structures of these compounds were prepared using ChemDraw software and saved in .pdb format. Further, all the ligands, including the positive control (BI2536; DrugBank ID: DB16107) and native ligand (DrugBank ID: DB07186), were converted into .pdbqt format using the OpenBabel tool [26].

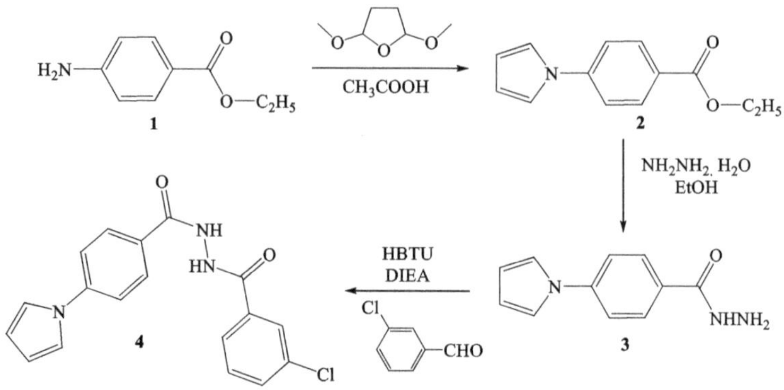

Scheme 1. Synthesis route of pyrrolyl benzohydrazide derivatives.

2.2.2. Target Preparation for Molecular Docking

The three-dimensional structure of the target protein PLK1 (PDBID: 2OWB) was retrieved from the Protein Data Bank database in .pdb format. Further, it was prepared for docking via the AutoDock 4.2 tool [27], which included the addition of polar hydrogen, Kollman charges, and solvation parameters. Moreover, the target protein was converted and saved in .pdbqt format.

2.2.3. Molecular Docking Interaction Study

AutoDock Vina was applied for molecular docking of all the ligands with the PLK1 target protein [28]. Prior to docking, grid co-ordinates were set on the specified active kinase domain of the PLK1 protein [29]. Grid center coordinates were kept as x = 0.069, y = 23.58, and z = 66.741, and the grid box was set at 40 × 40 × 40. The results showed affinity in terms of kcal/mol, and the algorithm divided the results in descending order of the 10 modes. Further, the Pymol tool was used to save the complex of best conformation based on the affinity results for each docked structure. Moreover, the Discovery Studio Visualization tool was used to analyze and visualize the complex in more detail.

2.2.4. Molecular Dynamics (MD) Simulation Study

Out of nineteen pyrrolyl benzohydrazide derivatives, two derivatives, i.e., **C8** [N'-(4-(1H-pyrrol-1-yl)benzoyl)-3-chlorobenzohydrazide] and **C18** [N'-(4-(1H-pyrrol-1-yl)benzoyl)-4-nitrobenzohydrazide] were screened out through molecular docking interactions, and MD simulations were performed on them to obtain better insight into **C8** and **C18** interactions with PLK1 under solvated states with respect to time. The GROMACS 5.1.5 [30] platform applied with a CHARMM27 [31] forcefield was used for executing simulation runs on PLK1 in an undocked native state and docked (with **C8** and **C18**) complex state. Ligand **C8** and **C18** topology files were created through the SwissParam server by applying all atoms of the CHARMM force field [32]. A cut-off distance of 1 nm was set for estimating Van der Waal and columbic interactions. However, neutrality of the system was maintained by adding counter ions, and the TIP3P water model was used to solvate the system. Periodic boundary conditions were applied by keeping a distance of 1 to 1.5 nm from the wall for the simulation run [33]. Energy minimization was performed with a 1000 kJ/mol/nm tolerance by applying the steepest descent algorithm, and position restrains were applied on the complex to equilibrate the system. NPT and NVT ensembles were used for 200 ps at 1 bar of pressure and a temperature of 300 K. Maxwell distribution was used to generate primary velocities, and a 0.1 ps coupling constant was used for velocity rescaling. The Parrinello–Rahman algorithm was used for temperature–pressure coupling with a 2 ps coupling constant. The system after equilibration was subjected to a 100 ns simulation run with a 2 fs time-step integration [34]. After each 500 steps, the trajectory was saved and analyzed using XMGRACE-5.1.22 and GROMACS analysis tools.

2.3. Wet Lab Investigations

2.3.1. Materials

The cancer cell lines (breast cancer MCF-7, lung cancer A549, and liver cancer HepG2) were procured from NCCS, India. Chemicals pertinent to cell culture were obtained from BD Biosciences (Franklin Lakes, NJ, USA). Solvents, chemicals, and MTT dye were purchased from HiMedia (Thane, India), whereas doxorubicin (standard drug) was procured from Sigma-Aldrich.

2.3.2. Cell Culture

A549, MCF-7, and HepG2 cell lines were cultured in DMEM medium, supplemented with 100 IU/mL penicillin, 100 µg/mL streptomycin, and 10% inactivated fetal bovine serum, in 5% CO_2 saturated conditions at 37 °C until confluence occurred. However, the viability of the cells was examined periodically.

2.3.3. Stock Solution of Tested Compounds

The stock solutions (20 mM) of pyrrolyl benzohydrazide derivatives and the positive control doxorubicin were prepared using a DMSO solvent.

2.3.4. Cytotoxic In Vitro MTT Assay

An MTT assay was applied to calculate the cytotoxic concentration of compounds (**C8** and **C18**) [35]. For this, 100 µL of cells (50,000 cells) was added to each well of a microtiter plate and treated with a medium containing 0.78, 1.56, 3.125, 6.25, 12.5, 25, 50, and 100 µM concentrations of **C8**, **C18**, and doxorubicin. Further, the plates were kept in an incubator (with 5% CO_2) for 24 h at 37 °C. After that, MTT dye, 20 µL from the stock (5 mg MTT in 1 mL PBS), was inoculated in each well and kept in an incubator under the same condition again for 4 h. The supernatant after treatment was collected and centrifuged, and DMSO (200 µL) was added to the pellet. Furthermore, this solution was added to its respective well, and formazan crystals were dissolved by shaking the plates. A microplate reader was used to measure the absorbance at 590 nm. The following formula was applied to calculate the % inhibition of growth for each cell line:

$$\%\text{Inhibition} = 100 - (\text{OD of Sample} \div \text{OD of Control}) \times 100$$
$$\%\text{Cell Viability} = 100 - \%\text{Inhibition}$$

2.3.5. Cell Cycle Analysis

A 6-well plate with a density of 2×10^5 cells/2 mL was incubated in a CO_2 incubator, which was kept overnight at 37 °C for 24 h. The cells educed were treated with **C8** (10 µM) in a 2 mL culture medium and incubated for 24 h. The medium was given a PBS wash, trypsinized, and harvested into a 5 mL storage vial. After 2 steps of PBS washes, the cells were fixed and permeabilized in 1 mL of pre-chilled 70% ethanol, added drop-wise with continuous stirring, to avoid the clumping of cells. The cells were incubated for 30 min in a −20 °C freezer. The cells educed were obtained and washed with PBS. Further, the cells were stained using 400 µL Propidium Iodide/RNase staining buffer that stains the DNA [36]. Again, the cells were incubated for 15 to 20 min at room temperature in the dark. The samples were analyzed using flow cytometry. A minimum of 10,000 cells was counted for each group.

2.3.6. Cell Apoptosis Assay

An apoptosis study was performed to understand Annexin V/PI expression using the A549 cell line [37]. A 6-well plate with a density of 0.5×10^6 cells/2 mL was incubated in a CO_2 incubator and kept overnight at 37 °C for 24 h. The cells educed were treated with **C8** (10 µM) in a 2 mL culture medium and incubated for 24 h. The medium was given a PBS wash; further, 200 µL of the trypsin–EDTA solution was added and again incubated for a few minutes. Subsequently, the cells were harvested in 12×75 mm polystyrene tubes with an additional 2 mL of culture media. The tubes were centrifuged for 5 min at 300× g at 25 °C. Later, the supernatant layer was decanted. Again, a PBS wash was given, and a further 5 µL of FITC Annexin V was added. Gentle stirring of the cells was performed, and they were incubated in the dark for 15 min at room temperature (25 °C). Then, 5 mL of PI and 400 µL of 1X Annexin Binding Buffer was added to each tube and stirred gently. The sample was analyzed using flow cytometry.

2.3.7. DAPI Assay

A 96-well glass-bottom plate with a density of 1×10^4 cells/200 µL was incubated in a CO_2 incubator and kept overnight at 37 °C for 24 h. The cells educed were treated with **C8** (10 mM) in 200 µL of culture medium and incubated for 24 h. The medium was given a PBS wash. Further, the cells were stained by adding 200 µL of DAPI staining solution for 10 min in the dark [38]. The cells were observed under a ZEISS, LSM 880 Fluorescence live-cell Imaging System (Confocal Microscopy, Jena, Germany) with a filter cube, with excitation at 358 nm and emission at 461 nm for DAPI.

2.3.8. Statistical Analysis

Statistical analysis was performed using one-way ANOVA and a Student t-test using Graph Pad Prism version 8.

3. Results and Discussion

De novo drug development for cancer is a tedious and multi-step process. This is due to the high heterogenicity and complexity associated with the cancer disease. In fact, cancer drug development is a time-, resource-, and labor- intensive job, and it has been observed that only a few drugs could pass the initial phases of the clinical trial after spending too much effort. Hence, drug repurposing has come up as a savior, wherein established drugs are proposed for new avenues in the field of cancer medication [5,39]. Even big pharma industries are investing in drug repurposing, and the drug repurposing market size has reached 25.2 billion US$ in the year 2021 [40]. Thus, this current research study attempted to assess the repurposing potential of anti-TB pyrrolyl benzohydrazide derivatives [12] (Figure 1) as anti-cancer agents.

3.1. Molecular Interaction of Pyrrolyl Benzohydrazide Derivatives with PLK1

Polo Like Kinase 1 is a well-established cancer target [41], and its overexpression is observed in several cancer cells, such as lung, pancreatic, ovarian, prostate, colorectal, and breast. Importantly, its expression is very low in normal cells, while it significantly increases in cancer cells [41,42]. In addition, PLK1 inhibition has been considered one of the potent strategies against cancer [43–45]. Thus, in the present study, nineteen pyrrolyl benzohydrazide derivatives (Table 1) that have been reported for anti-tuberculosis potential [12] were screened against the PLK1 enzyme.

Table 1. Docking results of pyrrolyl benzohydrazide derivative, control, and native ligand interactions with the target PLK1.

Compound Code	Name of Compound	Binding Affinity
C1	N′-(4-(1H-pyrrol-1-yl)benzoyl)-2,4-dichlorobenzohydrazide	−9 kcal/mol
C2	N′-(4-(1H-pyrrol-1-yl)benzoyl)-2-aminobenzohydrazide	−8.8 kcal/mol
C3	N′-(4-(1H-pyrrol-1-yl)benzoyl)-2-bromobenzohydrazide	−8.9 kcal/mol
C4	N′-(4-(1H-pyrrol-1-yl)benzoyl)-2-chlorobenzohydrazide	−9 kcal/mol

Table 1. *Cont.*

Compound Code	Name of Compound	Binding Affinity
C5	N′-(4-(1H-pyrrol-1-yl)benzoyl)-2-methylbenzohydrazide	−8.9 kcal/mol
C6	N′-(4-(1H-pyrrol-1-yl)benzoyl)-3-acetylbenzohydrazide	−9 kcal/mol
C7	N′-(4-(1H-pyrrol-1-yl)benzoyl)-3-aminobenzohydrazide	−7.8 kcal/mol
C8	N′-(4-(1H-pyrrol-1-yl)benzoyl)-3-chlorobenzohydrazide	−9.7 kcal/mol
C9	N′-(4-(1H-pyrrol-1-yl)benzoyl)-3-methylbenzohydrazide	−9.1 kcal/mol
C10	N′-(4-(1H-pyrrol-1-yl)benzoyl)-3-nitrobenzohydrazide	−9 kcal/mol
C11	N′-(4-(1H-pyrrol-1-yl)benzoyl)-4-aminobenzohydrazide	−8.8 kcal/mol
C12	N′-(4-(1H-pyrrol-1-yl)benzoyl)-4-bromobenzohydrazide	−8.9 kcal/mol
C13	N′-(4-(1H-pyrrol-1-yl)benzoyl)-4-chlorobenzohydrazide	−9 kcal/mol
C14	N′-(4-(1H-pyrrol-1-yl)benzoyl)-4-fluorobenzohydrazide	−8.8 kcal/mol
C15	N′-(4-(1H-pyrrol-1-yl)benzoyl)-4-hydroxybenzohydrazide	−8 kcal/mol
C16	N′-(4-(1H-pyrrol-1-yl)benzoyl)-4-methoxybenzohydrazide	−8.9 kcal/mol
C17	N′-(4-(1H-pyrrol-1-yl)benzoyl)-4-methylbenzohydrazide	−8.7 kcal/mol
C18	N′-(4-(1H-pyrrol-1-yl)benzoyl)-4-nitrobenzohydrazide	−9.6 kcal/mol
C19	N′-benzoyl-4-(1H-pyrrol-1-yl)benzohydrazide	−9 kcal/mol
Control (BI2536)	4-{[(7R)-8-cyclopentyl-7-ethyl-5-methyl-6-oxo-5,6,7,8-tetrahydropteridin-2-yl]amino}-3-methoxy-N-(1-methylpiperidin-4-yl)benzamide	−9.3 kcal/mol
Native Ligand	4-(4-methylpiperazin-1-yl)-N-{5-[2-(thiophen-2-yl)acetyl]-1H,5H-pyrrolo[3,4-c]pyrazol-3-yl}benzamide	−8.6 kcal/mol

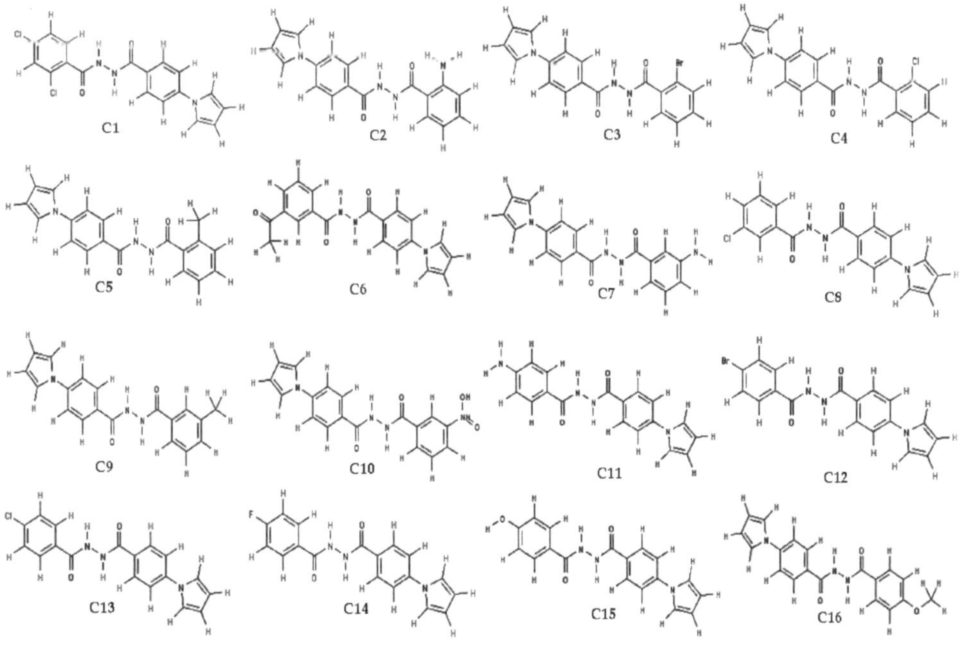

Figure 1. *Cont.*

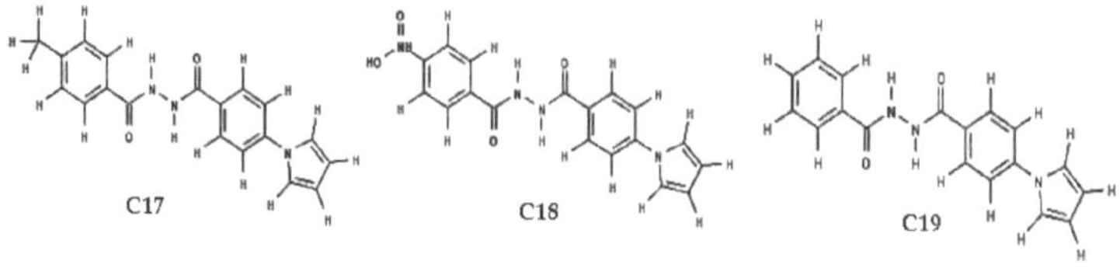

Figure 1. Structures of nineteen pyrrolyl benzohydrazide derivatives used in the present study.

The screening results depicted that N′-(4-(1H-pyrrol-1-yl)benzoyl)-3-chlorobenzohydrazide (**C8**) and N′-(4-(1H-pyrrol-1-yl)benzoyl)-4-nitrobenzohydrazide (**C18**) were the most potent among the nineteen tested derivatives against PLK1 (Table 1). Both **C8** and **C18** showed significant interactions with the 'kinase domain' of PLK1. The Gibbs free energy (ΔG) of the '**C8**-PLK1 interaction' was −9.7 kcal/mol, whereas ΔG of the '**C18**-PLK1 interaction' was −9.6 kcal/mol. To obtain a deeper insight into **C8** and **C18** interactions, the results were compared with the interactions of the positive control (BI2536) with PLK1 (Figure 2; Table 2). A redocking native ligand experiment was performed to validate the protocol, wherein the re-docked native ligand bound to the same vicinity of the PLK1 'active site' as the native ligand [46]. A superimposition image (Figure 2b) established the protocol standardization; in addition, all of **C8**, **C18**, and the positive control were also bound to the same domain of PLK1 (Figure 2a). However, the ΔG values (Table 2) suggested that **C8** and **C18** showed better interactions with PLK1 than the positive control (−9.3 kcal/mol) and native ligand (−8.6 kcal/mol). Insights into amino acids involved in the individual ligand interactions with PLK1 were shown through LigPlot analysis (Figure 2d). LigPlot analysis for both **C8** (Figure 2(d1)) and **C18** (Figure 2(d2)) showed that 13 amino acid residues, (i.e., Leu59, Cys67, Ala80, Val114, Leu130, Glu131, Leu132, Cys133, Arg134, Arg136, Phe183, Gly193, Asp194) interacted with the 'kinase domain' of PLK1. Here, Cys133 interacted through strong hydrogen bonding, while other amino acids showed hydrophobic interactions. However, the positive control (BI2536) displayed strong hydrogen bonding with Lys82, involving a total of 10 amino acid residues of PLK1 during the interaction (Figure 2(d3)). Strong hydrogen bonding interactions of **C8** and **C18** with the Cys133 amino acid residue of PLK1 (Figure 2(d1,d2)) have their due relevance, as Cys133 serves as a crucial part of the ATP-binding pocket, and it is considered a novel covalent site of PLK1 for drug discovery [41,47]. In addition, Shakil et al. [41] reported that Leu59, Cys67, Leu130, Cys133, Arg136, and Phe183 played an important role in PLK1 binding with different inhibitors. In fact, Leu132 formed the hinge region, and Cys67 and Phe183 configured the top/bottom of the ATP binding pocket. Importantly, both compounds **C8** and **C18** became associated with all these critical amino acid residues of the PLK1 ATP-binding pocket. The activation loop of PLK1 (2OWB) consists of Val210 (i.e., Thr210 a primary phosphorylation site of wild-type Plk1) and Ser137 (a secondary phosphorylation site). Neither of these two amino acids showed an interaction with **C8** and **C18**. However, to confirm their dynamic behavior with respect to time, both of these compounds were further subjected to molecular dynamics analysis.

Table 2. Interacting amino acids and binding energy of substrate docked with the active site of PLK1.

Ligands	Binding Energy	Interacting Amino Acids of PLK1
C8	−9.7 kcal/mol	Leu59, Cys67, Ala80, Val114, Leu130, Glu131, Leu132, **Cys133 ***, Arg134, Arg136, Phe183, Gly193, Asp194
C18	−9.6 kcal/mol	Leu59, Cys67, Ala80, Val114, Leu130, Glu131, Leu132, **Cys133 ***, Arg134, Arg136, Phe183, Gly193, Asp194

Table 2. *Cont.*

Ligands	Binding Energy	Interacting Amino Acids of PLK1
Positive control (BI2536)	−9.3 kcal/mol	Gly60, Lys61, Gly62, Gly63, Phe64, **Lys82** *, Val84, Lys97, Phe183, Asp194
Redocked Native ligand (DB07186)	−8.6 kcal/mol	Lys61, Gly62, Gly63, Phe64, Cys67, Lys82, Val114, Glu131, Cys133, Arg136, Phe183, Asp194, Gly 196

* Hydrogen bonded amino acids are represented in bold.

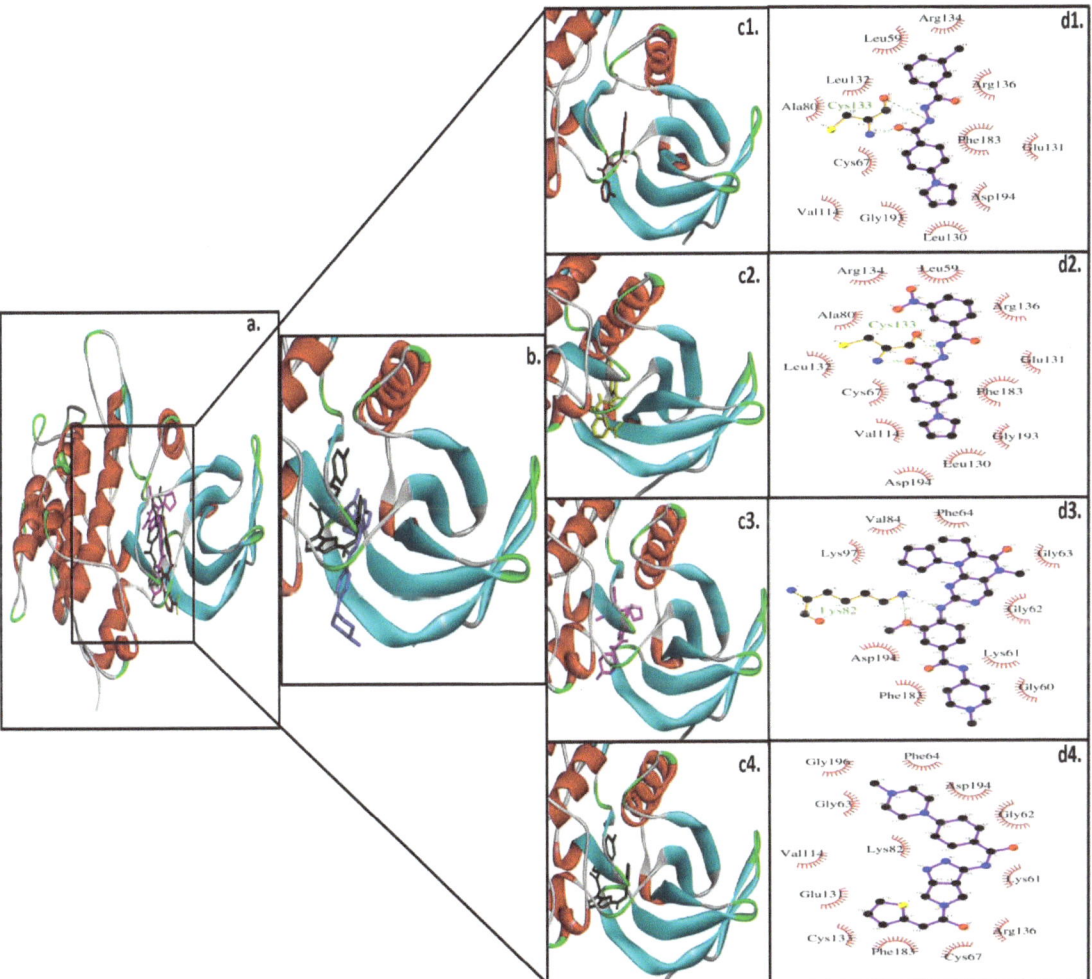

Figure 2. Ligand-docked active site images of PLK1 (PDB ID: 2OWB). (**a**) All the docked ligands (**C8**: red color; **C18**: yellow color; positive control (BI2536): magenta color; native ligand (DB07186): green color) in the catalytic active site of PLK1. (**b**) Enlarged overlay image of native ligand and redocked native ligand. (**c**) Enlarged image of (**c1**) C8 docking, (**c2**) C18 docking, (**c3**) BI2536 docking, and (**c4**) DB07186 docking. (**d**) Molecular interaction analysis of all the compounds ((**d1**): C8; (**d2**): C18; (**d3**): BI2536; (**d4**): DB07186) with PLK1 amino acid residues.

3.2. Molecular Dynamic (MD) Analysis of C8 and C18 with PLK1

The dynamic behavior of 'C8-PLK1' and 'C18-PLK1' complexes, under solvated conditions, was studied through an MD simulation/mimicking study with respect to time. The best docking pose for each complex was mapped for stability under a mimicable environment. The outcomes of the mimicking study, with various constraints helping us to understand the binding mode and stability, were reported in terms of the solvent accessible surface area (SASA), radius of gyration (R_g), number of hydrogen bonds, root mean square deviation (RMSD), and root mean square fluctuation (RMSF). All these parameters were mapped during the mimicking study time, and deviation of the secondary structure pattern between the protein and their complexes was measured.

Three mimicking studies with the protein (PLK1) alone (black color) and its complex with ligand C8 (red color) and C18 (green color) were executed for a 100 ns time duration. From the RMSD plot (Figure 3a), it was observed that the C8–PLK1 complex, after initial fluctuation, reached equilibrium at approximately 10 ns of time. After that, the complex displayed a constant trajectory with marginal deviation of ~0.1 nm, indicating that the structural stability of the protein was preserved while in complex with C8. Results also suggested that the unbound protein (PLK1 alone) also reached equilibrium after an initial fluctuation, and it showed a similar pattern of stable trajectory as C8 bound PLK1. On the other hand, C18-bound PLK1 was stable until 80 ns and started fluctuating in the range of ~0.3 nm until 90 ns. However, it also became stable at the end after this 10 ns fluctuation. The Rg plot (Figure 3b) showed that all the entries (including the innate protein (PLK1) and its complex forms with C8 and C18) exhibited a similar pattern of Rg during the entire simulation time with minimal (0.05 nm) variation in different distance ranges. Hydrogen bonding between the ligand and protein complex was evaluated, which in turn forecasted the focalization of the ligand into the binding cavity of the protein. All the intermolecular H-bonds among ligands and the protein were studied and plotted accordingly (Figure 3c). From the plot, it is clear that the number of H-bonds involved in the simulation runs fluctuated over time, but most strong H-bonds remained intact throughout the study time. The disappearance and then reappearance of a few H-bonds indicate the vital nature of the ligand inside the binding cavity. The solvent accessible surface area (SASA) determined the area surrounding the hydrophobic core developed between the protein–ligand complexes (Figure 3d). Reliable SASA values were obtained with a fluctuation of 10 nm^2 area for PLK1 and the C8–PLK1 complex, whereas more fluctuations of a 15 nm^2 area were observed in case of the C18–PLK1 complex. The SASA plots for PLK1 and C8–PLK1 almost overlapped with each other; however, C18–PLK1 complexes showed no overlap during 25 ns to 60 ns and after 90 ns until the end of the simulation run. The residue-wise variations were observed in the RMSF plot (Figure 3e,f), wherein the potentially interacting amino acids stiffened in the complex forms (C8–PLK1 and C18–PLK1) in comparison to the normal protein state (PLK1).

In addition, dynamic behavior of the 'PLK1-BI2536 (control)' complex under solvated conditions were also studied through an MD simulation study with respect to time (Figure S1 Supplementary Materials). From the RMSD plot (Figure S1a), it was observed that the BI2536–PLK1 complex, after initial fluctuation, reached equilibrium at approximately 10 ns of time. After that, the complex displayed constant trajectory with marginal deviation of ~0.09 nm, indicating that the structural stability of the protein was preserved while in complex with BI-2536. On the other hand, the Rg plot (Figure S1b) showed that the gyration of the protein–ligand complex (PLK1–BI2536) exhibited a similar pattern of Rg during the entire simulation time with minimal (0.025 nm) variation in different distance ranges after initial fluctuations. From the hydrogen bonding plot (Figure S1c), it was clear that the number of H-bonds involved in the simulation runs fluctuated over time but most strong H-bonds were intact during the study time. Furthermore, reliable SASA values (Figure S1d) were obtained with an initial fluctuation of a 15 nm^2 area for the PLK1–BI2536 complex up to 10 ns; however, minimal fluctuations of a 10 nm^2 area were observed after 10 ns until the end of the simulation run. The residue-wise variations were observed in the

RMSF plot (Figure S1e), where potentially interacting amino acids became stiffened in the complex form (PLK1-BI2536) similar to PLK1–C8 and PLK1–C18 complexes. In fact, from the findings of MD simulation results of PLK1–BI2536, it could be inferred that an almost similar pattern was observed for the control compound (BI2536) as in the case of the tested compounds (**C8** and **C18**).

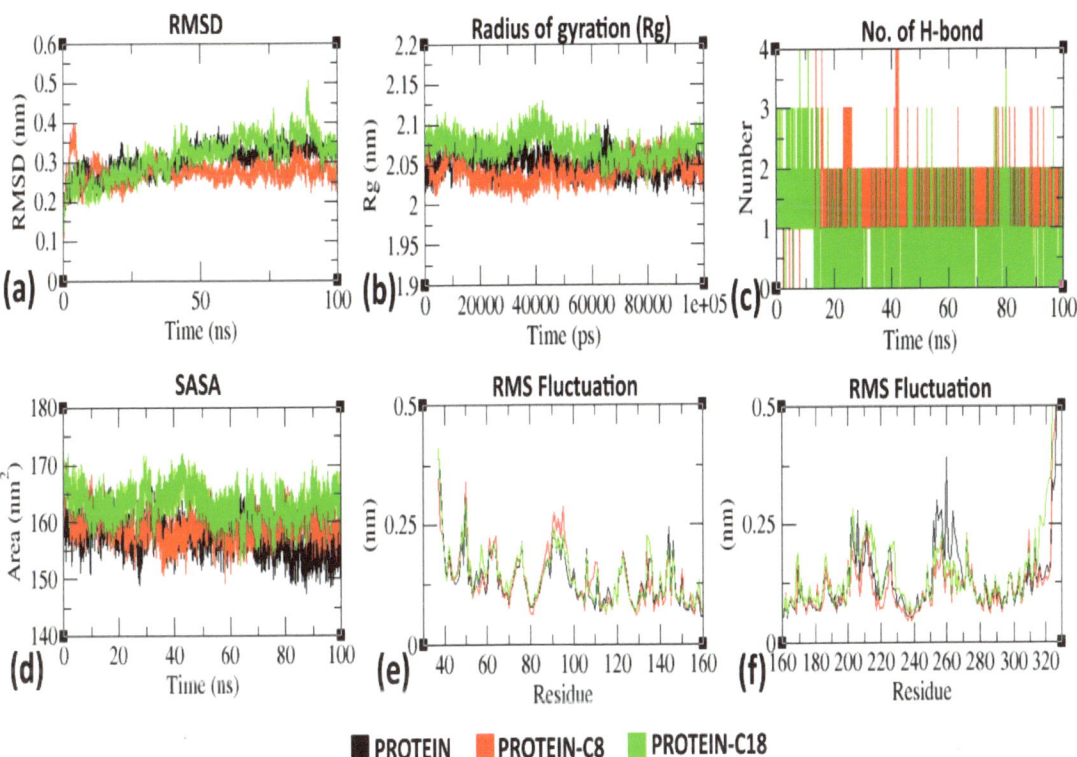

Figure 3. Analysis of MD simulation trajectories against the function of the RMSD, Rg, hydrogen bond, SASA, and RMSF of PLK1 (PDB ID: 2OWB) with synthetic compound **C8** and **C18** (ligand) complexes at 100,000 ps (100 ns). (**a**) RMSD; (**b**) radius of gyration (Rg); (**c**) hydrogen bonds; (**d**) SASA; (**e**,**f**) RMSF plot of the protein in the presence of **C8** and **C18**.

3.3. Cytotoxicity Analysis

Based on initial screening through molecular docking analysis and further confirmation of the stability of the PLK1 docked complex based on molecular dynamics, **C8** and **C18** appeared to be the most active compounds. Thus, the cytotoxicity of **C8** and **C18** was assessed against three cancer cell lines (A549, MCF 7, and HepG2) via MTT assays. As represented in Table 3 and Figure 4, compounds **C8** and **C18** exhibited significant inhibitory activities against A549 cells with IC_{50} values of 9.54 µM and 10.38 µM, respectively. However, the reference compound (doxorubicin) showed a better IC_{50} (8.20 µM) than the tested compounds. Moreover, the compounds **C8** and **C18** were tested on normal human lung epithelial BEAS-2B cells, and the IC_{50} values for both were found to be more than 200 µM. This showed a selectivity index of >10, which indicates that both **C8** and **C18** have more efficacy against tumor cells than the toxicity against normal cells. It can also be inferred from Table 2 that **C8** was more potent than **C18** against the tested cell lines. In addition, both **C8** and **C18** were less active against MCF7 and HepG2 cells than A549 cells. The lineage of A549 cells is the lung, MCF7 cells is the breast, and HepG2 cells is the liver; thus, the more potent activity of tested compounds against A549 cells has its due relevance.

There is a plethora of evidence that shows the correlation of tuberculosis with lung cancer, and tuberculosis is considered an important risk factor for lung cancer [48–50]. Hence, targeting lung cancer with anti-tubercular compound(s) seems to be an appealing strategy and could provide a boon to a tuberculosis-infected lung cancer patient in the future. Based on the cytotoxicity results, **C8** was selected further for cell cycle, cell apoptosis, and DAPI analysis against A549 cells to obtain deeper insight into the anticancer action.

Table 3. IC$_{50}$ values of compounds against different tumor cell lines.

Compounds	IC$_{50}$ (µM)		
	MCF7	A549	HepG2
C8	10.51 ± 1.9	9.54 ± 1.1	10.82 ± 1.3
C18	12.34 ± 0.9	10.38 ± 1.7	11.41 ± 2.5
Doxorubicin *	10.96 ± 1.6	8.20 ± 0.9	9.21 ± 1.0

* Doxorubicin was used as a positive control.

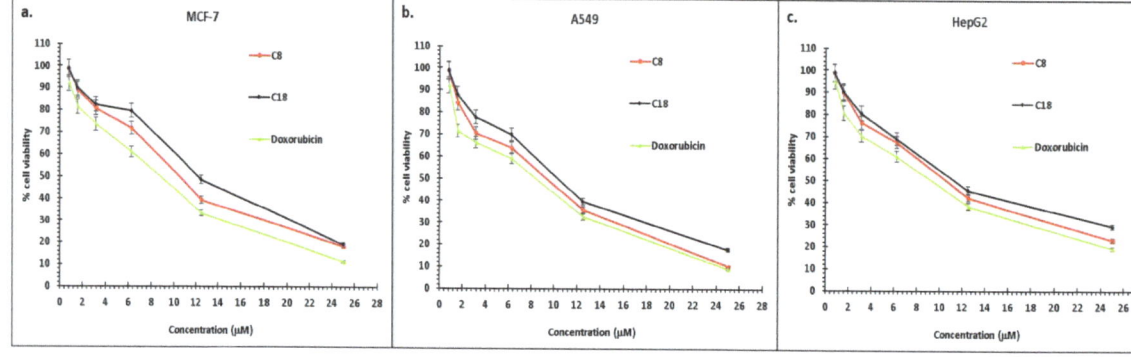

Figure 4. Cytotoxicity study of the test compounds **C8** and **C18** against MCF-7, A549, and HepG2 cells and their comparison with the positive control (doxorubicin). (**a**) Dose-response curve of test compounds for % cell viability against MCF-7 cell lines. (**b**) Dose-response curve of test compounds for % cell viability against A-549 cell lines. (**c**) Dose-response curve of test compounds for % cell viability against HepG2 cells.

3.4. Cell Cycle Analysis

Cell cycle arrest could be correlated well with the growth inhibition of cancer cells. Reports suggest that benzohydrazide derivatives stop cell progression at the G2/M phase of the cell cycle [51–53]. However, in the present study, to explain the action of **C8** on cell cycle distributions, A549 cells were treated with 10 µM (**C8**) for 24 h, and the distributions of A549 cells (treated and untreated) in various stages of the cell cycle were evaluated via flow cytometry (Figure 5). Consistent with the earlier findings [51–53], **C8** treatment led to maximum accumulation of A549 cells at the G2/M phase (39.48%); however, untreated A549 cells showed only 9.34% cells at the G2/M phase (Table 4). In addition, cell % was markedly reduced from 88.79% to 31.22% at G0/G1 phase when A549 cells were treated with **C8**. Obtained results suggested that **C8** demonstrated a significant antineoplastic effect and led to the stoppage A549 cell cycle progression at G2/M, metaphase, after the gestation period of 24 h. These results were in accordance with the other recent research conducted on A549 cells, wherein the anticancer effects were attributed to the blocking of the G2/M phase [54–56].

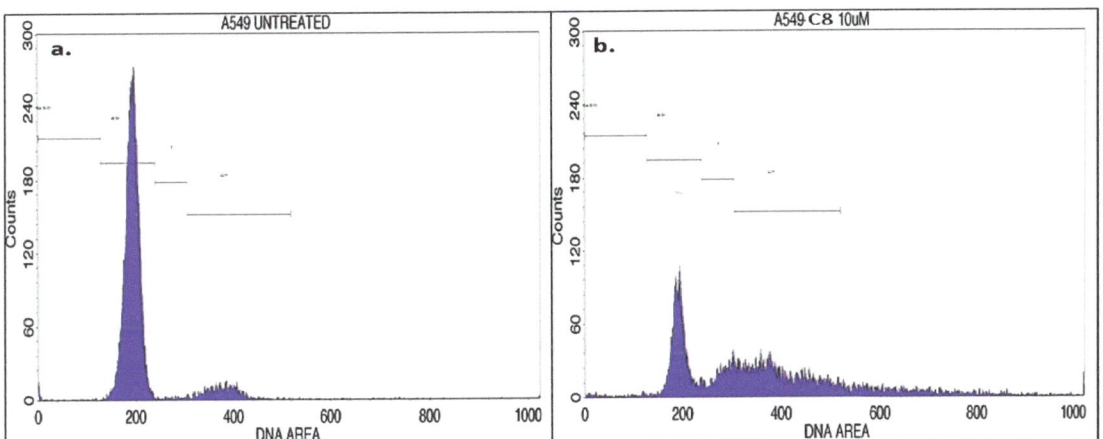

Figure 5. Flow cytometric histograms showing the phases of cell cycle distribution in the A549 cell line treated with (**a**) **C8** at a 10 μM concentration compared to the (**b**) untreated control.

Table 4. Effect of **C8** compound on cell cycle distributions of A549 cells.

Cell Cycle Stage	Untreated	C8 (10 μM)
Sub G0/G1	0.53	1.63
G0/G1	88.79	31.22
S	1.03	12.44
G2/M	9.34	39.48

3.5. Cell Apoptosis Analysis

To further understand the role of apoptosis in the anticancer properties of **C8**, FITC Annexin V/Propidium iodide staining was performed to evaluate the morphological changes upon treatment of A549 cells with **C8**. The quadrant plot (Figure 6) generated could distinguish live cells in the lower (left) quadrant (stained −ve for PI and FITC-annexin V), early apoptotic cells in the lower (right) quadrant (stained −ve for PI and +ve for FITC-annexin V), necrotic dead cells in the upper (left) quadrant (stained +ve for PI), and late apoptotic cells in the upper (right) quadrant (stained +ve for PI and FITC-annexin V). After treatment with **C8**, the percentage of apoptotic cells was moderately observed in early and late apoptotic states. The observations suggested that the test compound, **C8**, spurs reasonable apoptosis in human lung cancer A549 cells.

Figure 7 represents the bar graph for details of the percentage of cell stages observed in the quadrant layout in the apoptosis study. Here, the apoptosis rate was 33.21% (14.64% early apoptotic and 18.57% late apoptotic cells) in **C8**-treated A549 cells, whereas the percentage of viable cells was reduced from 99.88% to 60.52% after **C8** treatment of A549 cells, and 6.27% cells were reported as necrotic dead cells.

Moreover, Figure 8 shows the Annexin V histogram, obtained by using a BD FACS Calibur™ that differentiates cells at the M1 and M2 stages. Here, M1 denotes the negative expression/region, and M2 denotes the positive expression/region. The cells expressing Annexin V (M2 region) were considered apoptotic cells. Consequently, it can be concluded that the **C8** treatment of A549 cells triggered a shift in the cells towards apoptosis. Hence, it could be safely stated that **C8** not only arrested the G2/M stage of the cell cycle, but effectively induced apoptosis in A549 lung cancer cells.

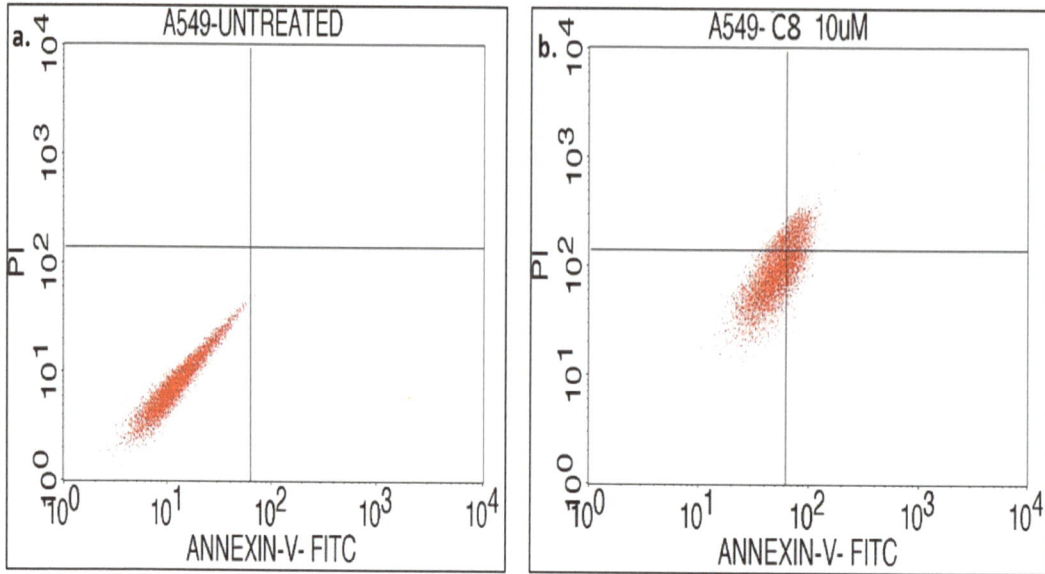

Figure 6. Quadrangular plot representing Annexin V/PI expression in A549 cells upon culture in the absence (**a**) and presence (**b**) of **C8** at a 10 µM concentration.

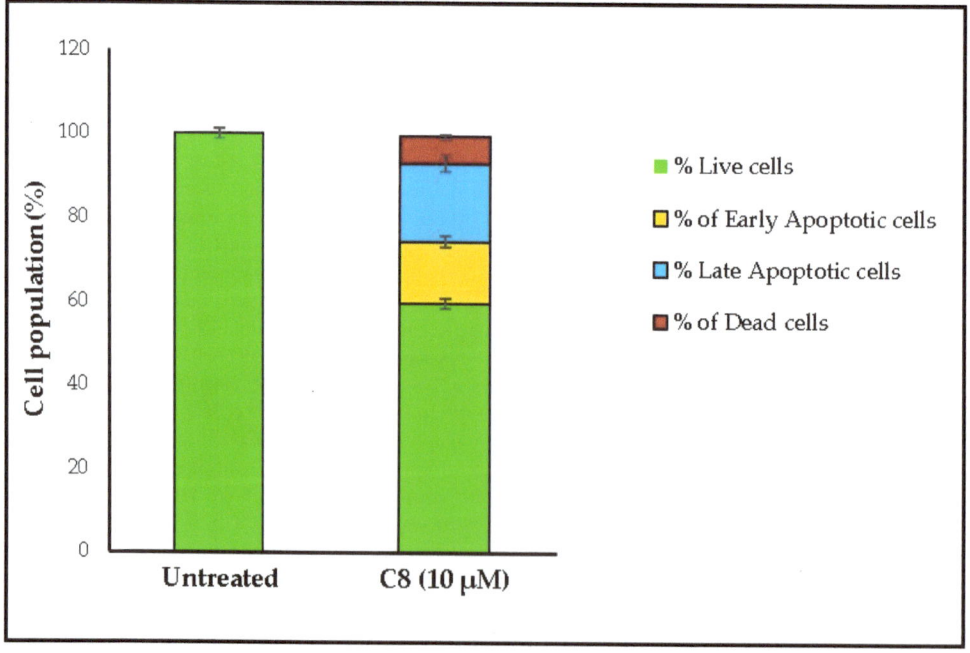

Figure 7. Bar graph showing the % of live, apoptotic, and dead cells in the absence and presence of **C8** at a 10 µM concentration.

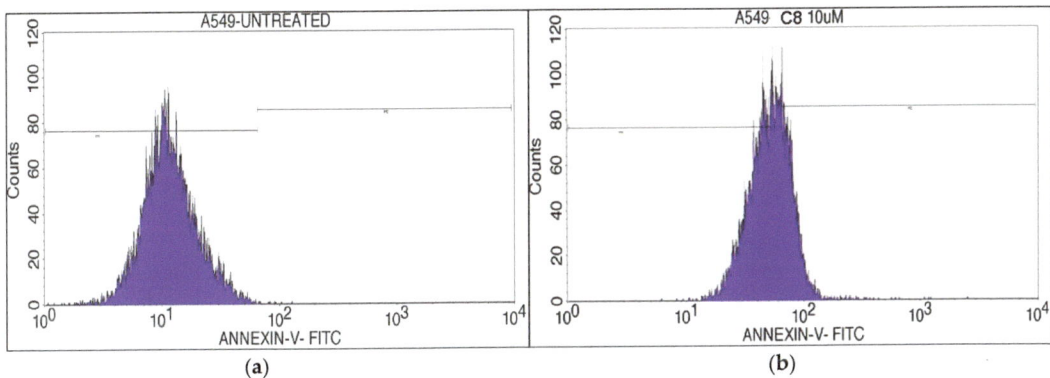

Figure 8. Histograms representing the Annexin V expression in A549 cells upon culture in the absence (**a**) and presence (**b**) of **C8** at a 10 μM concentration.

3.6. DAPI Assay

A DAPI staining assay was used to determine DNA fragmentation in **C8**-treated A549 lung cancer cells. Marked changes in the nuclear morphology and DNA fragmentation within the nucleus of the treated cells were observed (Figure 9). Here, cell nuclei were stained in blue, white arrows represent healthy DNA, and yellow arrows represent condensed and damaged DNA of the cells. In comparison to the untreated cells, **C8**-treated A549 cells showed significant DNA damage, blebbing, and condensing of the nucleus after the treatment period of 24 h; thus, confirming the DNA-damaging effect of **C8** against lung cancer A549 cells.

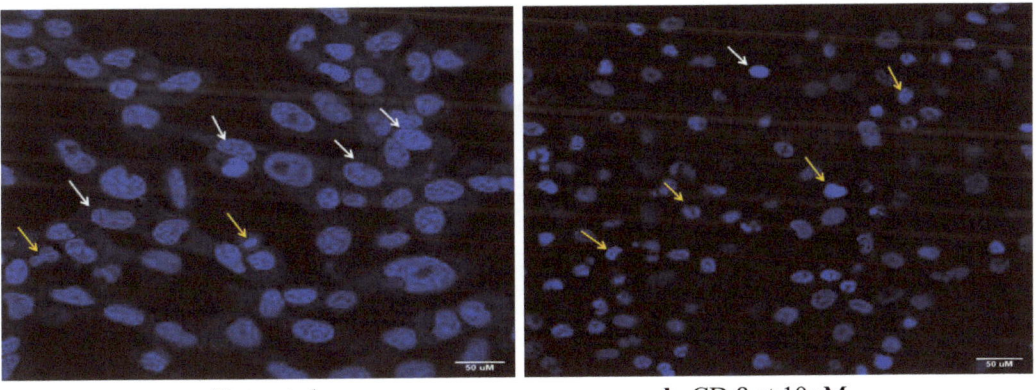

Figure 9. Fluorescent microscope images depicting the nuclear damage of DAPI-stained A549 cells at a magnification of 40×.

In the present investigation, compound **8** (**C8**) was found to be the most potent one among all the tested compounds during in silico screening against a cancer target (PLK1), which further showed a marked in vitro anticancer effect against A549 cell lines. Here, PLK1 was used as a biotarget for the initial screening of pyrrolyl benzohydrazide derivatives. In fact, PLK1 is overexpressed in different cancer cells [41–45] and plays an important role in mitosis initiation i.e., transition from G2 phase into the M phase [57]. The present study indicated that compound **C8**, screened on the basis of PLK1 inhibition and cell cytotoxicity, resulted in the marked arrest of A549 cells at the G2/M phase and induced apoptosis. In accordance with our findings, several earlier studies have also reported the cell cycle arrest of cancer cells at the DNA damage G2/M checkpoint and apoptosis after PLK1 inhibition [58–60]. In fact, strong PLK1 associations with the A549 cells [61–63] further strengthen the outcomes. However, it is too early to provide the conclusive remark on the applicability of **C8** as a dual therapeutic agent for tuberculosis and lung cancer. It is noteworthy to mention that the authors have already started to work on deciphering the exact molecular mechanism of the anticancer action and an in vivo evaluation of **C8**. Nevertheless, present outcomes might help in the development of new anti-cancer medications designed on anti-tubercular scaffolds, especially against lung cancer.

4. Conclusions

The present study evaluated the anti-cancer potential of anti-tubercular pyrrolyl benzohydrazide derivatives. The initial screening of different anti-tubercular pyrrolyl benzohydrazide derivatives was performed via computational approaches using docking and molecular dynamics studies. The compound N′-(4-(1H-pyrrol-1-yl) benzoyl)-3-chlorobenzohydrazide (named as **C8**) was screened out as the most potent one, among all the tested derivatives. However, an in vitro cytotoxicity assessment against cancer cell lines confirmed the computational findings. Further, to obtain insight into the anticancer activity of **C8** against human lung cancer A549 cells, cell cycle, apoptosis, and DAPI analyses were performed. Cell cycle and apoptosis analyses confirmed the arrest of the cell cycle at the G2/M phase and the induction of apoptosis in A549 cells after treatment with **C8**. Moreover, DAPI analysis confirmed the DNA fragmentation in **C8**-treated A549 cells. Still, more details of anti-cancer mechanistic aspects need to be studied along with in vivo assessments to bring these findings into reality. Nevertheless, an anti-tubercular compound showing potent anticancer potential, as well as against lung cancer, has its own due clinical relevance. This study might pave the way for a therapeutic strategy for tuberculosis-infected lung cancer patients in the near future.

Supplementary Materials: The following supporting information can be downloaded at: https://www.mdpi.com/article/10.3390/pr11071889/s1, Figure S1: Analysis of MD simulation trajectories against the functions of RMSD, Rg, hydrogen bond, SASA, and RMSF of PLK1 (PDB ID: 2OWB) with the control compound BI2536 (ligand) complex at 100000 ps (100 ns). (a) RMSD; (b) radius of gyration (Rg); (c) hydrogen bonds; (d) SASA; (e,f) RMSF plot of the protein in the presence of BI2536.

Author Contributions: Conceptualization, T.A.H., T.H. and A.M.; methodology, S.D. and N.V.G.; software, S.D., F.A. and S.M.D.R.; validation, S.D., N.V.G. and S.M.D.R.; formal analysis, F.A. and A.M.; resources, T.A.H. and A.M.; writing—original draft preparation, T.H., S.M.D.R. and N.V.G.; writing—review and editing, A.M., F.A. and T.A.H.; supervision, T.H. and T.A.H.; project administration, A.M. and T.A.H.; funding acquisition, T.A.H. All authors have read and agreed to the published version of the manuscript.

Funding: This research has been funded by a Scientific Research Deanship at the University of Ha'il—Saudi Arabia through project number BA-2102.

Institutional Review Board Statement: Not applicable.

Informed Consent Statement: Not applicable.

Data Availability Statement: Not applicable.

Acknowledgments: This research has been funded by a Scientific Research Deanship at the University of Ha'il—Saudi Arabia through project number BA-2102.

Conflicts of Interest: The authors declare no conflict of interest.

References

1. Albrecht, B.; Andersen, S.; Chauhan, K.; Graybosch, D.; Menu, P. Pursuing Breakthroughs in Cancer-Drug Development. Available online: https://www.mckinsey.com/industries/life-sciences/our-insights/pursuing-breakthroughs-in-cancer-drug-development (accessed on 25 January 2023).
2. Cancer. Available online: https://www.who.int/news-room/fact-sheets/detail/cancer (accessed on 25 January 2023).
3. Siegel, R.L.; Miller, K.D.; Wagle, N.S.; Jemal, A. Cancer Statistics, 2023. CA. *Cancer J. Clin.* **2023**, *73*, 17–48. [CrossRef] [PubMed]

4. Schein, C.H. Repurposing Approved Drugs for Cancer Therapy. *Br. Med. Bull.* **2021**, *137*, 13–27. [CrossRef]
5. Rodrigues, R.; Duarte, D.; Vale, N. Drug repurposing in cancer therapy: Influence of patient's genetic background in breast cancer treatment. *Int. J. Mol. Sci.* **2022**, *23*, 4280. [CrossRef] [PubMed]
6. Patil, S.M.; Sawant, S.S.; Kunda, N.K. Inhalable Bedaquiline-Loaded Cubosomes for the Treatment of Non-Small Cell Lung Cancer (NSCLC). *Int. J. Pharm.* **2021**, *607*, 121046. [CrossRef] [PubMed]
7. Parvathaneni, V.; Elbatanony, R.S.; Goyal, M.; Chavan, T.; Vega, N.; Kolluru, S.; Muth, A.; Gupta, V.; Kunda, N.K. Repurposing Bedaquiline for Effective Non-Small Cell Lung Cancer (NSCLC) Therapy as Inhalable Cyclodextrin-Based Molecular Inclusion Complexes. *Int. J. Mol. Sci.* **2021**, *22*, 4783. [CrossRef]
8. Choi, J.; Park, S.-J.; Jee, J.-G. Analogues of Ethionamide, a Drug Used for Multidrug-Resistant Tuberculosis, Exhibit Potent Inhibition of Tyrosinase. *Eur. J. Med. Chem.* **2015**, *106*, 157–166. [CrossRef] [PubMed]
9. Choi, J.; Jee, J.-G. Repositioning of Thiourea-Containing Drugs as Tyrosinase Inhibitors. *Int. J. Mol. Sci.* **2015**, *16*, 28534–28548. [CrossRef]
10. Falzon, D.; Hill, G.; Pal, S.N.; Suwankesawong, W.; Jaramillo, E. Pharmacovigilance and Tuberculosis: Applying the Lessons of Thioacetazone. *Bull. World Health Organ.* **2014**, *92*, 918–919. [CrossRef]
11. Lv, Q.; Wang, D.; Yang, Z.; Yang, J.; Zhang, R.; Yang, X.; Wang, M.; Wang, Y. Repurposing Antitubercular Agent Isoniazid for Treatment of Prostate Cancer. *Biomater. Sci.* **2019**, *7*, 296–306. [CrossRef]
12. Joshi, S.D.; Dixit, S.R.; Kulkarni, V.H.; Lherbet, C.; Nadagouda, M.N.; Aminabhavi, T.M. Synthesis, Biological Evaluation and in Silico Molecular Modeling of Pyrrolyl Benzohydrazide Derivatives as Enoyl ACP Reductase Inhibitors. *Eur. J. Med. Chem.* **2017**, *126*, 286–297. [CrossRef]
13. Wang, H.C.; Yan, X.Q.; Yan, T.L.; Li, H.X.; Wang, Z.C.; Zhu, H.L. Design, synthesis and biological evaluation of benzohydrazide derivatives containing dihydropyrazoles as potential EGFR kinase inhibitors. *Molecules.* **2016**, *21*, 1012. [CrossRef] [PubMed]
14. Basha, N.J.; Basavarajaiah, S.M.; Shyamsunder, K. Therapeutic Potential of Pyrrole and Pyrrolidine Analogs: An Update. *Mol. Divers.* **2022**, *26*, 2915–2937. [CrossRef]
15. Mateev, E.; Georgieva, M.; Zlatkov, A. Pyrrole as an Important Scaffold of Anticancer Drugs: Recent Advances. *J. Pharm. Pharm. Sci.* **2022**, *25*, 24–40. [CrossRef] [PubMed]
16. Tarzia, G.; Duranti, A.; Tontini, A.; Spadoni, G.; Mor, M.; Rivara, S.; Plazzi, P.V.; Kathuria, S.; Piomelli, D. Synthesis and Structure–Activity Relationships of a Series of Pyrrole Cannabinoid Receptor Agonists. *Bioorg. Med. Chem.* **2003**, *11*, 3965–3973. [CrossRef] [PubMed]
17. Chauhan, M.; Kumar, R. Medicinal Attributes of Pyrazolo[3,4-d]Pyrimidines: A Review. *Bioorg. Med. Chem.* **2013**, *21*, 5657–5668. [CrossRef]
18. Ansari, A.; Ali, A.; Asif, M.; Shamsuzzaman, S. Review: Biologically Active Pyrazole Derivatives. *New J. Chem.* **2017**, *41*, 16–41. [CrossRef]
19. Saleh, N.M.; El-Gazzar, M.G.; Aly, H.M; Othman, R.A. Novel Anticancer Fused Pyrazole Deriv Biologically active pyrazole derivatives atives as EGFR and VEGFR-2 Dual TK Inhibitors. *Front. Chem.* **2020**, *7*, 917 [CrossRef]
20. Arjun, H.A.; Elancheran, R.; Manikandan, N.; Lakshmithendral, K.; Ramanathan, M.; Bhattacharjee, A.; Lokanath, N.K.; Kabilan, S. Design, Synthesis, and Biological Evaluation of (E)-N'-((1-Chloro-3,4-Dihydronaphthalen-2-Yl)Methylene)Benzohydrazide Derivatives as Anti-Prostate Cancer Agents. *Front. Chem.* **2019**, *7*, 474. [CrossRef]
21. Morcoss, M.; Abdelhafez, E.S.; Abdel-Rahman, H.; Abdel-Aziz, M.; El-Ella, D.A. Novel Benzimidazole/Hydrazone Derivatives as Promising Anticancer Lead Compounds: Design, Synthesis, and Molecular Docking Study. *J. Adv. Biomed. Pharm. Sci.* **2020**, *3*, 45–52. [CrossRef]
22. Sarno, F.; Papulino, C.; Franci, G.; Andersen, J.H.; Cautain, B.; Melardo, C.; Altucci, L.; Nebbioso, A. 3-Chloro-N'-(2-Hydroxybenzylidene) Benzohydrazide: An LSD1-Selective Inhibitor and Iron-Chelating Agent for Anticancer Therapy. *Front. Pharmacol.* **2018**, *9*, 1006. [CrossRef]
23. Ohira, M.; Iwasaki, Y.; Tanaka, C.; Kuroki, M.; Matsuo, N.; Kitamura, T.; Yukuhiro, M.; Morimoto, H.; Pang, N.; Liu, B.; et al. A Novel Anti-Microtubule Agent with Carbazole and Benzohydrazide Structures Suppresses Tumor Cell Growth in Vivo. *Biochim. Biophys. Acta-Gen. Subj.* **2015**, *1850*, 1676–1684. [CrossRef]
24. Kamath, P.R.; Sunil, D.; Ajees, A.A.; Pai, K.S.R.; Biswas, S. N'-((2-(6-Bromo-2-Oxo-2H-Chromen-3-Yl)-1H-Indol-3-Yl)Methylene) Benzohydrazide as a Probable Bcl-2/Bcl-XL Inhibitor with Apoptotic and Anti-Metastatic Potential. *Eur. J. Med. Chem.* **2016**, *120*, 134–147. [CrossRef]
25. Radwan, A.A.; Al-Mohanna, F.; Alanazi, F.K.; Manogaran, P.S.; Al-Dhfyan, A. Target β-Catenin/CD44/Nanog Axis in Colon Cancer Cells by Certain N'-(2-Oxoindolin-3-Ylidene)-2-(Benzyloxy)Benzohydrazides. *Bioorg. Med. Chem. Lett.* **2016**, *26*, 1664–1670. [CrossRef]
26. O'Boyle, N.M.; Banck, M.; James, C.A.; Morley, C.; Vandermeersch, T.; Hutchison, G.R. Open Babel: An Open Chemical Toolbox. *J. Cheminform.* **2011**, *3*, 33. [CrossRef]
27. Rizvi, S.M.D.; Shakil, S.; Haneef, M. A Simple Click by Click Protocol to Perform Docking: AutoDock 4.2 Made Easy for Non-Bioinformaticians. *EXCLI J.* **2013**, *12*, 831–857.
28. Trott, O.; Olson, A.J. AutoDock Vina: Improving the Speed and Accuracy of Docking with a New Scoring Function, Efficient Optimization, and Multithreading. *J. Comput. Chem.* **2009**, *31*, 455–461. [CrossRef] [PubMed]

29. Rizvi, S.M.D.; Alshammari, A.A.A.; Almawkaa, W.A.; Ahmed, A.B.F.; Katamesh, A.; Alafnan, A.; Almutairi, T.J.; Alshammari, R.F. An Oncoinformatics Study to Predict the Inhibitory Potential of Recent FDA-Approved Anti-Cancer Drugs against Human Polo-like Kinase 1 Enzyme: A Step towards Dual-Target Cancer Medication. *3 Biotech* **2019**, *9*, 70. [CrossRef] [PubMed]
30. Hess, B.; Kutzner, C.; van der Spoel, D.; Lindahl, E. GROMACS 4: Algorithms for Highly Efficient, Load-Balanced, and Scalable Molecular Simulation. *J. Chem. Theory Comput.* **2008**, *4*, 435–447. [CrossRef] [PubMed]
31. Bjelkmar, P.; Larsson, P.; Cuendet, M.A.; Hess, B.; Lindahl, E. Implementation of the CHARMM Force Field in GROMACS: Analysis of Protein Stability Effects from Correction Maps, Virtual Interaction Sites, and Water Models. *J. Chem. Theory Comput.* **2010**, *6*, 459–466. [CrossRef] [PubMed]
32. Zoete, V.; Cuendet, M.A.; Grosdidier, A.; Michielin, O. SwissParam: A Fast Force Field Generation Tool for Small Organic Molecules. *J. Comput. Chem.* **2011**, *32*, 2359–2368. [CrossRef]
33. Mark, P.; Nilsson, L. Structure and dynamics of the TIP3P, SPC, and SPC/E water models at 298 K. *J. Phys. Chem. A.* **2001**, *105*, 9954–9960. [CrossRef]
34. Mandal, S.P.; Garg, A.; Prabitha, P.; Wadhwani, A.D.; Adhikary, L.; Kumar, B.R.P. Novel Glitazones as PPARγ Agonists: Molecular Design, Synthesis, Glucose Uptake Activity and 3D QSAR Studies. *Chem. Cent. J.* **2018**, *12*, 141. [CrossRef] [PubMed]
35. Murthy, S.S.; Narsaiah, T.B. Cytotoxic Effect of Bromelain on HepG2 Hepatocellular Carcinoma Cell Line. *Appl. Biochem. Biotechnol.* **2021**, *193*, 1873–1897. [CrossRef] [PubMed]
36. Crowley, L.C.; Chojnowski, G.; Waterhouse, N.J. Measuring the DNA content of cells in apoptosis and at different cell-cycle stages by propidium iodide staining and flow cytometry. *Cold Spring Harb. Protoc.* **2016**, *2016*, pdb-rot087247. [CrossRef] [PubMed]
37. Andree, H.A.; Reutelingsperger, C.P.; Hauptmann, R.; Hemker, H.C.; Hermens, W.T.; Willems, G.M. Binding of Vascular Anticoagulant Alpha (VAC Alpha) to Planar Phospholipid Bilayers. *J. Biol. Chem.* **1990**, *265*, 4923–4928. [CrossRef]
38. Hotz, M.A.; Gong, J.; Traganos, F.; Darzynkiewicz, Z. Flow Cytometric Detection of Apoptosis: Comparison of the Assays of in Situ DNA Degradation and Chromatin Changes. *Cytometry* **1994**, *15*, 237–244. [CrossRef]
39. Talevi, A.; Bellera, C.L. Challenges and Opportunities with Drug Repurposing: Finding Strategies to Find Alternative Uses of Therapeutics. *Expert Opin. Drug Discov.* **2020**, *15*, 397–401. [CrossRef]
40. Drug Repurposing Market-Global Market Share, Trends, Analysis and Forecast, 2023–2032. Available online: https://www.insightslice.com/drug-repurposing-market#:~:text=The%20global%20drug%20repurposing%20market,therapeutical%20uses%20for%20existing%20drugs (accessed on 7 February 2023).
41. Shakil, S.; Baig, M.H.; Tabrez, S.; Rizvi, S.M.D.; Zaidi, S.K.; Ashraf, G.M.; Ansari, S.A.; Khan, A.A.P.; Al-Qahtani, M.H.; Abuzenadah, A.M.; et al. Molecular and Enzoinformatics Perspectives of Targeting Polo-like Kinase 1 in Cancer Therapy. *Semin. Cancer Biol.* **2019**, *56*, 47–55. [CrossRef]
42. Cholewa, B.D.; Liu, X.; Ahmad, N. The Role of Polo-like Kinase 1 in Carcinogenesis: Cause or Consequence? *Cancer Res.* **2013**, *73*, 6848–6855. [CrossRef]
43. Chiappa, M.; Petrella, S.; Damia, G.; Broggini, M.; Guffanti, F.; Ricci, F. Present and Future Perspective on PLK1 Inhibition in Cancer Treatment. *Front. Oncol.* **2022**, *12*, 903016. [CrossRef]
44. Su, S.; Chhabra, G.; Singh, C.K.; Ndiaye, M.A.; Ahmad, N. PLK1 Inhibition-Based Combination Therapies for Cancer Management. *Transl. Oncol.* **2022**, *16*, 101332. [CrossRef] [PubMed]
45. Gutteridge, R.E.A.; Ndiaye, M.A.; Liu, X.; Ahmad, N. Plk1 Inhibitors in Cancer Therapy: From Laboratory to Clinics. *Mol. Cancer Ther.* **2016**, *15*, 1427–1435. [CrossRef] [PubMed]
46. Kothe, M.; Kohls, D.; Low, S.; Coli, R.; Cheng, A.C.; Jacques, S.L.; Johnson, T.L.; Lewis, C.; Loh, C.; Nonomiya, J.; et al. Structure of the Catalytic Domain of Human Polo-like Kinase 1. *Biochemistry* **2007**, *46*, 5960–5971. [CrossRef]
47. Liang, H.; Liu, H.; Kuang, Y.; Chen, L.; Ye, M.; Lai, L. Discovery of Targeted Covalent Natural Products against PLK1 by Herb-Based Screening. *J. Chem. Inf. Model.* **2020**, *60*, 4350–4358. [CrossRef] [PubMed]
48. Keikha, M.; Esfahani, B. The Relationship between Tuberculosis and Lung Cancer. *Adv. Biomed. Res.* **2018**, *7*, 58. [CrossRef]
49. Cabrera-Sanchez, J.; Cuba, V.; Vega, V.; van der Stuyft, P.; Otero, L. Lung Cancer Occurrence after an Episode of Tuberculosis: A Systematic Review and Meta-Analysis. *Eur. Respir. Rev.* **2022**, *31*, 220025. [CrossRef]
50. Qin, Y.; Chen, Y.; Chen, J.; Xu, K.; Xu, F.; Shi, J. The Relationship between Previous Pulmonary Tuberculosis and Risk of Lung Cancer in the Future. *Infect. Agent. Cancer* **2022**, *17*, 20. [CrossRef]
51. Fujita, M.; Oshima, T.; Morimoto, H. Benzohydrazide Derivative for Inducing g2/m Phase Arrest and Cell Death. Patent No WO2013061669A1, 2 May 2013.
52. Wang, G.; He, M.; Liu, W.; Fan, M.; Li, Y.; Peng, Z. Design, synthesis and biological evaluation of novel 2-phenyl-4,5,6,7-tetrahydro-1H- indole derivatives as potential anticancer agents and tubulin polymerization inhibitors. *Arab. J. Chem.* **2022**, *15*, 103504. [CrossRef]
53. Parrino, B.; Ullo, S.; Attanzio, A.; Spanò, V.; Cascioferro, S.; Montalbano, A.; Barraja, P.; Tesoriere, L.; Cirrincione, G.; Diana, P. New Tripentone Analogs with Antiproliferative Activity. *Molecules* **2017**, *22*, 2005. [CrossRef]
54. Zhang, Y.; Zhang, R.; Ni, H. Eriodictyol Exerts Potent Anticancer Activity against A549 Human Lung Cancer Cell Line by Inducing Mitochondrial-Mediated Apoptosis, G2/M Cell Cycle Arrest Vorinostat enhances the therapeutic potential of Erlotinib via MAPK in lung cancer cells and Inhibition of m-TOR/PI3K/Akt Signalling Pathway. *Arch. Med. Sci.* **2019**, *16*, 446–452. [CrossRef]

55. Song, Z.; Yin, Y.; Hao, S.; Wei, J.; Liu, B.; Huang, X.; Gao, C.; Zhu, R.; Liao, W.; Cai, D. JS-K induces G2/M phase cell cycle arrest and apoptosis in A549 and H460 cells via the p53/p21WAF1/CIP1 and p27KIP1 pathways. *Oncol. Rep.* **2019**, *41*, 3475–3487. [CrossRef]
56. Alqosaibi, A.I.; Abdel-Ghany, S.; Al-Mulhim, F.; Sabit, H. Vorinostat Enhances the Therapeutic Potential of Erlotinib via MAPK in Lung Cancer Cells. *Cancer Treat. Res. Commun.* **2022**, *30*, 100509. [CrossRef]
57. Liu, Z.; Sun, Q.; Wang, X. PLK1, a potential target for cancer therapy. *Transl. Oncol.* **2017**, *10*, 22–32. [CrossRef] [PubMed]
58. Schmit, T.L.; Zhong, W.; Setaluri, V.; Spiegelman, V.S.; Ahmad, N. Targeted depletion of Polo-like kinase (Plk) 1 through lentiviral shRNA or a small-molecule inhibitor causes mitotic catastrophe and induction of apoptosis in human melanoma cells. *J. Investig. Dermatol.* **2009**, *129*, 2843–2853. [CrossRef] [PubMed]
59. Jung, Y.; Kraikivski, P.; Shafiekhani, S.; Terhune, S.S.; Dash, R.K. Crosstalk between Plk1, p53, cell cycle, and G2/M DNA damage checkpoint regulation in cancer: Computational modeling and analysis. *Npj Syst. Biol. Appl.* **2021**, *7*, 46. [CrossRef] [PubMed]
60. Pezuk, J.A.; Brassesco, M.S.; Morales, A.G.; de Oliveira, J.C.; de Oliveira, H.F.; Scrideli, C.A.; Tone, L.G. Inhibition of polo-like kinase 1 induces cell cycle arrest and sensitizes glioblastoma cells to ionizing radiation. *Cancer Biother. Radiopharm.* **2013**, *28*, 516–522. [CrossRef] [PubMed]
61. Yan, W.; Yu, H.; Li, W.; Li, F.; Wang, S.; Yu, N.; Jiang, Q. Plk1 promotes the migration of human lung adenocarcinoma epithelial cells via STAT3 signaling. *Oncol. Lett.* **2018**, *16*, 6801–6807. [CrossRef] [PubMed]
62. Gunasekaran, P.; Lee, G.H.; Hwang, Y.S.; Koo, B.C.; Han, E.H.; Bang, G.; La, Y.K.; Park, S.; Kim, H.N.; Kim, M.H.; et al. An investigation of Plk1 PBD inhibitor KBJK557 as a tumor growth suppressor in non-small cell lung cancer. *J. Anal. Sci. Technol.* **2022**, *13*, 1–10. [CrossRef]
63. Zhang, R.; Xu, Z.; Ning, F.; Kong, Y.; Li, X.; Wang, X.; Yu, X. The effect of inhibition of Plk1 expression on the sensitivity and metastasis of cisplatin in lung cancer cell line A549. *Acta Med. Mediterr.* **2020**, *36*, 2833–2838.

Disclaimer/Publisher's Note: The statements, opinions and data contained in all publications are solely those of the individual author(s) and contributor(s) and not of MDPI and/or the editor(s). MDPI and/or the editor(s) disclaim responsibility for any injury to people or property resulting from any ideas, methods, instructions or products referred to in the content.

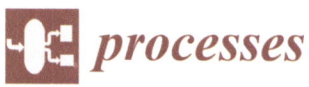

Article

Dipeptidyl Peptidase 4 Inhibitors in Type 2 Diabetes Mellitus Management: Pharmacophore Virtual Screening, Molecular Docking, Pharmacokinetic Evaluations, and Conceptual DFT Analysis

Daniela Istrate and Luminita Crisan *

"Coriolan Dragulescu" Institute of Chemistry, 24 M. Viteazu Avenue, 300223 Timisoara, Romania; istrate.dana@acad-icht.tm.edu.ro
* Correspondence: lumi_crisan@acad-icht.tm.edu.ro

Abstract: Dipeptidyl Peptidase 4 (DPP-4) expressed on the surface of many different cells is a promising target to develop new candidates for Type 2 diabetes mellitus (T2DM) management. In this light, we performed a computer-aided simulation involving 3-D pharmacophore screening, molecular docking, and drug-likeness assessment to identify novel potential DPP-4 inhibitors with an improved physicochemical profile to treat T2DM. In addition, global reactivity descriptors, including HOMO and LUMO energies, HOMO-LUMO gaps, and Fukui indices, were computed to confirm the essential structural features to achieve DPP-4 activity. The gathered outcomes recommend that eight out of 240 million compounds collected from eight pre-built databases (Molport, Chembl30, ChemDiv, ChemSpace, Mcule, Mcule-ultimate, LabNetwork, and ZINC) are drug-like and nontoxic, and may serve as starting points for designing novel, selective, and potent DPP-4 inhibitors. Furthermore, the success of the current workflow to identify DPP-4-potential inhibitors strengthens its potential efficiency to also predict natural compounds as novel adjutants or main therapy for T2DM or discover hit compounds of other targets.

Keywords: DPP-4; pharmacophore screening; docking; ADMETox; DFT; MLP; natural products

Citation: Istrate, D.; Crisan, L. Dipeptidyl Peptidase 4 Inhibitors in Type 2 Diabetes Mellitus Management: Pharmacophore Virtual Screening, Molecular Docking, Pharmacokinetic Evaluations, and Conceptual DFT Analysis. *Processes* **2023**, *11*, 3100. https://doi.org/10.3390/pr11113100

Academic Editor: Hoon Kim

Received: 26 September 2023
Revised: 23 October 2023
Accepted: 27 October 2023
Published: 28 October 2023

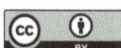

Copyright: © 2023 by the authors. Licensee MDPI, Basel, Switzerland. This article is an open access article distributed under the terms and conditions of the Creative Commons Attribution (CC BY) license (https:// creativecommons.org/licenses/by/ 4.0/).

1. Introduction

Type 2 diabetes (T2D), known as insulin resistance, is one of the most complex chronic metabolic disorders and is considered a major healthcare burden worldwide [1]. In general, T2D is marked by high blood sugar levels and in combination with other factors leads to chronic vascular complications [2], myocardial infarction [3], stroke (ischemic stroke, hemorrhagic stroke, transient ischemic attack) [4,5], atherosclerosis [6,7], microangiopathy [8], gangrene of the lower limbs [9,10], dental diseases [11], kidney diseases [12], etc. The most common oral medication for T2D (https://go.drugbank.com/drugs, accessed on 8 August 2023) is considered metformin [13] as an ingredient combined with other medications (DB00331) such as metformin-alogliptin, metformin-canagliflozin, metformin-dapagliflozin, metformin-empagliflozin, metformin-ertugliflozin, metformin-glyburide, metformin-linagliptin, metformin-pioglitazone, metformin-repaglinide, metformin-rosiglitazone, metformin-saxagliptin, metformin-sitagliptin, etc. Other oral drugs also prescribed in the treatment of T2DM that help the human body better manage insulin or remove extra glucose from the blood are (i) dopamine-2 agonist [14] (Bromocriptine, DB01200); (ii) dipeptidyl peptidase-4 (DPP-4) inhibitors [15,16] (alogliptin (DB06203), linagliptin (DB08882), linagliptin-empagliflozin, saxagliptin (DB06335), sitagliptin (DB01261), sitagliptin-simvastatin; (iii) Glucagon-like peptide-1 (GLP-1) receptor agonists [17,18] (dulaglutide (DB09045), exenatide (DB01276), liraglutide (DB06655), lixisenatide (DB09265), semaglutide (DB13928), tirzepatide (DB15171); (iv) sodium-glucose cotransporter-2 (SGLT2) inhibitors [19,20] (canagliflozin (DB08907), dapagliflozin (DB06292), dapagliflozin-metformin, dapagliflozin-saxagliptin, empagliflozin (DB09038), empagliflozin-linagliptin, ertugliflozin (DB11827); and (v) peroxisome proliferator-activated receptor (PPARγ) agonists [21,22] (rosiglitazone (DB00412), pioglitazone (DB01132), pioglitazone-alogliptin, pioglitazone-glimepiride, pioglitazone-metformin, etc. Additionally, diabetic patients (both type 1 and type 2 DM) have their immune responses disrupted and are more susceptible to many kinds of infections [23,24]. However, the global morbidity and mortality rates, which affect patients with T2D, ares on a continuous rise. In 2021, the International Diabetes Federation (IDF) Diabetes Atlas data (https://diabetesatlas.org/atlas/tenth-edition/, accessed on 8 August 2023), informed that 10.5% of the adult population between 20 and 79 years old have diabetes. Guariguata et al. [25] predict that more than 590 million people will be diagnosed with this disease by 2035. An alarming statistic shows that by 2045, approximately 46% of the population will be living with diabetes. Over 90% of these will have type 2 diabetes [26,27] and almost half of them do no know that they are living with the sickness. That is why essential projects (240 national diabetes associations across 160 countries (https://idf.org/our-network/regions-and-members/, accessed on 8 August 2023) are underway in the scientific community to prevent and control this disease. Thus, the scientific results play a significant role if they are made public and can be used as starting points for additional research. A total of 1,149,497 published papers were assembled in the Web of Science Core Collection (WoSCC) until June 2023 on the topics of "diabetes", 930,263 of which have been published after the year 2000. The scientific community's interest in the management of this disease has grown considerably (about 40%), observing a significant increase in scientific publications from approximately 17,000 in the year 2000 to approximately 70,000 in the year 2022 (Figure 1). So, in the early stage of drug design, in silico requirements have been managed by using various computational approaches, such as pharmacophore modeling [28–31], quantitative structure–activity relationships (QSAR) [32–35], molecular docking [36–39], molecular dynamics simulation [40–42], DFT simulation [35,43–46], etc. These techniques have generated notable interest by reducing the time required for experimental trials, as well as human and resource costs.

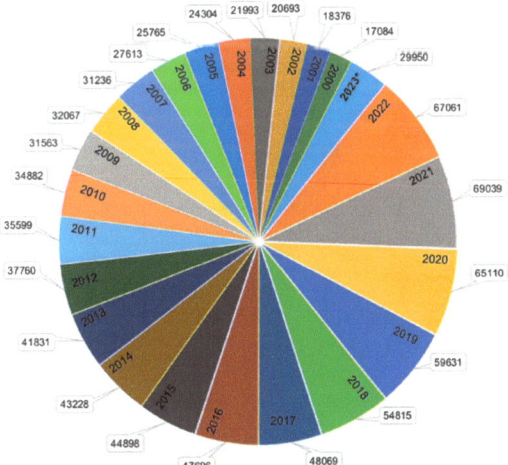

Figure 1. Number of publications indexed per year in the Web of Science Core Collection (WoSCC); 2023* (indexed before July).

DPP-4, also known as the T-cell activation antigen cluster of differentiation CD26, is an extensively investigated aminopeptidase, a member of the serine peptidase/prolyl oligopeptidase gene family. This aminopeptidase inactivates the incretin hormones glucagon-like peptide-1 (GLP-1) and glucose-dependent insulinotropic polypeptide (GIP) and its inhibition is believed to be a result of glucose-lowering therapy in T2D [35,47,48]. Following rapid development in the 2000s, DPP-4 inhibitors known as gliptins, approved by the Food and Drug Administration (FDA), by the European Medicines Agency (EMA), and by the Japanese Pharmaceuticals and Medical Devices Agency (PMDA), have been widely used in the management of T2D [15]. The gliptins as DPP-4 inhibitors appear to be very well tolerated, but some have been associated with different side effects, including severe joint pain (sitagliptin, vildagliptin, saxagliptin) [49], serious allergic and hypersensitivity reactions (sitagliptin) [50], dermal side effects/pruritus (aloglitin) [51], etc. Although gliptins have been associated with few short-term contraindications, the FDA conducts extensive follow-up evaluations of monitoring and reporting of adverse effects. Also, the scientific community pays special attention to finding inhibitors with fewer adverse effects in the fight against T2D disease.

Investigating the binding interactions of DPP-4 inhibitors at the binding site is essential for gaining insights into their effectiveness and for providing guidance in the exploration of new drug candidates. The crystal structure of DPP-4 displays a homodimeric configuration, with two chains, chain A and chain B, and it consists of four domains (a cytoplasmic domain (1–6), a transmembrane domain (TMD) (7–28), a flexible stalk segment (29–39), and the extracellular domain (40–766) with five subsites: S1 (SER630, VAL656, TRP659, TYR662, TYR666, ASN710, VAL711), S2 (ARG125, GLU205, GLU206, PHE357, ARG358, ARG669), S1' (PHE357, TYR547, PRO550, SER630, TYR631, TYR666), S2' (TYR547, TRP629, SER630, HIS740), and S2 extensive (VAL207, SER209, PHE357, ARG358) [52,53]. The mandatory ligand's interactions for DPP-4 inhibition with S1 and S2 subunits were observed both for alogliptin within the 3GB0 binding site, linagliptin within the 2RGU binding site, and sitagliptin within the 1×70 binding site. Moreover, alogliptin exhibited additional interactions with the S1' subunit, while linagliptin revealed additional interactions with both S1' and S2' subunits, and in the case of sitagliptin, the additional interactions were observed with the S2 extensive subunit [52,54–56]. The additional interactions between the ligand and DPP-4 subsites indicate an enhanced bioavailability potency and, consequently, encourage the exploration of diverse scaffold structures that can play a pivotal role in facilitating these interactions. This approach opens up avenues for the development of novel and potentially more effective DPP-4 inhibitors. Based on these observations, in the present work, we report a virtual screening experiment involving pharmacophore generation, drug-likeness evaluation, and molecular docking simulations to identify potential Dipeptidyl Peptidase 4 (DPP-4) inhibitors with an improved physicochemical profile for the management of type 2 diabetes mellitus (T2DM). To reach our goal, the virtual screening of eight (CHEMBL/ChemDiv/ChemSpace/MCULE/MCULE-ULTIMATE/MolPort/LabNetwork/ZINC) large compound databases (Table 1) using ligand- and structure/receptor-based protocols were engaged (Figure 2).

Table 1. The initial number of compounds from databases and the number of selected molecules as "hits".

Database	No of Molecules	Alogliptin (Molecules "Hits")	Sitagliptin (Molecules "Hits")	Linagliptin (Molecules "Hits")
MolPot	4,807,813	107	83	4
CHEMBL30	1,998,181	138	55	8
ChemDiv(2015)	1,456,120	16	8	1
ChemSpace	50,181,678	326	413	1
MCULE	45,257,086	190	718	1
MCULE-ULTIMATE	126,471,502	178	14	2
LabNetwork	1,794,286	58	11	2
ZINC	12,921,916	154	328	5
TOTAL	**244,888,582**	**1109**	**1619**	**24**

The bold of number represents the sum (TOTAL) of the number of compounds on each column.

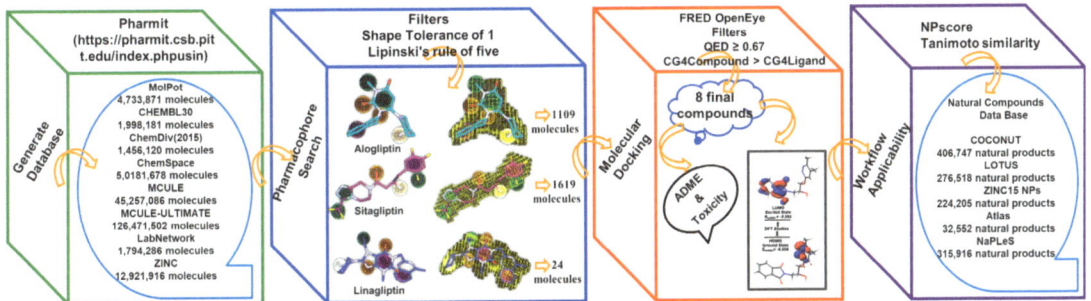

Figure 2. Methodological description of the present study.

2. Materials and Methods

Step 1—Pharmacophore generation. Pharmit [57] online program (https://pharmit.csb.pitt.edu/ accessed on 6 December 2022) was engaged to select potential inhibitors for DPP-4 taking into account the interactions between each ligand (alogliptin, sitagliptin, linagliptin) and their binding site (3G0B, 1X70, 2RGU), the structure similarity shape with query molecules, and the Lipinski's rule of five (molecular weight, MW < 500 g/mol; octanol-water partition coefficient, LogP < 5; rotatable bonds, RB < 10; polar surface area, PSA < 140 Å; hydrogen bond acceptor, nHA < 10; hydrogen bond donor, nHB < 5). The input for Pharmit was automatically generated using reference complex (protein–ligand): 3G0B—alogliptin, 1X70—sitagliptin, 2RGU—linagliptin). Using the RX protein structure, the energy minimization for each pose was available, and the root mean squared deviation (RMSD) between the query drug and the minimized selected compounds was analyzed. The value of shape tolerance was set to 1 for each simulation. The prioritized compounds by the pharmacophore model, were used in the docking procedure.

Step 2—Docking methodology. The co-crystal structures of DPP-4 with approved diabetes drugs: alogliptin, linagliptin, and sitagliptin were retrieved from the Protein Data Bank (https://www.rcsb.org/accessed on 11 January 2023). (PDB ID: 3G0B: Resolution: 2.25 Å; R-value free: 0.242; and R-value work: 0.207 [58], PDB ID: 1X70: Resolution: 2.1 Å; R-value free: 0.228; and R-value work: 0.193 [59], and PDB ID: 2RGU: Resolution: 2.6 Å; R-value free: 0.276; and R-value work: 0.217 [60]). The receptors were prepared for docking using the MakeReceptor (v.3.5.0.4) module from the OpenEye package [61]. The Chain A for each protein was selected, and the outer contour and box volume of 604 Å and 6226 Å for 3G0B, of 686 Å and 5029 Å for 1X70, and of 921 Å and 7114 Å for 2RGU [62] were generated. Additionally, one water molecule (HOH:1) for 3G0B structure, six water molecules (HOH:1551, HOH:1582, HOH:1605, HOH:1935, HOH:1957, HOH:1986) for 1X70, and two water molecules (HOH:1020, HOH:1041) were preserved for docking simulation. The prioritized compounds from step 1 were prepared for docking using the LigPrep module [63] for adding the hydrogen atoms and generating the ionization states at a pH range of 7.2 ± 0.2, and the Omega module (v.4.0.0.4) [64,65] for conformer generation. The docking protocol was validated in two steps. The first step debuted with the redocking of the approved drugs extracted from the crystal complex into the same binding site (3G0B, 1X70, 2RGU), followed by the second step with the RMSD calculating between the best-docked pose for alogliptin, sitagliptin, linagliptin, and corresponding X-ray structure. For this, the FRED program (v.3.5.0.4) [66–69] and the Superposition option of the Maestro module (v.13.4.134) of Schrödinger [70] were engaged.

Step 3—Quantitative Estimate of Drug-likeness (QED) score was calculated for all the compounds resulting from step 2 in order to quantify and categorize the chemical structures to properties of oral drugs (Equation (1)) [71].

$$QED = \exp\left(\frac{1}{n}\sum_{i=1}^{n} \ln d_i\right) \tag{1}$$

where d_i denotes the dth desirability function and $n = 8$ is the number of drug-likeness-related properties (molecular weight, MW; lipophilicity, logP; the number of aromatic rings, NAr; the number of hydrogen bond donors, nHD; the number of hydrogen bond acceptors, nHA; number of rotatable bonds, Nrotb; topological polar surface area, TPSA; and number of structural alerts, ALERTS).

Step 4—In silico predicted ADMETox Profile. The ADMETlab2.0 [72] online server (https://admetmesh.scbdd.com/, accessed on 25 May 2023) was used to predict the physicochemical (e.g., molecular weight, van der Waals volume, number of hydrogen bond acceptors, number of hydrogen bond donors, topological polar surface area, the n-octanol/water distribution coefficient, the aqueous solubility, etc.), medicinal chemistry (e.g., Lipinski Rule, Pfizer Rule, Pan Assay Interference Compounds (PAINS), etc.), and pharmacokinetic properties (absorption, distribution, metabolism, excretion and toxicity parameters) essential for all the compounds selected in the previous steps. These parameters are based on predictive models and are a viable alternative to experimental determinations of them. Additionally, the bioavailability radar plot outlines the physicochemical quality of the selected compounds, based on following parameters: molecular weight (MW), the logarithm of the n-octanol/water distribution coefficient (logP), the logarithm of aqueous solubility value (logS), the logarithm of the n-octanol/water distribution coefficients at pH = 7.4 (logD), number of hydrogen bond acceptors (nHA), number of hydrogen bond donors (nHD), topological polar surface area (TPSA), number of rotatable bonds (nRot), number of rings (nRings), number of atoms in the biggest ring (MaxRing), number of heteroatoms (nHet), formal charge (fChar), and number of rigid bonds (nRig) [72,73].

Step 5—Molecular Lipophilicity Potential (MLP). The Galaxy Visualizer (v.2022.11 beta, https://www.molinspiration.com/cgi-bin/galaxy, accessed on 17 August 2023) was employed to visualize the three-dimensional representation of molecular lipophilicity potential (MLP), which gives us information about the hydrophobic surface of compounds (violet and blue), and the hydrophilic surface of compounds (orange and red). Investigation of the 3D distribution of hydrophobicity on the molecular surface is very advantageous when presenting differences in predicted ADME parameters of compounds with the same/similar octanol-water partition coefficient values (logP). The 3D parameters offer considerably more information than logP parameter, which is represented by a single value [73–75]. For MLP prediction, the milogP parameter developed in-house by Molinspiration is used (https://www.molinspiration.com/services/logp.html, accessed on 17 August 2023). This parameter, named milogP2.2-2005, is calculated as a sum of fragment-based contributions and correction factors by including predicted and experimental logP values for a set of approximately 12,000 compounds, predominantly drug-like molecules [73–75].

Step 6—Electronic parameters. The final selected compounds from previous steps (1 to 4) were used as input for DFT studies. The Jaguar module (Schrödinger) [76,77] was engaged for compound optimization with the Becke three-parameter exchange potential and Lee–Yang–Parr correlation functional (B3LYP) [78,79] and 6-31G** basis set [80]. The highest occupied molecular orbital (HOMO), the lowest unoccupied molecular orbital (LUMO), the HOMO-LUMO gap energy (ΔE), and Fukui indices were explored to add new information about the reactive sites of compounds. The f_NN_HOMO parameter is associated with the Fukui function, $f-$, and it measures the atomic sites that are accessible for electrophilic attacks. Conversely, f_NN_LUMO is linked to the Fukui function, $f+$, it identifies the regions that are prone to nucleophilic attacks [81,82].

3. Results

The Pharmit tool generated the pharmacophoric points (Figure 3) for alogliptin, which includes three hydrogen acceptor (HA—orange), one hydrogen donor (HD—white), one aromatic (Ar—purple), and three hydrophobic features (Hy—green); for sitagliptin, which contains two hydrogen acceptors (HA—orange), one hydrogen donor (HD—white), one aromatic (Ar—purple), and three hydrophobic features (Hy—green); and for linagliptin, which comprises two hydrogen acceptors (HA—orange), one hydrogen donor (HD—white), two aromatics (Ar—purple), and one hydrophobic feature (Hy—green).

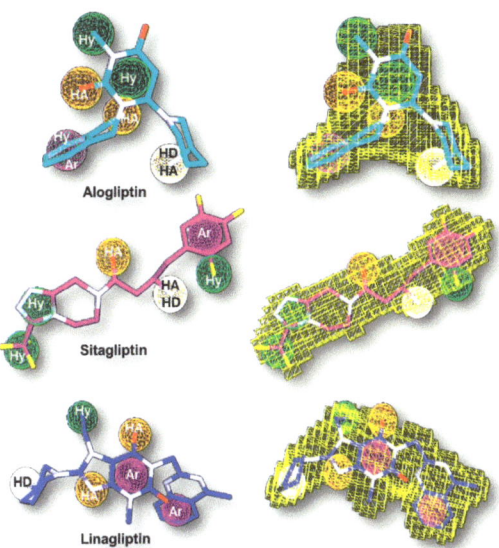

Figure 3. Pharmit pharmacophoric points: hydrogen acceptors (HA—orange), hydrogen donors (HD—white), aromatics (Ar—purple), and hydrophobic features (Hy—green); the shape tolerance is displayed in yellow; the carbon atoms are illustrated in cyan for alogliptin, purple in sitagliptin, and blue in linagliptin; the nitrogen atoms are displayed in white; the oxygen atoms are shown in red; the fluorine atoms are portrayed in yellow.

The virtual screening experiment based on pharmacophoric points, RMSD, and shape tolerance for alogliptin (3G0B), sitagliptin (1X70), and linagliptin (2RGU), set as reference molecules, generated 1109 compounds, 1619 compounds, and 24 compounds, respectively (Table 1), from a total number of 244,888,582 compounds. The RMSD range values for alogliptin and the 1109 selected compounds were between 0.160 and 0.935 Å, for sitagliptin and the 1619 selected compounds were between 0.218 and 0.934 Å, and for linagliptin and the 24 selected compounds were between 0.418 and 0.887 Å. All RMSD values are lower than 2 and are in agreement with the accepted threshold [83,84].

In order to improve the accuracy of screening, the high-performance molecular docking procedure was involved, by using Openeye's FRED (v.3.5.0.4) [66–69]. Thus, the best molecule "hits" (1109 for 3G0B, 1619 for 1X70, and 24 for 2RGU) were also downloaded and prepared (LigPrep and Omega) for the molecular docking studies. Preliminary to docking of all selected compounds, the native ligands (approved drugs: alogliptin, sitagliptin, and linagliptin) were redocked back into their active site (3GB0, 1X70, and 2RGU). The very low values of RMSD (0.430 Å for alogliptin, 0.618 Å for sitaglitin, and 1.056 Å for linagliptin), indicate the reliability of the docking procedure for the molecule "hits" against the selected targets. Also, the orientation of each RX ligand–receptor complex reproduced with significant accuracy. The docking analysis unveiled the following: (i) in the active binding site of 3GB0, 10 hydrogen bonds: HOH1, ARG125, GLU205, GLU206, SER630, TYR631, TRP629, TYR662, two with TYR547, and five hydrophobic: PHE357, TYR662, TYR666 and two with TYR547 for alogliptin; (ii) in the active binding site of 1X70, 10 hydrogen bonds: HOH1605, ARG125, SER209, ARG358, ASN710, GLU206, and two with GLU205 and TYR662, five halogen bonds: GLU205, GLU206, ASN710, and two with VAL207, six hydrophobic: ARG358, TYR662, TYR666, HIS740, and two with PHE357; and (iii) in the active binding site of 2RGU, 12 hydrogen bonds: HOH1020, GLU205, GLU206, SER630, TYR631, TYR662, TYR666, two with TYR547, and three with HOH1041, and nine hydrophobic: PHE357, VAL656, TRP627, VAL711, two with TYR547, and three with TRP629. These critical amino acid residue interactions of the alogliptin, sitagliptin, and linagliptin revealed comparable chemgauss4 (CG4) docking scores, of CG4 = −10.404, CG4 = −10.500, and CG4 = −9.771 in the active site of the targets 3G0B, 1X70, and 2RGU. Detailed results regarding the bond length, type of interactions, and the atoms implicated in these interactions are present in Figure 4 and Table S1.

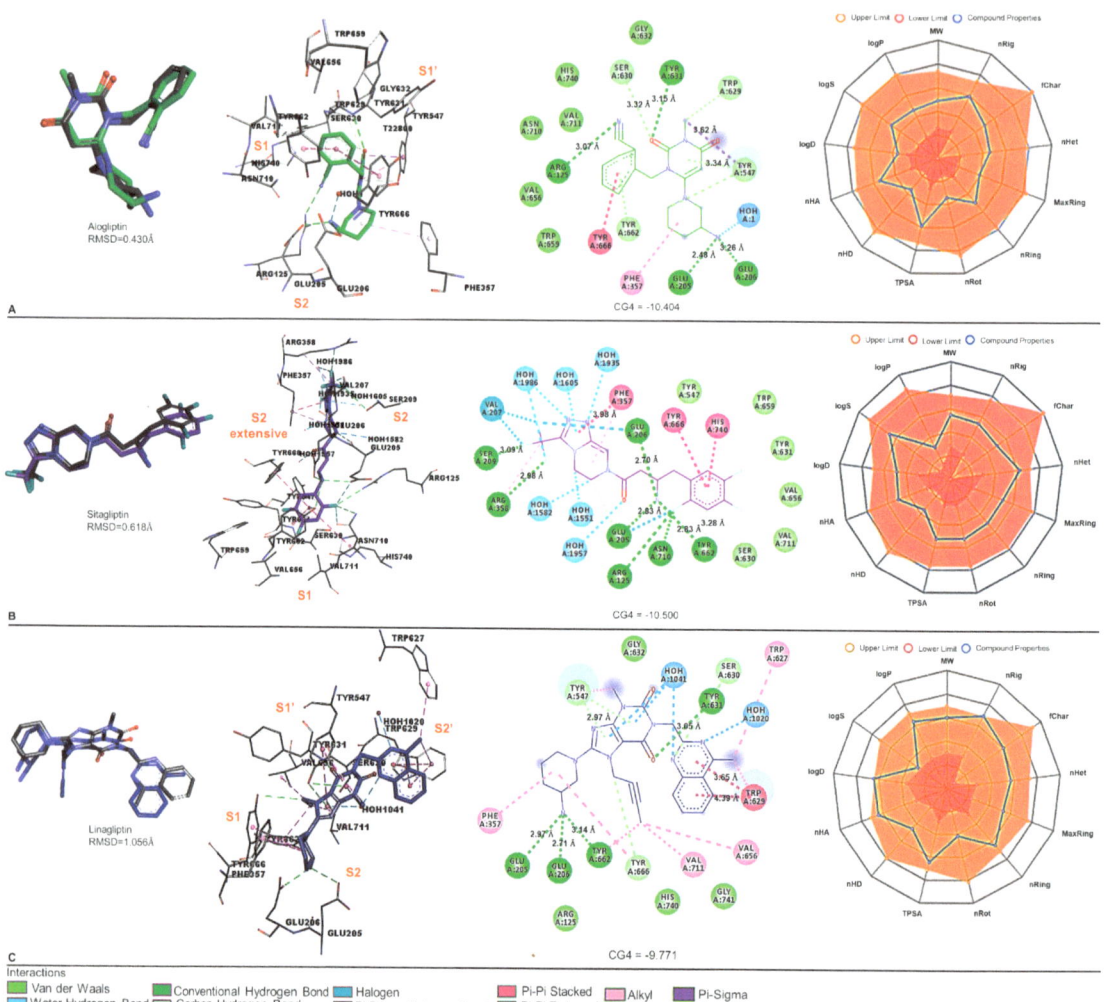

Figure 4. The best re-docked pose of the ligand superimposed on the co-crystallized one; docking view (3D and 2D representation) of the X-ray native alogliptin ((**A**), green), sitagliptin ((**B**), magenta), and linagliptin ((**C**), blue) and of the redocked pose in the active site of the target; the bioavailability radar for approved drugs is also depicted. In the bioavailability radar, the red and orange areas represent the lower and the upper limits of the physicochemical property values (MW = 100 ÷ 600, LogP = 0 ÷ 3, LogS = −4 ÷ 0.5, LogD = 1 ÷ 3; nHA = 0 ÷ 12; nHD = 0 ÷ 7; TPSA = 0 ÷ 140; nRot = 0 ÷ 11; NRing = 0 ÷ 6; MaxRing = 0 ÷ 18; nHet = 1 ÷ 15; fChar = −4 ÷ 4; nRig = 0 ÷ 30), while the blue area corresponds to the predicted values of the physicochemical properties of under-study compounds.

After validating the molecular docking procedure, the "hit" molecules resulting from step 1 were docked in the active site of the corresponding protein, following the same methodology. Then, a short analysis of the CG4 values, a search for possible IC50 values determined experimentally in the literature, and a visual analysis of the common fragment structures were performed (Figure 5).

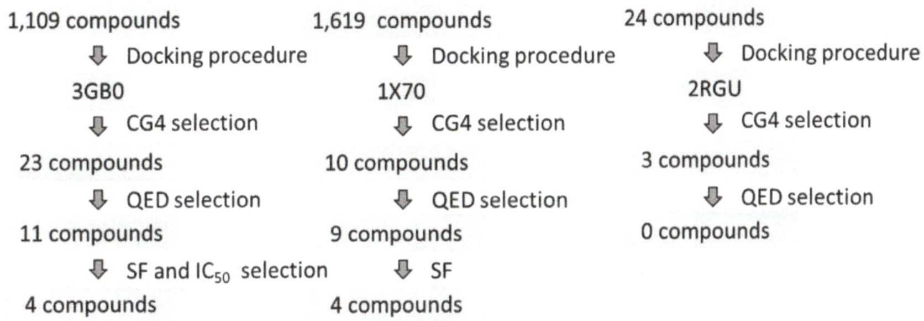

```
1,109 compounds          1,619 compounds          24 compounds
    ⇩ Docking procedure      ⇩ Docking procedure      ⇩ Docking procedure
3GB0                     1X70                     2RGU
    ⇩ CG4 selection          ⇩ CG4 selection          ⇩ CG4 selection
23 compounds             10 compounds             3 compounds
    ⇩ QED selection          ⇩ QED selection          ⇩ QED selection
11 compounds             9 compounds              0 compounds
    ⇩ SF and IC50 selection  ⇩ SF
4 compounds              4 compounds
```

Figure 5. The schematic representation of results from steps 2 and 3; CG4 = Chemgauss4 docking score; QED = Quantitative Estimate of Drug-likeness; SF = structure fragment; IC_{50} = the concentration of a drug/inhibitor needed to inhibit a biological process or response by 50%.

Thus, from the 1109 compounds docked in 3GB0, 23 compounds with CG4 higher than alogliptin were selected. Among them, only 11 present QED values higher than 0.67 (Tables 2 and S2). The analysis of these 11 compounds revealed six compounds (CHEMBL4162340, CHEMBL227676, CHEMBL1651766, CHEMBL3329689, CHEMBL1650443, CHEMBL1650449) that have IC50 values experimentally determined on DDP4; two compounds that have the same scaffold (PubChem-72845648 with CSC076365308); and three compounds that do not present experimentally determined IC50 values nor the same scaffold (CSC079167462, ZINC95941402, ZINC408512952). Based on the above, the four compounds named CSC076365308, ZINC95941402, ZINC408512952, and CSC079167462, similar to alogliptin, will be analyzed (Figure 6A). The results are shown in Figure 7 and Table 2. Also, the very low RMSD values between these compounds and alogliptin (https://pharmit.csb.pitt.edu/, accessed on 20 December 2022): 0.679 Å (CSC076365308), 0.601 Å (ZINC95941402), 0.857 Å (ZINC408512952), and 0.726 Å (CSC076365308) indicate a very good selection strategy in the search for new inhibitors for DPP-4.

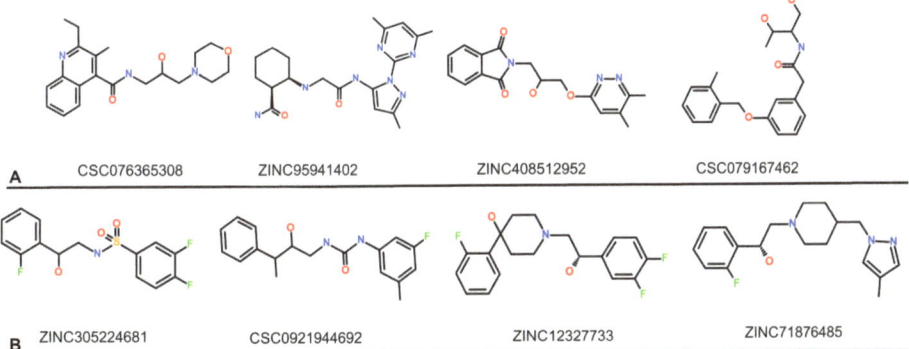

Figure 6. The 2D structure representation of selected compounds similar to alogliptin (**A**), and sitagliptin (**B**).

Table 2. Physicochemical parameters, QED, and CG4 values for the selected compounds similar to alogliptin (A) and sitagliptin (B) *.

(A)

	CSC076365308	ZINC95941402	ZINC408512952	CSC079167462	Alogliptin
MW	357.210	385.220	327.120	343.180	339.170
Volume	372.349	387.613	323.978	365.066	345.687
Density	0.959	0.994	1.010	0.940	0.981
nHA	6	9	7	5	7
nHD	2	4	1	3	2
nRot	7	6	5	9	3
nRing	3	3	3	2	3
MaxRing	10	6	9	6	6
nHet	6	9	7	5	7
fChar	0	0	0	0	0
nRig	18	20	18	13	21
Flexibility	0.389	0.300	0.278	0.692	0.143
Stereo Centers	1	2	1	2	1
TPSA	74.690	131.050	92.620	78.790	97.050
logS	−1.511	−1.832	−2.903	−2.535	−2.103
logP	1.740	0.78	1.63	2.128	1.185
logD	1.714	1.619	1.497	2.508	1.452
PAINS	0 alerts	0 alerts	0 alerts	0 alerts	0 alerts
Lipinski Rule	Accepted	Accepted	Accepted	Accepted	Accepted
Pfizer Rule	Accepted	Accepted	Accepted	Accepted	Accepted
Npscore	−1.407	−0.929	−1.042	−0.482	−1.318
QED	0.820	0.693	0.828	0.685	0.873
CG4	−11.248	−10.904	−10.783	−10.470	−10.404

(B)

	ZINC305224681	CSC092194469	ZINC12327733	ZINC71876485	Sitagliptin
MW	331.050	316.160	351.140	317.190	407.120
Volume	291.848	329.958	342.472	328.881	343.983
Density	1.134	0.958	1.025	0.964	1.184
nHA	4	4	3	4	6
nHD	2	3	2	1	2
nRot	5	7	4	5	6
nRing	2	2	3	3	3
MaxRing	6	6	6	6	9
nHet	8	5	6	5	12
fChar	0	0	0	0	0
nRig	14	13	18	17	17
Flexibility	0.357	0.538	0.222	0.294	0.353
Stereo Centers	1	2	1	1	1
TPSA	66.400	61.360	43.700	41.290	77.040
logS	−3.063	−4.277	−3.219	−1.797	−0.783
logP	2.518	3.453	2.664	2.314	0.694
logD	2.406	3.831	2.872	2.223	1.932
PAINS	0 alerts	0 alerts	0 alerts	0 alerts	0 alerts
Lipinski Rule	Accepted	Accepted	Accepted	Accepted	Accepted
Pfizer Rule	Accepted	Rejected	Accepted	Accepted	Accepted
Npscore	−1.854	−1.260	−0.950	−1.884	−1.404
QED	0.882	0.791	0.890	0.922	0.672
CG4	−11.107	−10.968	−10.712	−10.540	−10.500

* See Table S2 footer for parameter meanings.

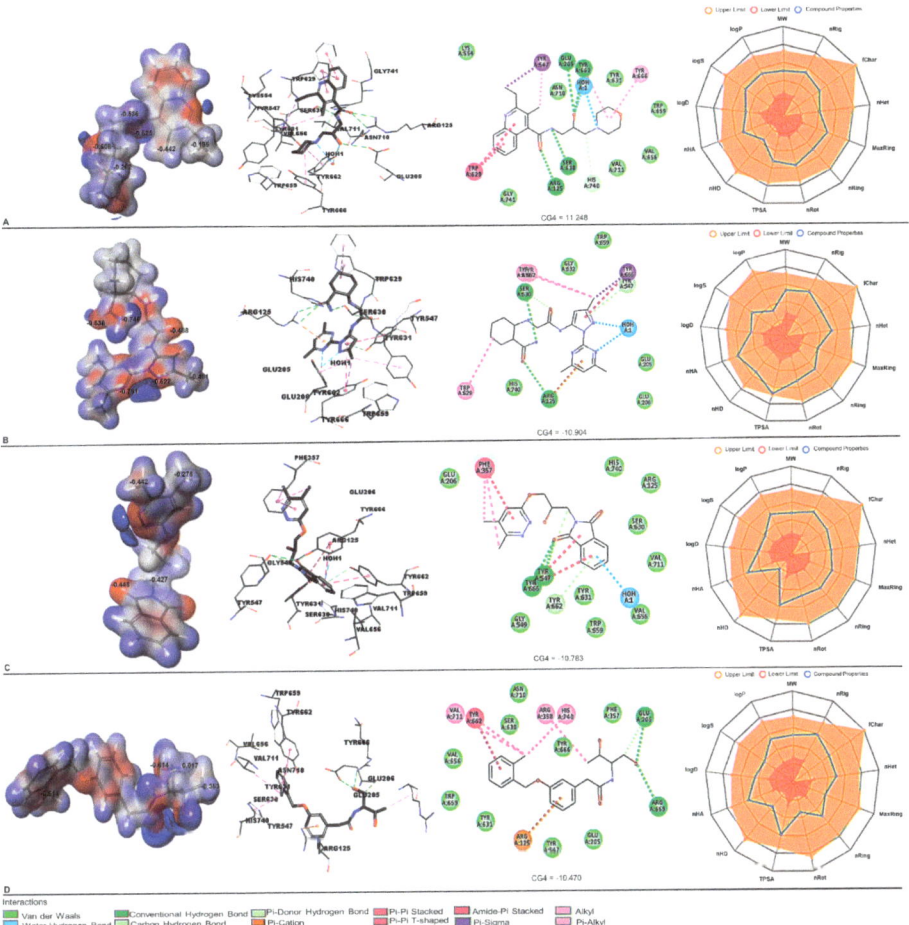

Figure 7. The electrostatic potential profiles; 3D and 2D representations of docking results and the bioavailability radar for selected compounds similar to alogliptin; CSC076365308 (**A**); ZINC95941402 (**B**); ZINC408512952 (**C**); and CSC079167462 (**D**); In the bioavailability radar the red and orange areas represent the lower and the upper limits of the physicochemical property values (MW = 100 ÷ 600, LogP = 0 ÷ 3, LogS = −4 ÷ 0.5, LogD = 1v3; nHA = 0 ÷ 12; nHD = 0 ÷ 7; TPSA = 0 ÷ 140; nRot = 0 ÷ 11; NRing = 0 ÷ 6; MaxRing = 0 ÷ 18; nHet = 1 ÷ 15; fChar = −4 ÷ 4; nRig = 0 ÷ 30), while the blue area corresponds to the predicted values of the physicochemical properties of compounds under study.

Exploring the binding interactions of potential DPP-4 inhibitors in the binding site is essential for understanding their action and also for further investigations to make them drug candidates. The selected compounds (Figure 6A) give more binding interactions in the active site of 3G0B and better values of CG4 scoring functions than alogliptin, as follows: (i) CSC076365308 arrayed a CG4 value of −11.248 and exhibited two water hydrogen bond interactions with HOH1, six conventional hydrogen bond interactions with SER630, GLU205, TYR662, ARG125 (two bonds), HIS740, and seven hydrophobic interactions with TYR547 (Pi-Sigma), TRP629 (Pi-Pi Stacked, three bonds), TYR547 (Pi-Alkyl), TYR662 (Pi-Alkyl), and TYR666 (Pi-Alkyl); (ii) ZINC95941402 showed a CG4 value of −10.904 and two water hydrogen bond interactions with HOH1, three conventional hydrogen bond interactions with SER630, ARG125 (two bonds), one carbon hydrogen bond interaction with SER630, one Pi-Donor hydrogen bond interaction with TYR547, one electrostatic interaction with ARG125 (Pi-Cation), and seven hydrophobic interactions with TYR666 (Pi-Sigma), TYR547 (Pi-Pi Stacked), TYR666 (Pi-Pi Stacked), TRP629 (Pi-Alkyl, two bonds), TYR631 (Pi-Alkyl), and TYR662 (Pi-Alkyl); (iii) ZINC408512952 led to a CG4 value of −10.783 and formed one water hydrogen bond interaction with HOH1, two conventional hydrogen bond interactions with TYR547, TYR666, carbon hydrogen bond interaction with TYR547, one Pi-Donor hydrogen bond interaction with TYR662 and six hydrophobic interactions with TYR662 (Pi-Pi Stacked), PHE357 (Pi-Pi Stacked), TYR666 (Pi-Pi T-shaped, two bonds), and PHE357 (Pi-Alkyl, two bonds); and (iv) CSC079167462 conducted to a CG4 value of −10.449 and displayed two conventional hydrogen bond interactions with GLU206, ARG669, one carbon hydrogen bond interaction with GLU206, one electrostatic interaction with ARG125 (Pi-Cation), and five hydrophobic interactions with TYR662 (Pi-Pi Stacked), VAL711 (Alkyl), ARG358 (Alkyl, TYR662 (Pi-Alkyl), and HIS740 (Pi-Alkyl). Figure 6 portrays the binding modes of each "hit" molecule into the active of 3GB0. Also, the bond length, type of interactions, and the atoms implicated in interactions are present in detail in Table S3.

From the 1619 compounds docked in 1×70, 10 compounds with CG4 higher than sitagliptin were selected. Among them, only nine present QED values higher than the threshold value of 0.67 (Tables 2, S4 and S5). The analysis of these nine compounds revealed five compounds that have the same scaffold (SC078285176, CSC088278900, CSC073335161, CSC091579518 with CSC092194469 and CSC102344798 with ZINC305224681) and four compounds that do not present experimentally determined IC50 values nor the same scaffold (ZINC305224681, CSC092194469, ZINC12327733, ZINC718764852—Figure 6B). In view of this, the four compounds named ZINC305224681, CSC092194469, ZINC12327733, and ZINC71876485 will be analyzed (Figure 6B). The results are shown in Figure 8 and Table 2. Likewise, the very low RMSD values between these compounds and sitagliptin (https://pharmit.csb.pitt.edu/, accessed on 28 December 2022): 0.570 Å (ZINC305224681), 0.597 Å (CSC092194469), 0.856 Å (ZINC12327733), and 0.702 Å (ZINC71876485) demonstrate a very good selection technique in the search for new DPP-4 inhibitors. The selected compounds (Figures 6B and 8) give more binding interactions in the active site of 1×70 and better values of CG4 scoring functions than sitagliptin, as follows: (i) ZINC305224681 with a CG4 value of −11.107 displayed three water hydrogen bond interactions with HOH1551, HOH1582, HOH1605, HOH1957, five conventional hydrogen bond interactions with GLU206, ARG125, TYR547, GLU205 (two bonds), one Pi-Donor hydrogen bond interaction with TYR662, one Halogen (Fluorine) with ARG125, and three hydrophobic interactions with TYR662 (Pi-Pi Stacked), PHE357 (Pi-Pi T-shaped), and TYR666 (Pi-Pi T-shaped); (ii) CSC092194469 exhibited a CG4 value of −10.968 and formed three water hydrogen bond interactions with HOH1957, HOH1551, HOH1605, HOH1957, three conventional hydrogen bond interactions with GLU206, GLU205, TYR662, one Pi-Donor hydrogen bond interaction with TYR662, and three hydrophobic interactions with TYR662 (Pi-Pi Stacked), PHE357 (Pi-Pi Stacked), TYR666 (Pi-Pi T-shaped) and HIS740 (Pi-Alkyl); (iii) ZINC12327733 revealed a CG4 value of −10.712 and established one water hydrogen bond interaction with HOH1605, five conventional hydrogen bond interactions with SER209, GLU205 (two bonds), ASN710 (two bonds), one Pi-Donor hydrogen bond interaction with TYR662, one Halogen (Fluorine) with SER630, two electrostatic interactions with GLU206 (Attractive Charge, Salt Bridge), and one hydrophobic interaction with TYR666 (Pi-Pi T-shaped); and (iv) ZINC71876485 showed a CG4 value of −10.540 and displayed one water hydrogen bond interaction with HOH1605, two electrostatic interactions with GLU206 (Attractive Charge), GLU205 (Salt Bridge), two conventional hydrogen bond interactions with GLU205, ASN710, two carbon hydrogen bond interactions with SER209, GLU206, one Halogen (Fluorine) with HIS740, two Pi-Donor hydrogen bond interaction with SER209, TYR662, and three hydrophobic interactions with TYR666 (Pi-Pi T-shaped), ARG358 (Alkyl), and PHE357 (Pi-Alkyl).

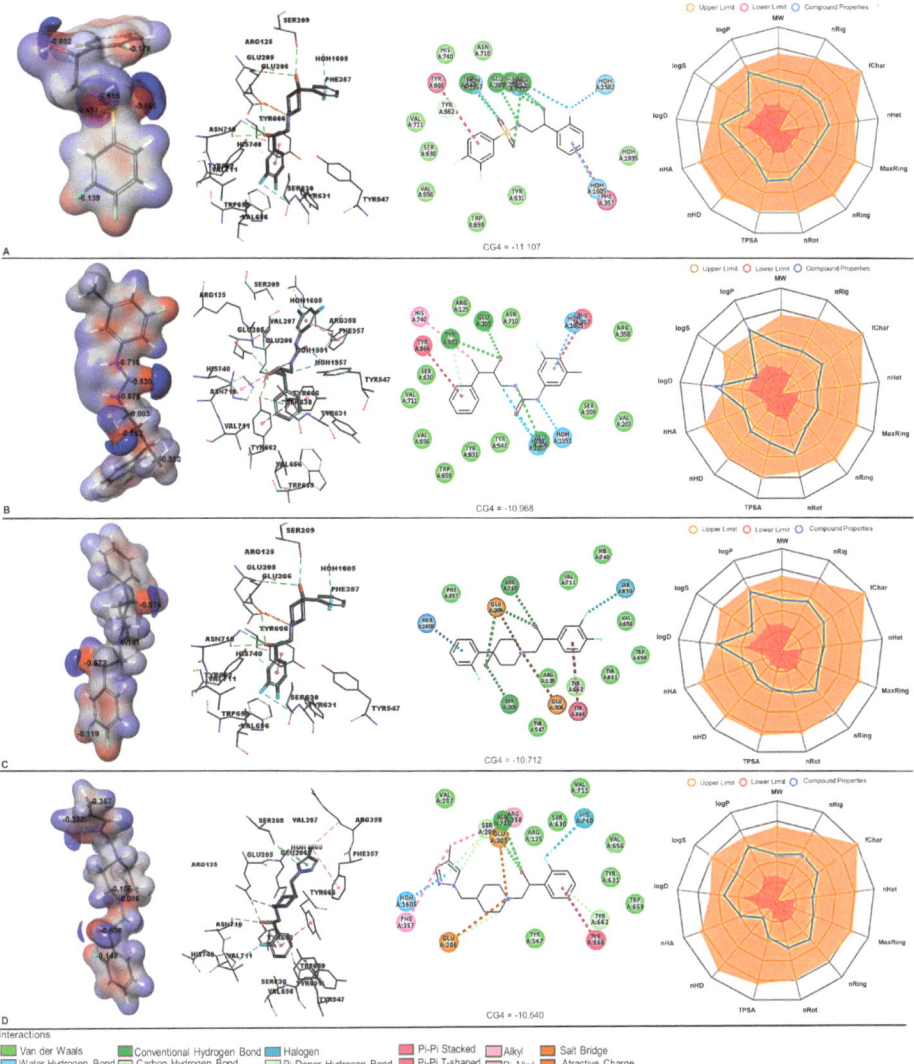

Figure 8. The electrostatic potential profiles; 3D and 2D representations of docking results and the bioavailability radar for selected compounds similar to sitagliptin; ZINC305224681 (**A**), CSC092194469 (**B**), ZINC12327733 (**C**), and ZINC7187648 (**D**); In the bioavailability radar the red and orange areas represent the lower and the upper limits of the physicochemical property values (MW = 100 ÷ 600, LogP = 0 ÷ 3, LogS = −4 ÷ 0.5, LogD = 1v3; nHA = 0 ÷ 12; nHD = 0 ÷ 7; TPSA = 0 ÷ 140; nRot = 0 ÷ 11; NRing = 0 ÷ 6; MaxRing = 0 ÷ 18; nHet = 1 ÷ 15; fChar = −4 ÷ 4; nRig = 0 ÷ 30), while the blue area corresponds to the predicted values of the physicochemical properties of compounds understudy.

The term PAINS (Pan Assay INterference compoundS) is associated with promiscuous bioactivity and assay interference in all virtual high-throughput screening (vHTS) simulations. The selected compounds show zero PAINS alerts and are assumed not to give false positive results and, thus, will not be flagged as suspicious compounds in the screening compound databases. In addition, it was found that all selected compounds meet the Pfizer criteria with one exception, compound CSC092194469, which presents logP = 3.453 and TPSA = 61.360 (Table 2). Regarding Lipinski's rule (molecular weight (MW) less than 500 Da, no more than 10 hydrogen bond acceptors (nHA), no more than five hydrogen bond donors (nHD), and an octanol–water partition coefficient (logP) not greater than 5), it can be seen that all the criteria to predict drug-like properties for selected compounds are satisfied (Table 2). Therefore, all selected compounds named CSC076365308, ZINC95941402, ZINC408512952, and CSC079167462 are similar to alogliptin, and ZINC305224681, CSC092194469, ZINC12327733, and ZINC71876485 are similar to Sitagliptin and will be further analyzed by molecular docking and the DFT approaches (Figure 6).

The Absorption, Distribution, Metabolism, Excretion, and Toxicity (ADMET) parameters related to the bioavailability of the eight best-selected compounds (Figure 6) are also reported in Tables S6–S10. The green color displays an excellent predicted value, the yellow color indicates a medium predicted value, and the red color portrays a poor predicted value for each parameter. "How much drug is absorbed if administered orally?" "How much is absorbed in the gastrointestinal tract?" "How are distribution and metabolism affected by poor absorption?" and "Which properties lead to toxicity?" are the most important questions to which researchers try to find answers to understand the disposition of a drug within a human body. Thus, this step is one of the most essential parts of in silico drug design because it can predict the applicability of the compounds as a drug. The predicted absorption parameters (Table S6) show that Caco-2 Permeability (the human colon adenocarcinoma cell lines) has an excellent score for all four compounds (CSC076365308, ZINC95941402, ZINC408512952, CSC079167462) versus alogliptin. For this parameter, excellent values are predicted, and for ZINC305224681, CSC09219446, ZINC12327733, ZINC71876485, and sitagliptin. The human intestinal absorption parameter has excellent values for all compounds except CSC076365308. The computed distribution parameters are presented in Table S7. The same trend, from poor for the blood–brain barrier (BBB) permeation to excellent for volume distribution VDss, was observed for all compounds. The metabolism parameters are related to the cytochrome P450, which is a necessary detoxification enzyme in the human body. The five isozymes of CYP450, named 1A2, 3A4, 2C9, 2C19, and 2D6 are responsible for metabolizing approximately two-thirds of known drugs. The values presented in Table S8 show the compound's probability of being a substrate/inhibitor. The excretion parameters (Table S9) for CL (hepatic and renal clearance of a drug) have excellent values for CSC076365308 and CSC079167462 versus alogliptin. AMES Toxicity parameter, which is related to mutagenicity and with a close relationship to carcinogenicity, has excellent values for ZINC95941402 and ZINC40851295, and medium values for CSC076365308 and CSC079167462 versus aloglitin, which has poor value. Related to the sitagliptin, which displays a poor value for the AMES Toxicity parameter, the excellent value for ZINC305224681, CSC092194469, and ZINC12327733, and medium value for ZINC71876485 were observed. All toxicity-predicted parameters together with toxicity rules (Skin Sensitization Rule, Acute Toxicity Rule, Genotoxic Carcinogenicity Rule, NonGenotoxic Carcinogenicity Rule, and FAF-Drugs4 Rule) are presented in Table S10.

Knowledge of hydrophobicity is very important for evaluating ligand–protein and protein–protein/membrane interactions but also for characterizing molecules. The Molecular Lipophilicity Potential (MLP) of the molecular surface is estimated from atomic hydrophobicity contributions and delivers valuable information about the hydrophobicity distribution for compounds that have even the same/very similar logP values. Thus, the CSC079167462 exhibit very different 3D hydrophobicity distribution versus alogliptin, the CSC092194469 and ZINC12327733, which display very different 3D hydrophobicity distributions versus sitagliptin and are expected to easily penetrate membranes, while ZINC95941402, ZINC408512952 and CSC076365308 show a large hydrophilic region similar to alogliptin and prefer the transcellular route versus intracellular [85,86]. The MLP representation delivers a pathway to understanding the influence of a particular atom or fragment on hydrophobicity. In this way, an accurate representation is very useful to explore the substituent effects of each compound (Figures 9, S3 and S4). This structural information is completed with the chemical reactivity and kinetic stability data of each selected compound by analysis of HOMO and LUMO orbitals resulting from DFT optimization (Figure 10) [44,45,76,77]. For further investigation, the HOMO and LUMO energy values expressed in hartree were transformed into Electron-volt (Ev).

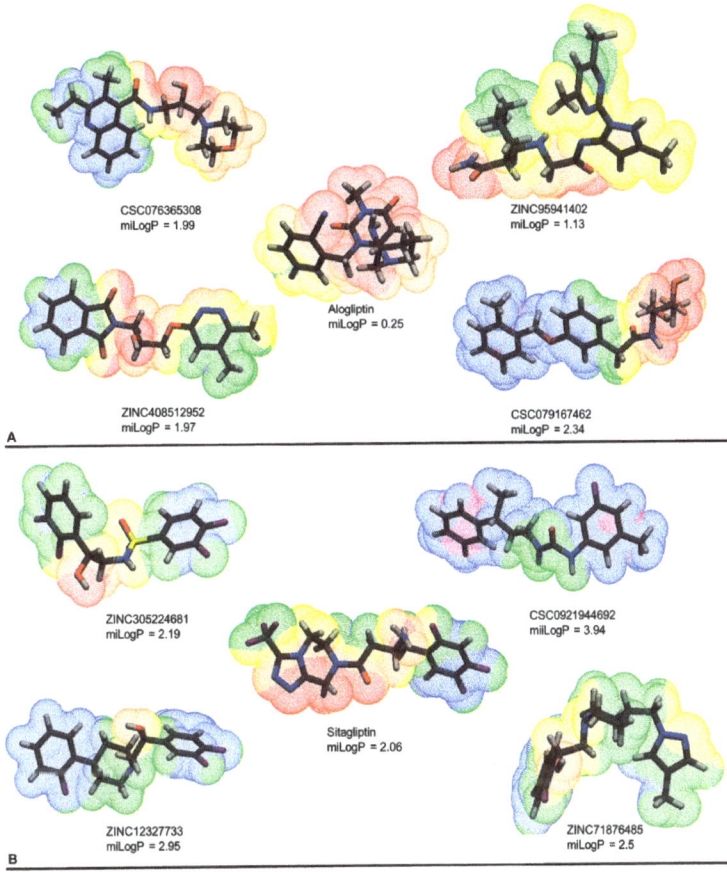

Figure 9. The Molecular Lipophilicity Potential of the molecular surface; the hydrophobic surface is pictured in violet and blue; the hydrophilic surface is portrayed in orange and red; compounds similar to alogliptin (**A**), and compounds similar to sitagliptin (**B**).

The density functional theory (DFT) calculations incorporating the B3LYP-D3/6-31G** basis set were performed in the gas phase. The HOMO energy values were found between −5.890 (CSC079167462) and −9.516 (ZINC12327733), while the LUMO energy values were found between −0.241 (CSC079167462) and −4.013 (ZINC95941402). The difference between energy values (energy gap between the HOMO and LUMO, ΔE) was found between 3.754 (ZINC408512952) and 5.945 (ZINC12327733). The large ΔE value for ZINC12327733 indicates that this molecule is stable and less reactive, while the low ΔE value for ZINC408512952 shows a substantial potential for charge transfer interactions within this molecule (Figure 10). The biggest differences in the HOMO (the donor) and the LUMO (the acceptor) distribution are observed for ZINC408512952, CSC079167462, ZINC305224681, ZINC12327733, and ZINC71876485 (Figure 10). For these compounds, the distinct localization of orbitals displays its tendency to bind with the DPP-4 receptor because the HOMO-donor/LUMO-acceptor of the compound and the LUMO-acceptor/HOMO-donor of the receptor's residues could share orbital interactions during the binding steps.

For ZINC408512952, the influence of the HOMO energy on the biological activity can be characterized in terms of Pi-Pi charge transfer with PHE357 and pyridazine rings of it. In a similar way, the influence of the HOMO energy for CSC079167462 is related in terms of the Pi-Cation charge transfer with ARG125 and its phenyl ring, for ZINC305224681, it is related in terms of the Pi-Pi charge transfer with PHE357 and its phenyl ring, for ZINC12327733, it is related in terms of Pi-Donor HB with HOH1605 and the phenyl ring substituted with an F atom, and for ZINC71876485, it is related in terms of Pi-Donor HB with HOH1605 and SER209 and its pyrazole ring. Instead, the LUMO orbitals localization suggests the susceptibility of the selected molecules toward nucleophilic attack. This is in agreement with the molecular docking results (Figure 7, Tables S3 and S5).

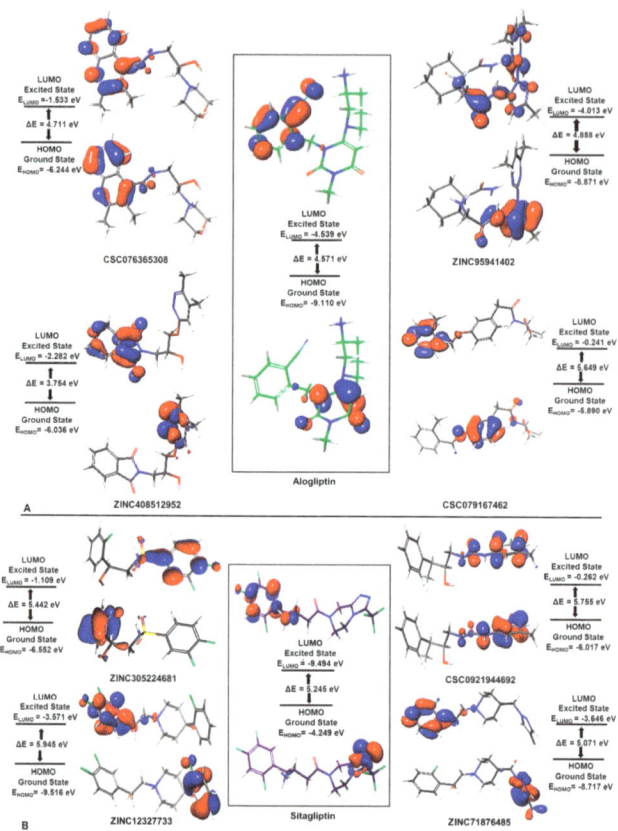

Figure 10. The highest occupied molecular orbital (HOMO) and the lowest unoccupied molecular orbital (LUMO) for selected compounds similar to alogliptin (**A**); the highest occupied molecular orbital (HOMO) and the lowest unoccupied molecular orbital (LUMO) for selected compounds similar to sitagliptin (**B**); the blue and red color of orbitals denotes a positive and a negative phase distribution in the molecular orbital wave function.

In addition, to pinpoint the most reactive sites within each selected molecule for both electrophilic and nucleophilic reactions, the Fukui indices were computed and displayed (Figure 11). The sites favored for electrophilic attacks are indicated by the highest positive values of $f-$, while the preferred centers for nucleophilic attacks are denoted by the highest positive values of $f+$ [87,88]. The f_NN indices named f_NN HOMO and f_NN LUMO were assessed, and are generally of interest because they do not require any changes in either the spin density or the spin multiplicity. A high positive value of f_NN HOMO suggests the atom's ability to donate electrons, and, therefore, acts as a nucleophile, while a high positive value of f_NN LUMO indicates the atom's ability to accept electrons, and, thus, acts as an electrophile. According to the computations, the most significant positive values of f_NN HOMO indices, which are associated with the $f-$, and f_NN LUMO indices, which are associated with the $f-$, for carbon, nitrogen and oxygen atoms, were displayed and highlighted in Figure 11.

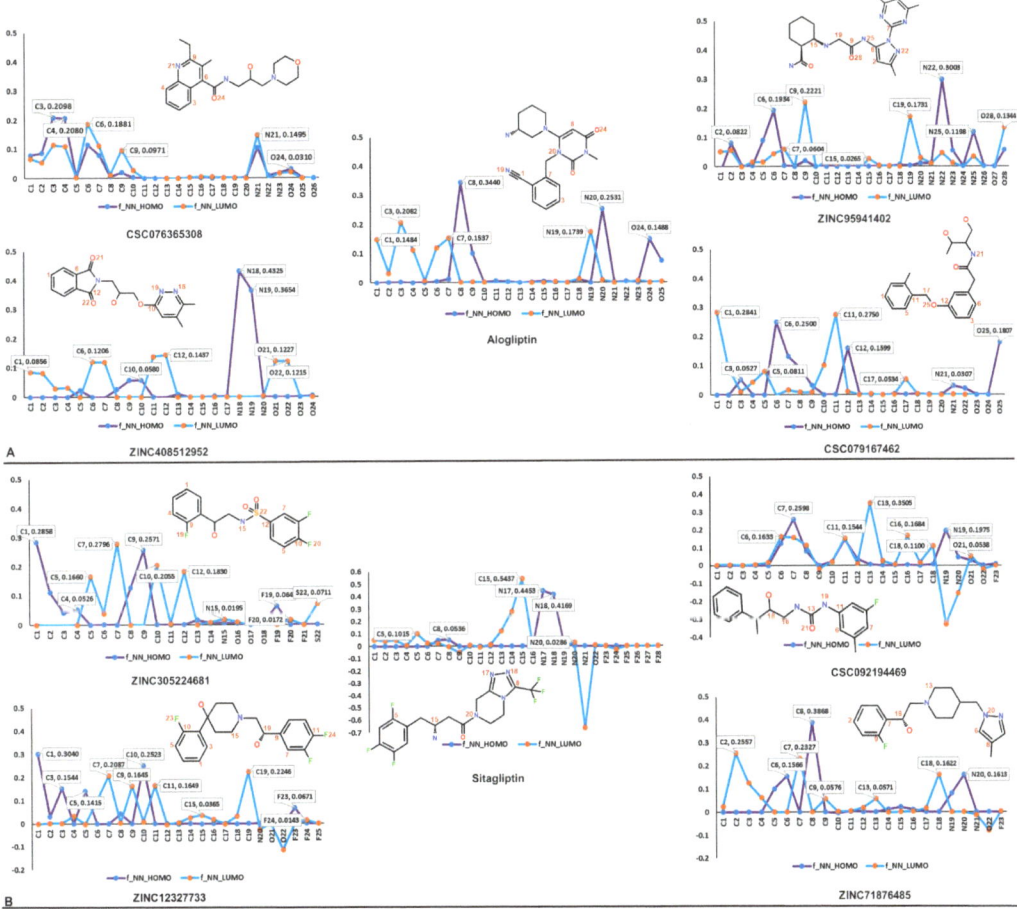

Figure 11. Plots of the reactivity Fukui indices for selected compounds similar to alogliptin (**A**) and sitagliptin (**B**).

The most relevant values are in the atom N18 (0.4325), N19 (0.3654) of the pyridazine ring (interactions with PHE357) of ZINC408512952; C8 (0.3868) of the pyrazole ring (interactions with PHE357, GLN209) of ZINC7187648; C1 (0.3040), C10 (0.2523) of phenyl ring substituted with one fluorine atom (interactions with HOH1605) of ZINC12327733; N22 (0.3003) of the pyrazole ring (interactions with TYR547, TYR666, HOH1) of ZINC95941402; C1 (0.2858), C9 (0.2571) of phenyl ring substituted with one fluorine and methyl (interactions with PHE357, HOH1605) of ZINC305224681; C7 (0.2598) of phenyl ring substituted with fluorine atom (interactions with PHE357, HOH1605), N19 (0.1975) of the urea group (interactions with HOH1551) of CS092194469; C6 (0.2500) of phenyl ring (interactions with ARG125) of CSC079167462; and C3 (0.2098), C4 (0.2080) of quinolone ring (interactions with TRP629) of CSC076365308 for electrophilic attack. The most relevant values are in the atom C13 (0.3505) of urea group of CS092194469; C1 (0.2841) and C11 (0.2750) of phenyl ring (interactions with TYR662) of CSC079167462; C7 (0.2796), C10 (0.2055) of phenyl ring substituted with two fluorine atoms (interactions with TYR666) of ZINC305224681; C2 (0.2557), C7 (0.2327) of phenyl ring substituted with one fluorine at-om (interactions with TYR662, TYR666) of ZINC7187648; C19 (0.2246), C7 (0.2087) of phenyl ring substituted with two fluorine atoms (interactions with TYR662, TYR666) of ZINC12327733; C9 (0.2221) of acetamide group of ZINC95941402; C6 (0.1881), N21 (0.1495) of quinolone ring (interactions with TRP629) of CSC076365308; and O21 (0.1227), O22 (0.1215) of isoindoline-dione ring (interactions with TRP547, TYR666) of ZINC408512952 for nucleophilic attack. These outcomes reinforce those previously mentioned and also demonstrate the involvement of these molecular fragments in the essential ligand–receptor interactions, confirming the connection between the electronic properties and possible potency of these compounds. It is therefore important to explore these eight compounds as potential, non-toxic DPP4 inhibitors in the management of T2DM.

4. Workflow Applicability and Future Research Direction

The applicability of the current workflow lies in the successful use of complementary computational methods in the prediction of DPP-4 inhibitors with improved properties compared to approved drugs for T2DM. The current workflow, with the inherent limitations of a purely theoretical simulation, will be effectively used to screen databases of natural compounds to select new NPs as adjuvants or even as primary therapy for T2DM. For this, the first steps were performed, and the Natural product-likeness score (NPscore) [72] for selected compounds was investigated. The NPscore is a helpful measure based on fragments from natural products' chemical space that can help to guide the design of new compounds with bioactive areas. The best NPscore of −0.482 for CSC079167462 and −0.950 for ZINC12327733 were identified. Thus, these two compounds were involved in a similarity search (Tanimoto coefficient greater than 0.85 [89] in the COCONUT (COlleCtion of Open Natural ProdUcTs) natural products database (https://coconut.naturalproducts.net/, accessed on 30 August 2023) [90] and 22 NPs were selected (Table S11). These NPs will be the subject of a new investigation that continues the topic presented here and may open new avenues to guide the quick design and prediction of NPs from natural resources with improved properties in T2DM management. Also, the selective inhibition of the DPP-4 enzyme in relation to other DPP family members (enzymes with high-sequence homology e.g., DPP-8 and DPP-9 [53,91,92] will be investigated.

5. Conclusions

In summary, in the present work, we developed a trustworthy in silico workflow involving a pharmacophore virtual screening search, molecular docking, ADMETox, and DFT simulations to identify the key structural characteristics responsible for DPP-4 inhibitors' activity. The study was initiated by conducting virtual screening using pharmacophores, molecular shape, and energy minimization, directly providing the ligand–receptor complex structure from the PDB (alogliptin—3G0B, sitagliptin—1X70, and linagliptin-2RGU) in the online platform Pharmit [57]. The pharmacophore search was performed using eight large pre-built databases (CHEMBL30/ChemDiv/ChemSpace/MCULE/MCULE-ULTIMATE/MolPort/LabNetwork/ZINC). The in silico analysis revealed that eight compounds (CSC076365308, ZINC95941402, ZINC40851295, CSC079167462 similar to alogliptin, and ZINC305224681, CSC092194469, ZINC12327733, ZINC71876485 similar to sitagliptin) fulfilled all the parameters investigated here. The selected molecules have strong hydrogen bonds and hydrophobic interactions with the most important amino acids from the binding site, GLN205, GLN206, TYR547 and SER630, and implicitly superior docking scores to that of the FDA-approved drugs for diabetes, alogliptin and sitagliptin. These findings were supported by the HOMO-LUMO gap energy, which was used to investigate the stability of the molecular interactions for the selected compounds. The present study provided here will be a trustworthy theoretical basis for chemists who are interested in designing, predicting, and synthesizing new potent DPP-4 inhibitors. This methodology will be applied to identify new NPs from extended natural compounds' libraries both for DPP-4 and for other targets involved in appropriate diseases.

Supplementary Materials: The following supporting information can be downloaded at: https://www.mdpi.com/article/10.3390/pr11113100/s1, Figure S1: 2D representation and docking view (3D and 2D representation) of the selected compounds similar to alogliptin; the bioavailability radar for the selected compounds is also depicted; Figure S2: 2D representation and docking view (3D and 2D representation) of the selected compounds similar to sitagliptin; the bioavailability radar for the selected compounds is also depicted; Figure S3: The Molecular Lipophilicity Potential of the molecular surface for selected compounds similar to alogliptin; the hydrophobic surface are pictured in the violet and blue; the hydrophilic surface are portrayed in orange and red; Figure S4: The Molecular Lipophilicity Potential of the molecular surface for selected compounds similar to sitagliptin; the hydrophobic surface are pictured in the violet and blue; the hydrophilic surface are portrayed in orange and red; Table S1: Docked interaction analysis of approved drugs with target proteins alogliptin—3G0B, sitagliptin—1X70, and linagliptin—2RGU; Table S2: Physicochemical parameters, QED and CG4 values for the selected compounds similar to alogliptin; Table S3: Docked interaction analysis of selected compounds similar to alogliptin—3G0B; Table S4: Physicochemical parameters, QED and CG4 values for the selected compounds similar to sitagliptin; Table S5: Docked interaction analysis of selected compounds similar to sitagliptin—1X70; Table S6: Absorption parameters for the selected compounds similar to alogliptin (A) and to sitagliptin (B); Table S7: Distribution parameters for the selected compounds similar to alogliptin (A) and to sitagliptin (B); Table S8: Metabolism parameters for the selected compounds similar to alogliptin (A) and to sitagliptin (B); Table S9: Excretion parameters for the selected compounds similar to alogliptin (A) and to sitagliptin (B); Table S10: Toxicity parameters for the selected compounds similar to alogliptin (A) and to sitagliptin (B); Table S11: Twenty-two NPs were selected from COCONUT (COlleCtion of Open Natural ProdUcTs) natural products database (https://coconut.naturalproducts.net/, accessed on 30 August 2023).

Author Contributions: Conceptualization, L.C. and D.I.; methodology, L.C.; validation, L.C. and D.I.; formal analysis, L.C. and D.I.; investigation, L.C. and D.I.; resources, L.C.; writing—original draft preparation, L.C. and D.I.; writing—review and editing, L.C.; visualization, L.C. and D.I.; supervision, L.C., project administration, L.C.; funding acquisition, L.C. All authors have read and agreed to the published version of the manuscript.

Funding: This research received no external funding. The APC was funded by L.C.

Data Availability Statement: Not applicable.

Acknowledgments: The authors thank OpenEye Ltd., and BIOVIA software Inc. (Discovery Studio Visualizer) for providing academic license. This work was supported by Project No. 1.2 from the "Coriolan Dragulescu" Institute of Chemistry, Timisoara, Romania.

Conflicts of Interest: The authors declare no conflict of interest.

Abbreviations

The following abbreviations are mentioned in this manuscript: ADMETox, Absorption, Distribution, Metabolism, Excretion, and Toxicity; DFT, Density Functional Theory; DPP-4, Dipeptidyl Peptidase 4; Hy, hydrophobic; HOMO, highest occupied molecular orbital; LUMO, lowest unoccupied molecular orbital; MLP, Molecular Lipophilicity Potential; nHA, Hydrogen Bond Acceptor; nHD, Hydrogen Bond Donor; NPs, natural products; PAINS, Pan Assay INterference compoundS; PDB, Protein Data Bank; RA, ring aromatic; RMSD, Root Mean Squared Deviation; T2DM, Type 2 diabetes mellitus; QED, Quantitative Estimate of Drug-likeness.

References

1. Berbudi, A.; Rahmadika, N.; Tjahjadi, A.I.; Ruslami, R. Type 2 Diabetes and its Impact on the Immune System. *Curr. Diabetes Rev.* **2020**, *16*, 442–449. [PubMed]

2. Skyler, J.S.; Bergenstal, R.; Bonow, R.O.; Buse, J.; Deedwania, P.; Gale, E.A.; Howard, B.V.; Kirkman, M.S.; Kosiborod, M.; Reaven, P.; et al. Intensive glycemic control and the prevention of vardiovascular events: Implications of the ACCORD, ADVANCE, and VA Diabetes Trials: A position statement of the American Diabetes Association and a Scientific Statement of the American College of Cardiology Foundation and the American Heart Association. *J. Am. Coll. Cardiol.* **2009**, *53*, 298–304. [PubMed]
3. Cui, J.; Liu, Y.; Li, Y.; Xu, F.; Liu, Y. Type 2 Diabetes and Myocardial Infarction: Recent Clinical Evidence and Perspective. *Front. Cardiovasc. Med.* **2021**, *24*, 644189. [CrossRef] [PubMed]
4. Putaala, J.; Liebkind, R.; Gordin, D.; Thorn, L.M.; Haapaniemi, E.; Forsblom, C.; Groop, P.-H.; Kaste, M.; Tatlisumak, T. Diabetes mellitus and ischemic stroke in the young: Clinical features and long-term prognosis. *Neurology* **2011**, *76*, 1831–1837. [CrossRef]
5. Chen, R.; Ovbiagele, B.; Feng, W. Diabetes and Stroke: Epidemiology, Pathophysiology, Pharmaceuticals and Outcomes. *Am. J. Med. Sci.* **2016**, *351*, 380–386. [CrossRef]
6. La Sala, L.; Prattichizzo, F.; Ceriello, A. The Link between Diabetes and Atherosclerosis. *Eur. J. Prev. Cardiol.* **2019**, *26*, 15–24. [CrossRef]
7. Ye, J.; Li, L.; Wang, M.; Ma, Q.; Tian, Y.; Zhang, Q.; Liu, J.; Li, B.; Zhang, B.; Liu, H.; et al. Diabetes Mellitus Promotes the Development of Atherosclerosis: The Role of NLRP3. *Front. Immunol.* **2022**, *29*, 900254. [CrossRef]
8. Zhang, L.; Jiang, F.; Xie, Y.; Mo, Y.; Zhang, X.; Liu, C. Diabetic endothelial microangiopathy and pulmonary dysfunction. *Front. Endocrinol.* **2023**, *14*, 1073878. [CrossRef]
9. Gutman, M.; Kaplan, O.; Skornick, Y.; Klausner, J.M.; Lelcuk, S.; Rozin, R.R. Gangrene of the lower limbs in diabetic patients: A malignant complication. *Am. J. Surg.* **1987**, *154*, 305–308. [CrossRef]
10. Gao, L.; Li, T.; Wang, S.; Wang, J. Comprehensive treatment of diabetic hallux gangrene with lower extremity vascular disease: A case report. *J. Int. Med. Res.* **2019**, *47*, 6374–6384. [CrossRef]
11. Casanova, L.; Hughes, F.; Preshaw, P. Diabetes and periodontal disease: A two-way relationship. *Br. Dent. J.* **2014**, *217*, 433–437. [CrossRef] [PubMed]
12. Yu, S.M.-W.; Bonventre, J.V. Acute Kidney Injury and Progression of Diabetic Kidney Disease. *Adv. Chronic Kidney Dis.* **2018**, *25*, 166–180. [CrossRef] [PubMed]
13. Hotta, N. A new perspective on the biguanide, metformin therapy in type 2 diabetes and lactic acidosis. *J. Diabetes Investig.* **2019**, *10*, 906–908. [CrossRef] [PubMed]
14. Tavares, G.; Marques, D.; Barra, C.; Rosendo-Silva, D.; Costa, A.; Rodrigues, T.; Gasparini, P.; Melo, B.F.; Sacramento, J.F.; Seiça, R.; et al. Dopamine D2 receptor agonist, bromocriptine, remodels adipose tissue dopaminergic signalling and upregulates catabolic pathways, improving metabolic profile in type 2 diabetes. *Mol. Metabol.* **2021**, *51*, 101241. [CrossRef] [PubMed]
15. Saini, K.; Sharma, S.; Khan, Y. DPP-4 inhibitors for treating T2DM-hype or hope? an analysis based on the current literature. *Front. Mol. Biosci.* **2023**, *10*, 1130625. [CrossRef]
16. Röhrborn, D.; Wronkowitz, N.; Eckel, J. DPP4 in diabetes. *Front. Immunol.* **2015**, *6*, 386. [CrossRef]
17. Hinnen, D. Glucagon-Like Peptide 1 Receptor Agonists for Type 2 Diabetes. *Diabetes Spectr.* **2017**, *30*, 202–210. [CrossRef]
18. Zhao, X.; Wang, M.; Wen, Z.; Lu, Z.; Cui, L.; Fu, C.; Xue, H.; Liu, Y.; Zhang, Y. GLP-1 Receptor Agonists: Beyond Their Pancreatic Effects. *Front. Endocrinol.* **2021**, *12*, 721135. [CrossRef]
19. Xu, B.; Li, S.; Kang, B.; Zhou, J. The current role of sodium-glucose cotransporter 2 inhibitors in type 2 diabetes mellitus management. *Cardiovasc. Diabetol.* **2022**, *21*, 83. [CrossRef]
20. Zhang, S.; Qi, Z.; Wang, Y.; Song, D.; Zhu, D. Effect of sodium-glucose transporter 2 inhibitors on sarcopenia in patients with type 2 diabetes mellitus: A systematic review and meta-analysis. *Front. Endocrinol.* **2023**, *14*, 1203666. [CrossRef]
21. Chiarelli, F.; Di Marzio, D. Peroxisome proliferator-activated receptor-gamma agonists and diabetes: Current evidence and future perspectives. *Vasc. Health. Risk Manag.* **2008**, *4*, 297–304.
22. Frkic, R.L.; Richter, K.; Bruning, J.B. The therapeutic potential of inhibiting PPARγ phosphorylation to treat type 2 diabetes. *J. Biol. Chem.* **2021**, *297*, 101030. [CrossRef]
23. Zhou, K.; Lansang, M.C. Diabetes Mellitus and Infections. In *Endotext*; MDText.com: South Dartmouth, MA, USA, 2000. Available online: https://www.ncbi.nlm.nih.gov/books/NBK569326/ (accessed on 30 August 2023).
24. Casqueiro, J.; Janine, C.; Alves, C. Infections in patients with diabetes mellitus: A review of pathogenesis. *Indian J. Endocrinol. Metab.* **2012**, *16*, S27–S36. [PubMed]
25. Guariguata, L.; Whiting, D.R.; Hambleton, I.; Beagley, J.; Linnenkamp, U.; Shaw, J.E. Global estimates of diabetes prevalence for 2013 and projections for 2035. *Diabetes Res. Clin. Pract.* **2014**, *103*, 137–149. [CrossRef] [PubMed]
26. Ozougwu, J.C.; Obimba, K.C.; Belonwu, C.D.; Unakalamba, C.B. The pathogenesis and pathophysiology of type 1 and type 2 diabetes mellitus. *J. Physiol. Pathophysiol.* **2013**, *4*, 46–57. [CrossRef]
27. Weyer, C.; Bogardus, C.; Mott, D.M.; Pratley, R.E. The natural history of insulin secretory dysfunction and insulin resistance in the pathogenesis of type 2 diabetes mellitus. *J. Clin. Investig.* **1999**, *104*, 787–794. [CrossRef]
28. Rahman, S.U.; Ali, H.S.; Jafari, B.; Zaib, S.; Hameed, A.; Al-Kahraman, Y.M.S.A.; Langer, P.; Iqbal, J. Structure-Based Virtual Screening of Dipeptidyl Peptidase 4 Inhibitors and their In vitro Analysis. *Comput. Biol. Chem.* **2021**, *91*, 107326–107353. [CrossRef]
29. Meduru, H.; Wang, Y.-T.; Tsai, J.J.P.; Chen, Y.-C. Finding a Potential Dipeptidyl Peptidase-4 (DPP-4) Inhibitor for Type-2 Diabetes Treatment Based on Molecular Docking, Pharmacophore Generation, and Molecular Dynamics Simulation. *Int. J. Mol. Sci.* **2016**, *17*, 920. [CrossRef]

30. Crisan, L.; Avram, S.; Pacureanu, L. Pharmacophore-based screening and drug repurposing exemplified on glycogen synthase kinase-3 inhibitors. *Mol. Divers.* **2017**, *21*, 385–405. [CrossRef]
31. Pacureanu, L.; Bora, A.; Crisan, L. New Insights on the Activity and Selectivity of MAO-B Inhibitors through In Silico Methods. *Int. J. Mol. Sci.* **2023**, *24*, 9583. [CrossRef]
32. Hermansyah, O.; Bustamam, A.; Yanuar, A. Virtual screening of dipeptidyl peptidase-4 inhibitors using quantitative structure–activity relationship-based artificial intelligence and molecular docking of hit compounds. *Comput. Biol. Chem.* **2021**, *95*, 107597–107608. [CrossRef] [PubMed]
33. Ivan, D.; Crisan, L.; Funar-Timofei, S.; Mracec, M. A quantitative structure–activity relationships study for the anti-HIV-1 activities of 1-[(2-hydroxyethoxy)methyl]-6-(phenylthio)thymine derivatives using the multiple linear regression and partial least squares methodologies. *J. Serb. Chem. Soc.* **2013**, *78*, 495–506. [CrossRef]
34. Crisan, L.; Pacureanu, L.; Avram, S.; Bora, A.; Avram, S.; Kuruncziu, L. PLS and shape-based similarity analysis of maleimides–GSK-3 inhibitors. *J. Enzym. Inhib. Med. Chem.* **2014**, *29*, 599–610. [CrossRef] [PubMed]
35. Syam, Y.M.; Anwar, M.M.; Abd El-Karim, S.S.; Elseginy, S.A.; Essa, B.M.; Sakr, T.M. New quinoxaline compounds as DPP-4 inhibitors and hypoglycemics: Design, synthesis, computational and bio-distribution studies. *RSC Adv.* **2021**, *11*, 36989–37011. [CrossRef] [PubMed]
36. Alsamghan, A.S.; Alwabli, A.S.; Abadi, M.; Alsaleem, S.A.; Anbari, D.M.; Alomari, A.S.; Alzahrani, O.; Alam, Q.; Tarique, M. From sequence analysis of DPP-4 to molecular docking based searching of its inhibitors. *Bioinformation* **2020**, *16*, 444–451. [PubMed]
37. Crisan, L.; Istrate, D.; Bora, A.; Pacureanu, L. Virtual screening and drug repurposing experiments to identify potential novel selective MAO-B inhibitors for Parkinson's disease treatment. *Mol. Div.* **2021**, *25*, 1775–1794. [CrossRef]
38. Crisan, L.; Bora, A. Small Molecules of Natural Origin as Potential Anti-HIV Agents: A Computational Approach. *Life* **2021**, *11*, 722. [CrossRef]
39. Pantaleão, S.Q.; Maltarollo, V.G.; Araujo, S.C.; Gertrudesc, J.C.; Honorio, K.M. Molecular docking studies and 2D analyses of DPP-4 inhibitors as candidates in the treatment of diabetes. *Mol. Biosyst.* **2015**, *11*, 3188–3193. [CrossRef]
40. Qi, J.-H.; Chen, P.-y.; Cai, D.-y.; Wang, Y.; Wei, Y.-l.; He, S.-p.; Zhou, W. Exploring novel targets of sitagliptin for type 2 diabetes mellitus: Network pharmacology, molecular docking, molecular dynamics simulation, and SPR approaches. *Front. Endocrinol.* **2023**, *13*, 1096655–1096668. [CrossRef]
41. Zhao, L.; Zhang, M.; Pan, F.; Li, J.; Dou, R.; Wang, X.; Wang, Y.; He, Y.; Wang, S.; Cai, S. In silico analysis of novel dipeptidyl peptidase-IV inhibitory peptides released from Macadamia integrifolia antimicrobial protein 2 (MiAMP2) and the possible pathways involved in diabetes protection. *Curr. Res. Nutr. Food Sci.* **2021**, *4*, 603–611. [CrossRef]
42. Singh, A.; Mishra, A. Molecular dynamics simulation and free energy calculation studies of Coagulin L as dipeptidyl peptidase-4 inhibitor. *J. Biomol. Struct. Dyn.* **2022**, *40*, 1128–1138. [CrossRef] [PubMed]
43. Shoombuatong, W.; Prachayasittikul, V.; Anuwongcharoen, N.; Songtawee, N.; Monnor, T.; Prachayasittikul, S.; Prachayasittikul, V.; Nantasenamat, C. Navigating the chemical space of dipeptidyl peptidase-4 inhibitors. *Drug Des. Devel. Ther.* **2015**, *9*, 4515–4549. [PubMed]
44. Visa, A.; Plesu, N.; Maranescu, B.; Ilia, G.; Borota, A.; Crisan, L. Combined Experimental and Theoretical Insights into the Corrosion Inhibition Activity on Carbon Steel Iron of Phosphonic Acids. *Molecules* **2021**, *26*, 135. [CrossRef] [PubMed]
45. Crisan, L.; Borota, A.; Bora, A.; Pacureanu, P. Diarylthiazole and Diarylimidazole Selective COX-1 Inhibitors Analysis through Pharmacophore Modeling, Virtual Screening, and DFT-Based Approaches. *Struct. Chem.* **2019**, *30*, 2311–2326. [CrossRef]
46. Mohammad, B.D.; Baig, M.S.; Bhandari, N.; Siddiqui, F.A.; Khan, S.L.; Ahmad, Z.; Khan, F.S.; Tagde, P.; Jeandet, P. Heterocyclic Compounds as Dipeptidyl Peptidase-IV Inhibitors with Special Emphasis on Oxadiazoles as Potent Anti-Diabetic Agents. *Molecules* **2022**, *27*, 6001. [CrossRef]
47. Deacon, C.F. Physiology and Pharmacology of DPP-4 in Glucose Homeostasis and the Treatment of Type 2 Diabetes. *Front. Endocrinol.* **2019**, *10*, 80. [CrossRef]
48. Makrilakis, K. The Role of DPP-4 Inhibitors in the Treatment Algorithm of Type 2 Diabetes Mellitus: When to Select, What to Expect. *Int. J. Environ. Res. Public Health* **2019**, *16*, 2720. [CrossRef]
49. Tarapués, M.; Cereza, G.; Figueras, A. Association of musculoskeletal complaints and gliptin use: Review of spontaneous reports. *Pharmacoepidemiol. Drug Saf.* **2013**, *22*, 1115–1118. [CrossRef]
50. Nader, M.A. Inhibition of anaphylaxis like reaction and mast cell activation by Sitagliptin. *Int. Immunopharmacol.* **2011**, *11*, 1052–1056. [CrossRef]
51. Rendell, M.; Drincic, A.; Andukuri, R. Alogliptin benzoate for the treatment of type 2 diabetes. *Expert Opin. Pharmacother.* **2012**, *13*, 553–563. [CrossRef]
52. Nabeno, M.; Akahoshi, F.; Kishida, H.; Miyaguchi, I.; Tanaka, Y.; Ishii, S.; Kadowaki, T. A comparative study of the binding modes of recently launched dipeptidyl peptidase IV inhibitors in the active site. *Biochem. Biophys. Res. Comm.* **2013**, *434*, 191–196. [CrossRef]
53. Arulmozhiraja, S.; Matsuo, N.; Ishitsubo, E.; Okazaki, S.; Shimano, H.; Tokiwa, H. Comparative Binding Analysis of Dipeptidyl Peptidase IV (DPP-4) with Antidiabetic Drugs-An Ab Initio Fragment Molecular Orbital Study. *PLoS ONE* **2016**, *11*, e0166275. [CrossRef] [PubMed]

54. Lambeir, A.M.; Durinx, C.; Scharpé, S.; De Meester, I. Dipeptidyl-peptidase IV from bench to bedside: An update on structural properties, functions, and clinical aspects of the enzyme DPP IV. *Crit. Rev. Clin. Lab. Sci.* **2003**, *40*, 209–294. [CrossRef] [PubMed]
55. Mathur, V.; Alam, O.; Siddiqui, N.; Jha, M.; Manaithiya, A.; Bawa, S.; Sharma, N.; Alshehri, S.; Alam, P.; Shakeel, F. Insight into Structure Activity Relationship of DPP-4 Inhibitors for Development of Antidiabetic Agents. *Molecules* **2023**, *28*, 5860. [CrossRef]
56. Pan, J.; Zhang, Q.; Zhang, C.; Yang, W.; Liu, H.; Lv, Z.; Liu, J.; Jiao, Z. Inhibition of Dipeptidyl Peptidase-4 by Flavonoids: Structure–Activity Relationship, Kinetics and Interaction Mechanism. *Front. Nutr.* **2022**, *9*, 892426. [CrossRef]
57. Sunseri, J.; Koes, D.R. Pharmit: Interactive exploration of chemical space. *Nucleic Acids Res.* **2016**, *44*, W442–W448. [CrossRef]
58. Zhang, Z.; Wallace, M.B.; Feng, J.; Stafford, J.A.; Skene, R.J.; Shi, L.; Lee, B.; Aertgeerts, K.; Jennings, A.; Xu, R.; et al. Design and Synthesis of Pyrimidinone and Pyrimidinedione Inhibitors of Dipeptidyl Peptidase IV. *J. Med. Chem.* **2011**, *54*, 510–524. [CrossRef] [PubMed]
59. Kim, D.; Wang, L.; Beconi, M.; Eiermann, G.J.; Fisher, M.H.; He, H.; Hickey, G.J.; Kowalchick, J.E.; Leiting, B.; Lyons, K.; et al. (2R)-4-Oxo-4-[3-(Trifluoromethyl)-5,6-dihydro[1,2,4]triazolo[4,3-a]pyrazin-7(8H)-yl]-1-(2,4,5-trifluorophenyl)butan-2-amine: A Potent, Orally Active Dipeptidyl Peptidase IV Inhibitor for the Treatment of Type 2 Diabetes. *J. Med. Chem.* **2005**, *48*, 141–151. [CrossRef]
60. Eckhardt, M.; Langkopf, E.; Mark, M.; Tadayyon, M.; Thomas, L.; Nar, H.; Pfrengle, W.; Guth, B.; Lotz, R.; Sieger, P.; et al. 8-(3-(R)-Aminopiperidin-1-yl)-7-but-2-ynyl-3-methyl-1-(4-methyl-quinazolin-2-ylmethyl)-3,7-dihydropurine-2,6-dione (BI 1356), a Highly Potent, Selective, Long-Acting, and Orally Bioavailable DPP-4 Inhibitor for the Treatment of Type 2 Diabetes. *J. Med. Chem.* **2007**, *50*, 6450–6453. [CrossRef]
61. *MakeReceptor*, v. 3.5.0.4; OpenEye Scientific Software Inc.: Santa Fe, NM, USA, 2020.
62. Istrate, D.; Crisan, L. Natural Compounds as DPP-4 Inhibitors: 3D-Similarity Search, ADME Toxicity, and Molecular Docking Approaches. *Symmetry* **2022**, *14*, 1842. [CrossRef]
63. *Schrödinger Release 2022-4: LigPrep*; Schrödinger LLC: New York, NY, USA, 2022.
64. *OMEGA*, 4.0.0.4; OpenEye Scientific Software: Santa Fe, NM, USA, 2019. Available online: http://www.eyesopen.com (accessed on 30 August 2023).
65. Hawkins, P.C.D.; Skillman, A.G.; Warren, G.L.; Ellingson, B.A.; Stahl, M.T. Conformer Generation with OMEGA: Algorithm and Validation Using High Quality Structures from the Protein Databank and Cambridge Structural Database. *J. Chem. Inf. Model.* **2010**, *50*, 572–584. [CrossRef] [PubMed]
66. *FRED*, 3.5.0.4; OpenEye Scientific Software: Santa Fe, NM, USA. Available online: http://www.eyesopen.com (accessed on 30 August 2023).
67. Kelley, B.P.; Brown, S.P.; Warren, G.L.; Muchmore, S.W. POSIT: Flexible Shape-Guided Docking for Pose Prediction. *J. Chem. Inf. Model.* **2015**, *55*, 1771–1780. [CrossRef]
68. McGann, M. FRED Pose Prediction and Virtual Screening Accuracy. *J. Chem. Inf. Model.* **2011**, *51*, 578–596. [CrossRef] [PubMed]
69. McGann, M. FRED and HYBRID docking performance on standardized datasets. *J. Comput. Aided Mol. Des.* **2012**, *26*, 897–906. [CrossRef] [PubMed]
70. *Schrödinger Release 2022-4: Maestro*, v. 13.4.134; Schrödinger LLC: New York, NY, USA, 2022.
71. Bickerton, G.R.; Paolini, G.V.; Besnard, J.; Muresan, S.; Hopkins, A.L. Quantifying the chemical beauty of drugs. *Nat. Chem.* **2012**, *4*, 90–98. [CrossRef] [PubMed]
72. Xiong, G.; Wu, Z.; Yi, J.; Fu, L.; Yang, Z.; Hsieh, C.; Yin, M.; Zeng, X.; Wu, C.; Lu, A.; et al. ADMETlab 2.0: An integrated online platform for accurate and comprehensive predictions of ADMET properties. *Nucleic Acids Res.* **2021**, *49*, W5–W14. [CrossRef]
73. Veber, D.F.; Johnson, S.R.; Cheng, H.Y.; Smith, B.R.; Ward, K.W.; Kopple, K.D. Molecular properties that influence the oral bioavailability of drug candidates. *J. Med. Chem.* **2002**, *45*, 2615–2623. [CrossRef]
74. Ertl, P.; Rohde, B.; Selzer, P. Fast calculation of molecular polar surface area as a sum of fragment-based contributions and its application to the prediction of drug transport properties. *J. Med. Chem.* **2000**, *43*, 3714–3717. [CrossRef]
75. Lipinski, C.A.; Lombardo, F.; Dominy, B.W.; Feeney, P.J. Experimental and computational approaches to estimate solubility and permeability in drug discovery and development settings. *Adv. Drug. Delivery Rev.* **1997**, *23*, 4–25. [CrossRef]
76. *Schrödinger Release 2022-4: Jaguar*; Schrödinger LLC: New York, NY, USA, 2022.
77. Bochevarov, A.D.; Harder, E.; Hughes, T.F.; Greenwood, J.R.; Braden, D.A.; Philipp, D.M.; Rinaldo, D.; Halls, M.D.; Zhang, J.; Friesner, R.A. Jaguar: A high-performance quantum chemistry software program with strengths in life and materials sciences. *Int. J. Quantum Chem.* **2013**, *113*, 2110–2142. [CrossRef]
78. Gill, P.M.W.; Johnson, B.G.; Pople, J.A.; Frisch, M.J. The performance of the Becke—Lee—Yang—Parr (B—LYP) density functional theory with various basis sets. *Chem. Phys. Lett.* **1992**, *197*, 499–505. [CrossRef]
79. Stephens, P.J.; Devlin, F.J.; Chabalowski, C.F.; Frisch, M.J. Ab Initio Calculation of Vibrational Absorption and Circular Dichroism Spectra Using Density Functional Force Fields. *J. Phys. Chem.* **1994**, *98*, 11623–11627. [CrossRef]
80. Lee, C.; Yang, W.; Parr, R.G. Development of the Colle-Salvetti correlation-energy formula into a functional of the electron density. *Phys. Rev.* **1988**, *B37*, 785–789. [CrossRef] [PubMed]
81. Fukui, K. Role of Frontier Orbitals in Chemical Reactions. *Science* **1982**, *218*, 747–754. [CrossRef]
82. Martínez-Araya, J.I. Why is the dual descriptor a more accurate local reactivity descriptor than Fukui functions? *J. Math. Chem.* **2015**, *53*, 451–465. [CrossRef]

83. Alves, M.J.; Froufe, H.J.C.; Costa, A.F.T.; Santos, A.F.; Oliveira, L.G.; Osório, S.R.M.; Abreu, R.M.V.; Pintado, M.; Ferreira, I.C.F. Docking studies in target proteins involved in antibacterial action mechanisms: Extending the knowledge on standard antibiotics to antimicrobial mushroom compounds. *Molecules* **2014**, *19*, 1672–1684. [CrossRef]
84. Houston, D.R.; Walkinshaw, M.D. Consensus docking: Improving the reliability of docking in a virtual screening context. *J. Chem. Inf. Model.* **2013**, *53*, 384–390. [CrossRef]
85. Barnes, T.M.; Mijaljica, D.; Townley, J.P.; Spada, F.; Harrison, I.P. Vehicles for Drug Delivery and Cosmetic Moisturizers: Review and Comparison. *Pharmaceutics* **2021**, *12*, 2012. [CrossRef]
86. Ng, K.W.; Lau, W.M. Skin Deep: The basics of Human Skin Structure and Drug Penetration. In *Percutaneous Penetration Enhancers Chemical Methods in Penetration Enhancement*, 1st ed.; Dragicevic, N., Maibach, H., Eds.; Springer: Berlin/Heidelberg, Germany, 2015; pp. 3–11.
87. Faver, J.; Merz, K.M., Jr. The Utility of the HSAB Principle via the Fukui Function in Biological Systems. *J. Chem. Theory Comput.* **2010**, *9*, 548–559. [CrossRef]
88. Zamora, P.P.; Bieger, K.; Cuchillo, A.; Tello, A.; Muena, J.P. Theoretical determination of a reaction intermediate: Fukui function analysis, dual reactivity descriptor and activation energy. *J. Mol. Struct.* **2021**, *1227*, 129369. [CrossRef]
89. Martin, Y.C.; Kofron, J.L.; Traphagen, L.M. Do Structurally Similar Molecules Have Similar Biological Activity? *J. Med. Chem.* **2002**, *45*, 4350–4358. [CrossRef] [PubMed]
90. Sorokina, M.; Merseburger, P.; Rajan, K.; Yirik, M.A.; Steinbeck, C. COCONUT online: Collection of Open Natural Products database. *J. Cheminform.* **2021**, *13*, 2. [CrossRef] [PubMed]
91. Huan, Y.; Jiang, Q.; Liu, J.; Shen, Z. Establishment of a dipeptidyl peptidases (DPP) 8/9 expressing cell model for evaluating the selectivity of DPP4 inhibitors. *J. Pharmacol. Toxicol. Methods* **2015**, *71*, 8–12. [CrossRef] [PubMed]
92. Feng, J.; Zhang, Z.; Wallace, M.B.; Stafford, J.A.; Kaldor, S.W.; Kassel, D.B.; Navre, M.; Shi, L.; Skene, R.J.; Asakawa, T.; et al. Discovery of alogliptin: A potent, selective, bioavailable, and efficacious inhibitor of dipeptidyl peptidase IV. *J. Med. Chem.* **2007**, *50*, 2297–2300. [CrossRef]

Disclaimer/Publisher's Note: The statements, opinions and data contained in all publications are solely those of the individual author(s) and contributor(s) and not of MDPI and/or the editor(s). MDPI and/or the editor(s) disclaim responsibility for any injury to people or property resulting from any ideas, methods, instructions or products referred to in the content.

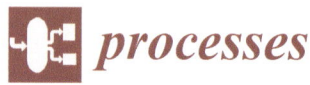 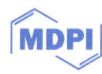

Article

Novel Betulin-1,2,4-Triazole Derivatives Promote In Vitro Dose-Dependent Anticancer Cytotoxicity

Alexandra Prodea [1,2], Andreea Milan [1,2], Marius Mioc [1,2], Alexandra Mioc [2,3], Camelia Oprean [4,5], Roxana Racoviceanu [1,2], Roxana Negrea-Ghiulai [2,3], Gabriel Mardale [2,3], Ștefana Avram [2,6], Mihaela Balan-Porcărașu [7,*], Slavița Rotunjanu [2,3], Cristina Trandafirescu [1,2], Irina Șoica [8] and Codruța Șoica [2,3]

[1] Department of Pharmaceutical Chemistry, Faculty of Pharmacy, Victor Babes University of Medicine and Pharmacy, Eftimie Murgu Square, No. 2, 300041 Timișoara, Romania; alexandra.ulici@umft.ro (A.P.); andreea.milan@umft.ro (A.M.); marius.mioc@umft.ro (M.M.); babuta.roxana@umft.ro (R.R.); trandafirescu.cristina@umft.ro (C.T.)

[2] Research Centre for Pharmaco-Toxicological Evaluation, Victor Babes University of Medicine and Pharmacy, Eftimie Murgu Square, No. 2, 300041 Timișoara, Romania; alexandra.mioc@umft.ro (A.M.); roxana.ghiulai@umft.ro (R.N.-G.); mardale.gabriel@umft.ro (G.M.); stefana.avram@umft.ro (Ș.A.); slavita.rotunjanu@umft.ro (S.R.); codrutasoica@umft.ro (C.Ș.)

[3] Department of Pharmacology-Pharmacotherapy, Faculty of Pharmacy, Victor Babes University of Medicine and Pharmacy, Eftimie Murgu Square, No. 2, 300041 Timișoara, Romania

[4] Department of Drug Analysis, Environmental Chemistry, Hygiene and Nutrition, Faculty of Pharmacy, Victor Babes University of Medicine and Pharmacy, Eftimie Murgu Square, No. 2, 300041 Timișoara, Romania; camelia.oprean@umft.ro

[5] Department of Chemistry and Toxicology, OncoGen Centre, County Hospital 'Pius Branzeu', Blvd. Liviu Rebreanu 156, 300736 Timișoara, Romania

[6] Department of Pharmacognosy, Faculty of Pharmacy, Victor Babes University of Medicine and Pharmacy, 2nd Eftimie Murgu Sq., 300041 Timișoara, Romania

[7] Institute of Macromolecular Chemistry 'Petru Poni', 700487 Iasi, Romania

[8] Medical School, University College London, 74 Huntley St., London WC1E 6DE, UK; irina.soica.20@ucl.ac.uk

* Correspondence: mihaela.balan@icmpp.ro

Citation: Prodea, A.; Milan, A.; Mioc, M.; Mioc, A.; Oprean, C.; Racoviceanu, R.; Negrea-Ghiulai, R.; Mardale, G.; Avram, Ș.; Balan-Porcărașu, M.; et al. Novel Betulin-1,2,4-Triazole Derivatives Promote In Vitro Dose-Dependent Anticancer Cytotoxicity. Processes 2024, 12, 24. https://doi.org/10.3390/pr12010024

Academic Editors: Alina Bora and Luminita Crisan

Received: 28 November 2023
Revised: 19 December 2023
Accepted: 20 December 2023
Published: 21 December 2023

Copyright: © 2023 by the authors. Licensee MDPI, Basel, Switzerland. This article is an open access article distributed under the terms and conditions of the Creative Commons Attribution (CC BY) license (https:// creativecommons.org/licenses/by/ 4.0/).

Abstract: Betulin is a birch bark-derived lupane-type pentacyclic triterpene with a wide spectrum of biological activities. Given their enhanced antiproliferative potential and enhanced pharmacological profile, betulin derivatives are continuously investigated in scientific studies. The objective of the current study was to in vitro assess the antiproliferative properties of novel synthesized 1,2,4-triazole derivatives of diacetyl betulin. The compounds were investigated using three cancer cell lines: A375 (melanoma), MCF-7 (breast cancer), HT-29 (colorectal cancer), and HaCaT (human keratinocytes). Bet-TZ1 had the lowest recorded IC_{50} values (ranging from 22.41 to 46.92 μM after 48 h of exposure) than its precursor and other tested compounds in every scenario, with the highest cytotoxicity against the A375 cell line. Bet-TZ3 demonstrated comparable cytotoxicity to the previously mentioned compound, with an IC_{50} of 34.34 μM against A375. Both compounds caused apoptosis in tested cells, by inducing specific nuclear morphological changes and by increasing the expression of caspase 9, indicating significant cytotoxicity, which was consistent with the literature and viability evaluation. Bet-TZ1 and Bet-TZ3 inhibit cancer cell migration, with the former having a stronger effect than the latter. The HET−CAM test indicated that all compounds have no irritative potential, suggesting that they can be used locally.

Keywords: triazole derivatives; betulin; cytotoxicity; melanoma; colorectal cancer; breast cancer

1. Introduction

The structural diversity and the high number of phytocompounds found in nature have always exceeded the representatives found in the synthetic libraries developed by chemists. As a consequence, several phytocompounds with therapeutic effects, such as morphine, codeine, and artemisinin, among many others, have been successfully used in therapy [1]. In particular, approximately 50% of all approved anticancer drugs since the 1940s originated from natural compounds; they act through a wide range of mechanisms involving a variety of molecular targets and signaling pathways [2]. Simultaneously, organic synthesis has produced an array of small molecules with cytotoxic properties that are currently used as systemic chemotherapy; unfortunately, this approach comes with severe side effects due to non-selective cytotoxicity, multidrug resistance, and high risk of cancer relapse [3]. Finding new therapeutic alternatives is therefore critical in cancer management in order to improve the therapeutic outcome and the patient's life quality as well; a promising solution to such challenges is the continuous investigation of phytocompounds which may come with increased efficacy and milder side effects [4,5]. Despite many phytocompounds displaying clear therapeutic potential, their application is currently limited by their innate physico-chemical properties and toxicity [6].

Betulin (Bet; lup-20(29)-ene-3b,28-diol) is a lupane-derived pentacyclic triterpene isolated predominantly from the birch bark [7]. Bet has numerous documented biological activities including anticancer, anti-inflammatory, and anti-HIV [8]; these effects were attributed to the modulation of several signaling pathways such as NF-kB (Nuclear factor kappa-light-chain-enhancer of activated B cells), Nrf-2 (Nuclear factor erythroid 2-related factor 2), and COX-2 (cyclooxygenase-2) [9]. The anticancer effect of Bet, in particular, has been explained through cell viability and angiogenesis inhibition, cell migration suppression, and cell cycle arrest in the G_0/G_1 phase [10]. As the structure of Bet consists of four six-membered rings, an additional five-membered ring, one isopropenyl group at C_{19}, and two hydroxyl groups at C_3 and C_{28} [11], the compound exhibits high lipophilicity which greatly reduces its bioavailability [12]. A frequently employed strategy in drug development combines the potential of phytocompounds with the advantages of chemical derivatization with the resulting semisynthetic compounds usually displaying enhanced selectivity and biological activity as well as improved pharmacokinetic properties [13]. For betulin, its complex structure allows for various modifications in different positions, such as C_3 [14], C_{28} [15], C_{30} [16], and ring A [17] (Figure 1) that may result in semisynthetic derivatives with optimized pharmacological profiles.

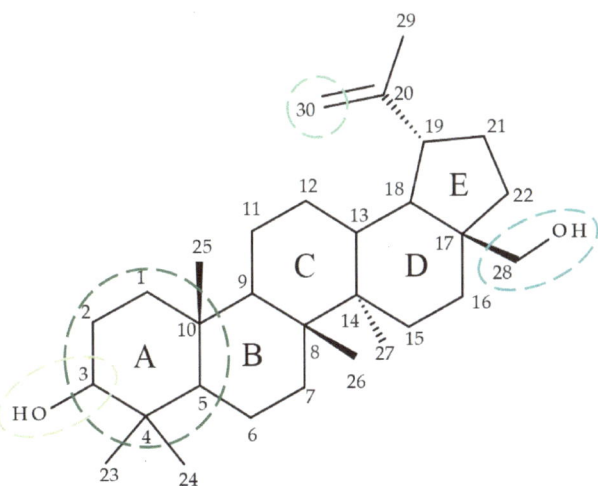

Figure 1. Target positions frequently employed for betulin derivatization.

Currently, heterocyclic scaffolds are included in the structure of more than 85% of the approved drugs, with the majority being represented by nitrogen-containing heterocycles, such as triazoles [18]. Triazoles are five-membered heterocycles that can be divided given the position of the two nitrogen atoms into two isomers, 1,2,3-triazoles and 1,2,4-triazoles [19]. They have been extensively used in drug design as they increase the stability of molecules, and can act as linkers [20] and bioisosteres of amide bonds [21]. Additionally, both isomers are highly water soluble and, together with their derivatives, display a wide spectrum of biological properties including anticancer, antioxidative, and anti-inflammatory [22].

As an example, this approach was previously used to develop novel Bet-1,2,3-triazole derivatives with improved cytotoxicity against human ductal carcinoma (T47D), human adenocarcinoma (MCF-7), and glioblastoma (SNB-19) cell lines [23]. Considering the intrinsic limitations of betulin as a therapeutic agent, such as low bioavailability, as well as the advantages provided by triazoles in terms of pharmacological effects, the synthesis of **Bet-triazoles** derivatives should lead to a significant improvement in the pharmacologic potential of the unmodified compound.

The current study expands on the synthesis of diacetylbetulin derivatives containing a 5-substituted-1,2,4-TZ at C_{30} (**Bet-TZ1-4**) followed by their cytotoxicity assessment in several cancer cells such as melanoma (A375), breast cancer (MCF-7), and colorectal cancer (HT-29) as well as in human keratinocytes (HaCaT). A preliminary toxicity assessment was conducted through HET−CAM assay regarding their irritant potential.

2. Results

2.1. Chemistry

Figure 2 depicts the synthetic route as well as the reaction conditions required to synthesize betulin-triazole derivatives (**Bet-TZ1-4**). By using slightly modified methods previously reported [24], high yields (above 50%) of triazole derivatives (**TZ1-4**) and brominated diacetyl-betulin (**Br-Bet**) were obtained. The subsequent alkylation of the SH group on the triazole ring (**TZ1-4**) with **Br-Bet** in dimethylformamide (DMF)/K_2CO_3 produced moderate yields (32–41%) of betulin-triazole derivatives (**Bet-TZ1-4**). Despite the purity of the precursors, TLC examination revealed that the reaction produced additional lipophilic side products that were easily separated by column chromatography using $CHCl_3$:ethyl acetate 1:1 as eluent for **Bet-TZ2-4** or $CHCl_3$:ethyl acetate 2:1 for **Bet-TZ1**, due to the significant Rf value differences. During TLC (thin layer chromatography) analysis, there was also an additional spot of low intensity above the reference spot for each compound. This spot migrated with the main one, regardless of the eluents used. As a result, after separation by column chromatography, only fractions with a faint trace were retained, resulting in yield values below 50%. Following NMR (nuclear magnetic resonance) tests, it was discovered that the respective spot corresponds to a tautomer. As a result, if it was previously known that this tautomerism occurs, all the discarded fractions containing the tautomer would have been kept, producing compounds with higher yields. All synthesized compounds' structures were confirmed using ^1H, ^{13}C NMR, and FTIR spectroscopy. All spectral results are available in the Supplementary Materials section of the manuscript.

The deacetylation of Bet was successful and its ^1H and ^{13}C NMR spectra confirm the structure according to the existing literature [25]. Moreover, the bromination of diacetyl-Bet (**Br-Bet**) led to a mixture of allylic and vinylic bromine derivatives, as previously reported in the literature [26]. The ^1H NMR spectra of **Bet-TZ1-4** show the peaks for the betulin scaffold in the 5.1–0.6 ppm region. The peaks for C(30)H_2, C(29)H_2, and H3 from the betulin backbone resonate at about 3.8 ppm, 4.9–5.0 ppm, and 4.3–4.4 ppm, respectively. Their integral ratio is 2:2:1, suggesting that only the allylic bromine derivative reacted with the triazole derivatives.

When analyzing the aromatic region corresponding to the ^1H NMR spectra for **Bet-TZ1-4**, where the protons of the triazole derivatives resonate, we observed that the peaks were doubled, but if integrated, the integral values were in appropriate ratios compared to the protons from Bet. We attributed this behavior to the existence of a slow exchange tautomeric equilibrium that can occur in 3,5-disubstituted 1,2,4-triazoles [27,28]. Out of the three tautomeric forms possible, two tautomers with long enough stability to be individually detected by NMR spectroscopy were observed (Table 1).

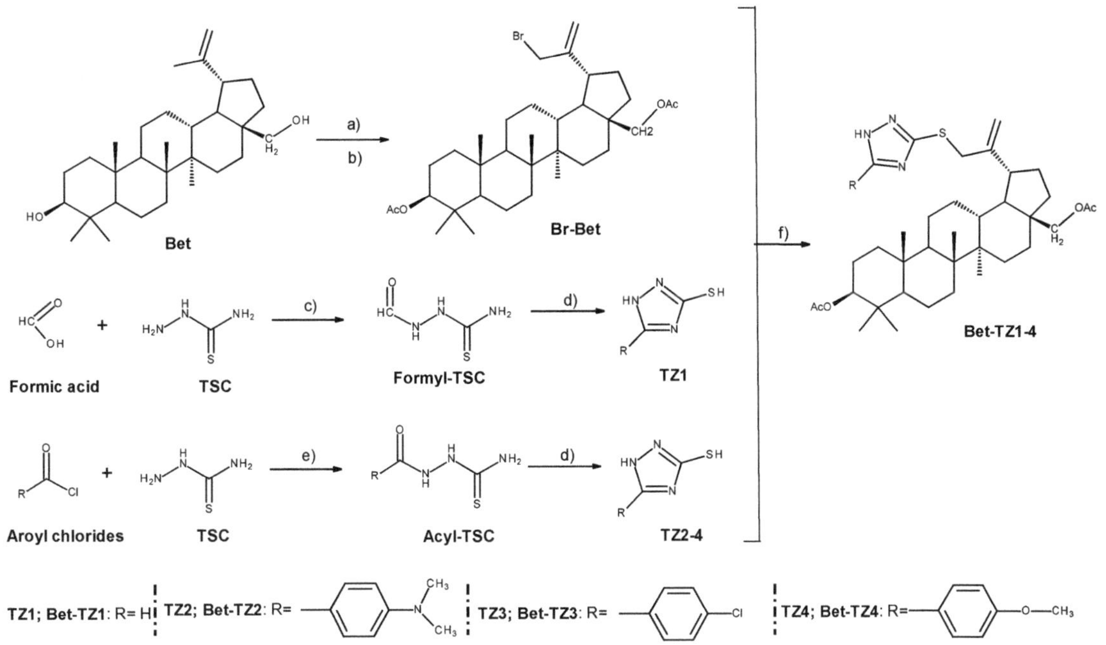

Figure 2. Synthesis of betulin-triazole derivatives (**Bet-TZ1**₋₄); Bet (betulin); Br-Bet (3,28-O-diacetyl-30-bromo-betulin); TSC (thiosemicarbazide); **TZ1** (1H-1,2,4-triazole-3-thiol); **TZ2** (5-[4-(dimethylamino) phenyl]-1H-1,2,4-triazole-3-thiol); **TZ3** (5-(4-chlorophenyl)-1H-1,2,4-triazole-3-thiol); **TZ4** (5-(4-methoxyphenyl)-1H-1,2,4-triazole-3-thiol); **Bet-TZ1** 3,28-O-diacetyl-30-(1H-1,2,4-triazole-3-yl-sulfanyl)-betulin); **Bet-TZ2** (3,28-O-diacetyl-30-{5-[4-(dimethylamino) phenyl]-1H-1,2,4-triazole-3-yl-sulfanyl}-betulin); **Bet-TZ3** (3,28-O-diacetyl-30-[5-(4-chlorophenyl)-1H-1,2,4-triazole-3-yl-sulfanyl]-betulin); **Bet-TZ4** (3,28-O-diacetyl-30-[5-(4-methoxyphenyl)-1H-1,2,4-triazole-3-yl-sulfanyl]-betulin). Reaction conditions: (**a**) acetic anhydride, pyridine, DMAP, r.t., 12 h; (**b**) NBS, CCl₄, r.t., 48 h; (**c**) reflux, 30 min; (**d**) H₂O, NaOH, reflux, 1 h; (**e**) pyridine/DMF, 1 h, 50 °C; (**f**) DMF, K₂CO₃, r.t., 72 h.

Table 1. Percentage of triazole tautomers, as calculated from the ^{1}H NMR integral values for the H36 peaks (**Bet-TZ1**) or the NH peaks (**Bet-TZ2-4**).

Compound	Bet-TZ1	Bet-TZ2	Bet-TZ3	Bet-TZ4
Tautomer percentage	25%	19%	41%	26%
	75%	81%	59%	74%

In order to prove beyond any doubt that the doubling of the triazole derivative peaks is due to the existence of a tautomeric equilibrium, to each solution of **Bet-TZ1-4** in DMSO-d₆, for which the initial experiments were recorded, we added a drop of trifluoroacetic acid (TFA) and then recorded all the NMR spectra again. Adding TFA speeded up the tautomeric equilibrium leading to a fast exchange system and the NMR spectra show only one set of peaks for the triazole derivatives in appropriate integral ratios compared to the protons from Bet.

The ^{13}C NMR spectra of **Bet-TZ1-4** show broad peaks for C19 (44–45 ppm), C20 (149–150 ppm), C29 (110–112 ppm), and C30 (35–36 ppm) of the Bet residue. The H, C-HMBC spectra of **Bet-TZ2-4** show long range correlation peaks, over three bonds, between the triazole's C35 and H30 from betulin (Figures S10, S16, S22 and S28), proving that the reactions took place. The complete assignment of the peaks is given in the experimental section and all the 1D and 2D NMR spectra are available in the Supporting Information. In the case of **Bet-TZ2**, where the two tautomeric forms are almost in a 1:1 ratio, we can observe peaks (broad) for C36 and C35 from each isomer (Figure 3) and doubled peaks for the carbons of the p-chlorophenyl residue for C20 and C29. After adding TFA, we can observe that the peaks are no longer doubled and are noticeably narrower.

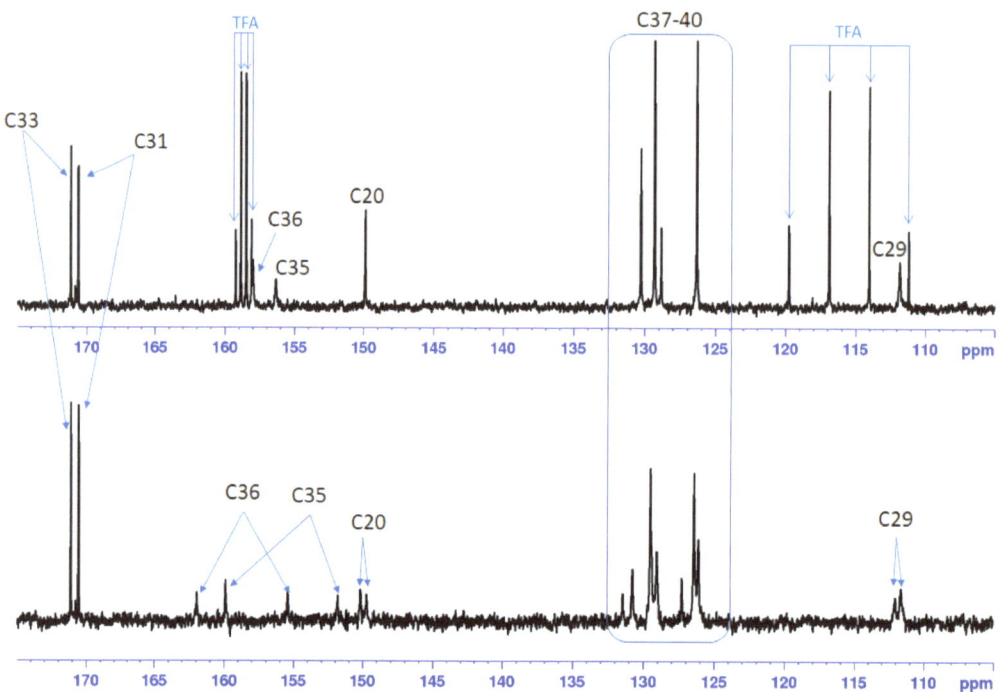

Figure 3. ^{13}C NMR spectra (175–105 ppm region) of **Bet-TZ3** in DMSO-d_6 (bottom) and in DMSO-d_6 with one drop of TFA (top) indicating the loss of signals corresponding to the tautomer form after acid addition.

2.2. Evaluation of Diacetylbetulin Derivatives Cytotoxic Effect

The viability of HaCaT, A375, MCF-7, and HT-29 cells, after a 48-h treatment period with the novel synthesized compounds (10, 25, 50, 75, and 100 µM), was assessed using the Alamar blue assay. Incubation of HaCaT cells with the tested compounds revealed significant inhibition of cell viability at 48 h after **Bet-TZ1** was used in the highest concentrations (100 and 75 µM). This inhibitory effect at 48 h was stronger compared to the effect of 5-FU (positive control) and to the parent compound (Bet) at the corresponding concentrations, as follows: 9.44 ± 6.90% (**Bet-TZ1** 100 µM) and 14.76 ± 9.84% (**Bet-TZ1** 75 µM) vs. 21.57 ± 14.62% (5-FU 100 µM), 27.25 ± 14.90% (5-FU 75 µM), (42.00 ± 7.79% Bet 100 µM) (46.26 ± 7.64% Bet 75 µM) (Figure 4A). A 48-h incubation of A375 cells with 100, 75, and 50 µM **Bet-TZ1** and **Bet-TZ3** promoted a significant reduction of cell viability in a concentration-dependent manner vs. Bet, as follows: 1.22 ± 1.09%, 3.83 ± 2.68%, 19.78 ± 7.36% (**Bet-TZ1**), 22.78 ± 18.44%, 29.65 ± 8.98%, 35.58 ± 6.92% (**Bet-TZ3**) vs. 17.04 ± 1.71%, 30.83 ± 9.01%, 45.64 ± 10.63% (**Bet**) (Figure 4B). **Bet-TZ1** also produced a cytotoxic effect on MCF-7 cells at 100, 75, and 50 µM (1.73 ± 5.48%, 16.47 ± 8.93%, 27.85 ± 5.74%) compared to Bet alone (42.78 ± 6.47%, 47.54 ± 7.00%, 48.92 ± 5.05%) (Figure 4C). The other tested compounds did not influence the cell viability of HaCaT, A375, MCF-7, and HT-29 in a statistically significant manner.

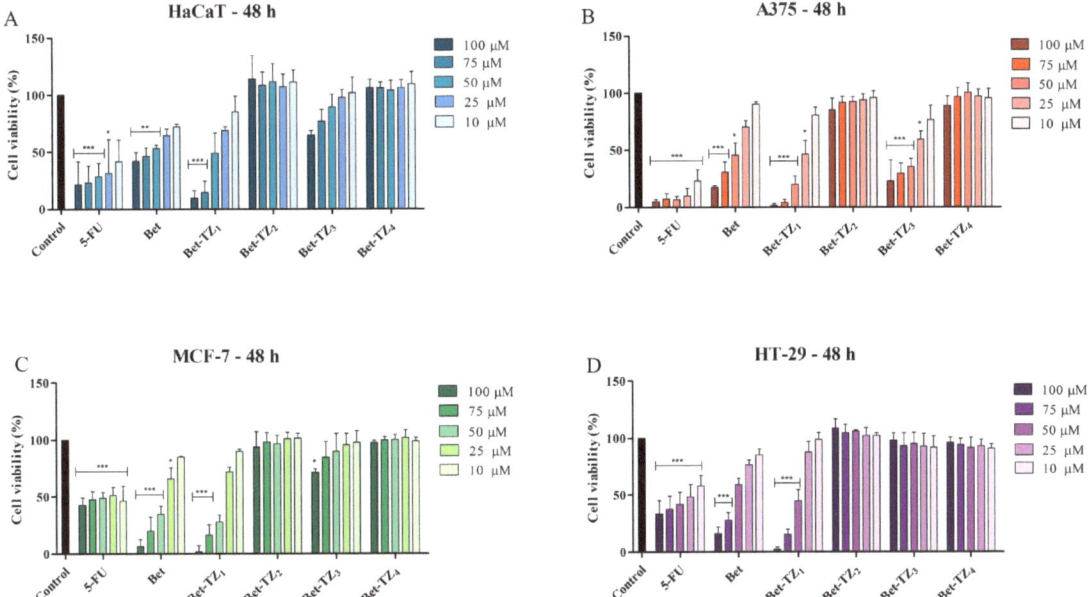

Figure 4. Cell viability after 48-h treatment with 5-FU, Bet, **Bet-TZ1-4** (100, 75, 50, 25, and 10 μM) of HaCaT (**A**), A375 (**B**), MCF-7 (**C**), and HT-29 (**D**) cells. The results represent viability percentages compared to the control group, considered 100% (* $p < 0.05$, ** $p < 0.01$, and *** $p < 0.001$). The results represent the mean values ± SD of three separate experiments executed in triplicate.

Table 2 presents the calculated IC_{50} values (μM) after 48-h treatment with 5-FU, Bet, **Bet-TZ1**, and **Bet-TZ3** on HaCaT, A375, MCF-7, and HT-29 cell lines.

Table 2. The calculated IC_{50} values (μM) of 5-FU, Bet, **Bet-TZ1**, and **Bet-TZ3** on HaCaT, A375, MCF-7, and HT-29 cell lines; the compounds deemed ineffective have IC_{50} values above 100 μM.

	5-FU	Bet	Bet-TZ1	Bet-TZ3
	48 h	48 h	48 h	48 h
HaCaT	15.25	60.75	42.52	>100
A375	1.06	46.19	22.41	34.34
MCF-7	38.01	37.29	33.52	>100
HT-29	29.80	55.67	46.92	>100

2.3. Diacetylbetulin Derivatives Effect on Cell Morphology

In HaCaT cells, no significant morphological changes were recorded in terms of confluence and aspect between the control group and the **Bet**, **Bet-TZ2**, **Bet-TZ3**, and **Bet-TZ4**-treated cells. However, **Bet-TZ1** treatment decreased the number of cells, rendering them rounder and detached, in a similar manner to the 5-FU positive control (Figure 5). In A375 cells, treatment with both **Bet-TZ1** and **Bet-TZ3**, respectively, at their IC_{50} induced morphological changes (rounder and detached cells) and a decreased number of cells, in agreement with the results of cell viability testing (Figure 5).

Treatment with **Bet-TZ1** (IC_{50}) induced similar changes in MCF-7 and HT-29 cells, in terms of number and cell morphology, changes comparable to those caused by 5-FU used as a positive control (Figure 6).

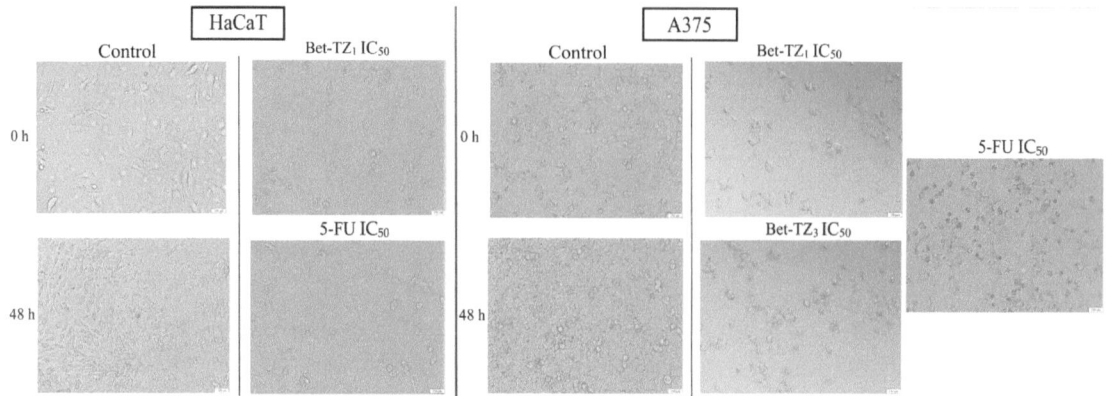

Figure 5. The evaluation of morphological changes of HaCaT and A375 cells after a 48-h treatment with **Bet-TZ1**, **Bet-TZ3**, and 5-FU (IC$_{50}$); the scale bar was 150 µm.

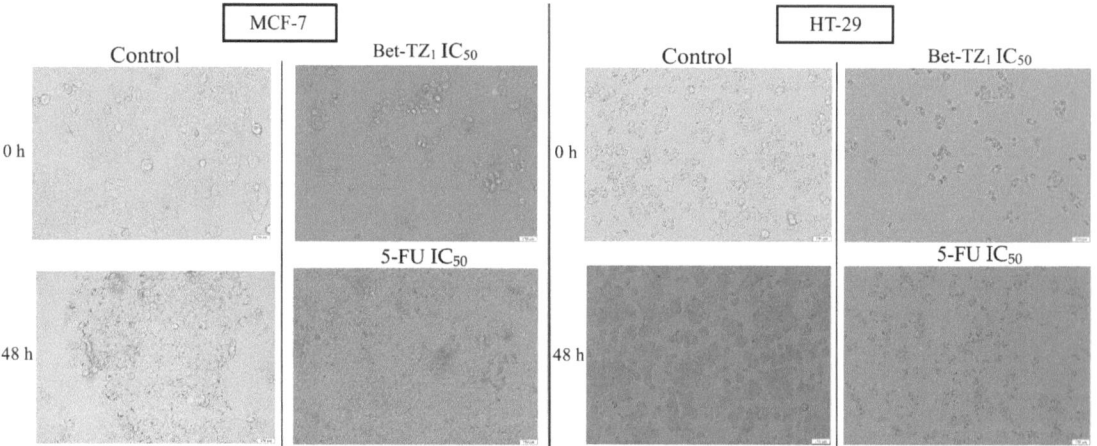

Figure 6. The evaluation of morphological changes of MCF-7 and HT-29 cells after 48-h treatment with **Bet-TZ1** and 5-FU (IC$_{50}$); the scale bar was 150 µm.

The cells' cytoskeleton and nuclei undergo characteristic morphological changes during apoptosis. To determine whether the cytotoxic effects recorded in HaCaT, A375, MCF-7, and HT-29 cells after a 48-h treatment with **Bet-TZ1** (IC$_{50}$) and **Bet-TZ3** (IC$_{50}$—A375 and 100 µM—MCF-7 and HT-29), respectively, occurred as a result of apoptotic cell death induction, cells' nuclei were stained with Hoechst solution, while the cytoskeleton was labeled with beta-tubulin antibody and Alexa fluor 488. Treatment with both **Bet-TZ1** and **Bet-TZ3**, respectively, induced morphological changes in A375 cells that are consistent with apoptosis. Specific observed hallmarks included small and bright nuclei indicative of nuclear condensation, nuclear fragmentation, and small, round-shaped cells whose membrane start to disorganize, thus leading to the formation of apoptotic bodies (Figure 7). In contrast, the necrotic cell death induced by staurosporine used as a positive control was mainly accompanied by morphological changes of the cell shape that occur due to cell membrane disruption (Figure 7).

Similar morphological changes, consistent with apoptosis, occurred in HaCaT, MCF-7, and HT-29 cell lines, after treatment with **Bet-TZ1** (IC$_{50}$) (Figure 8).

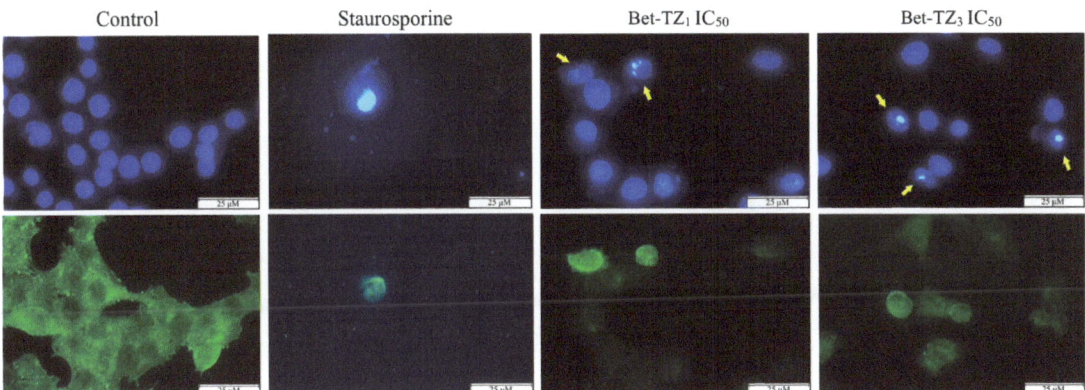

Figure 7. The impact of 48-h treatment with **Bet-TZ1** and **Bet-TZ3** (IC$_{50}$) on A375 nuclei; blue—Hoechst staining was used for the nuclei while beta-tubulin—green staining—was used to highlight the cytoskeleton. Staurosporine (5 μM) was used as a control (positive) for necrotic cell death. The scale bar was 50 μm. Yellow arrows indicate specific apoptotic-related morphological changes.

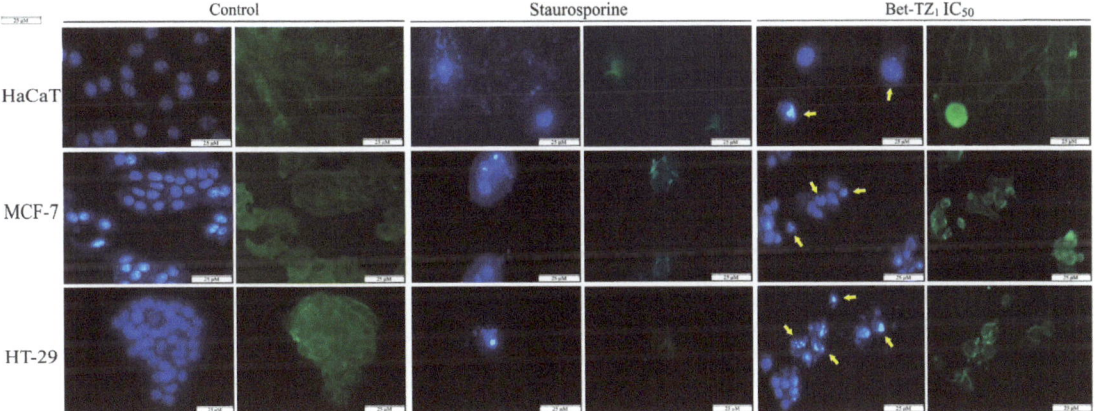

Figure 8. The impact of a 48-h treatment with **Bet-TZ1** (IC$_{50}$) on HaCaT, MCF-7, and HT-29 nuclei; blue—Hoechst staining was used for the nuclei while beta-tubulin—green staining—was used to highlight the cytoskeleton. The effect of staurosporine (5 μM) was recorded as a control (positive) for necrotic cell death. The scale bar was 50 μm. Yellow arrows indicate specific apoptotic-related morphological changes.

2.4. Real-Time PCR Quantification of Apoptotic Markers

To further establish the proapoptotic effect of **Bet-TZ1** and **Bet-TZ3**, RT-PCR (reverse transcription polymerase chain reaction) was employed to quantify caspase 9 expression in all three **Bet-TZ1**-treated cell lines, and the A375 cell line treated with **Bet-TZ3**, at a sub-cytotoxic concentration (10 μM). Betulin increased caspase 9 expression in all treated cells, according to the results (Figure 9). **Bet-TZ1** and **Bet-TZ3** both promote caspase 9 expression in the A375 cell line, outperforming their parent compound, with **Bet-TZ1** being the most active. This scenario also occurs in the MCF-7 and HT-29 cell lines, where **Bet-TZ1** increases caspase 9 expression compared to both control and Bet.

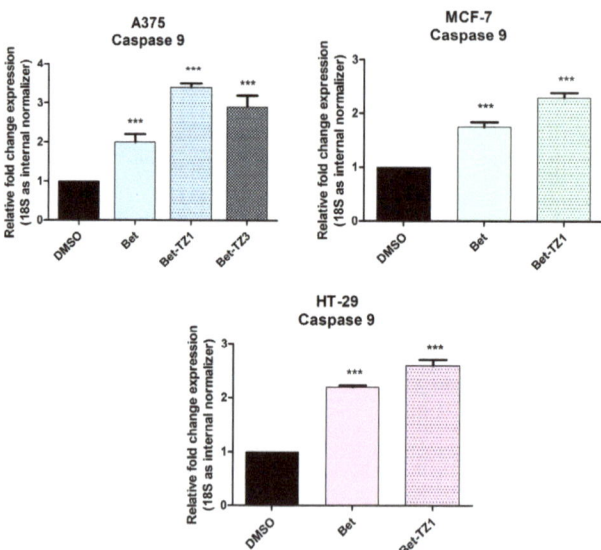

Figure 9. The recorded fold change expression in mRNA of caspase 9 in cells treated with a 10 µM concentration of Bet, **Bet-TZ1** (A375, MCF-7, HT-29), and **Bet-TZ3** showing an increase in caspase 9 expression as a result of compound stimulation of cancer cells. The results were normalized to 18 S and DMSO was used as control. Data represent the mean values ± SD of three separate experiments. One-way ANOVA with Dunnett's post hoc test was applied to determine the statistical differences compared to control (*** $p < 0.001$).

2.5. Scratch Assay

The antimigratory potential on HaCaT, A375, HT-29, and MCF-7 was assessed after 48-h treatment with **Bet-TZ1** at 10 µM (Figures 10–13) and on HaCaT and A375 after 48-h treatment with **Bet-TZ3** at 10 µM (Figures 10 and 11).

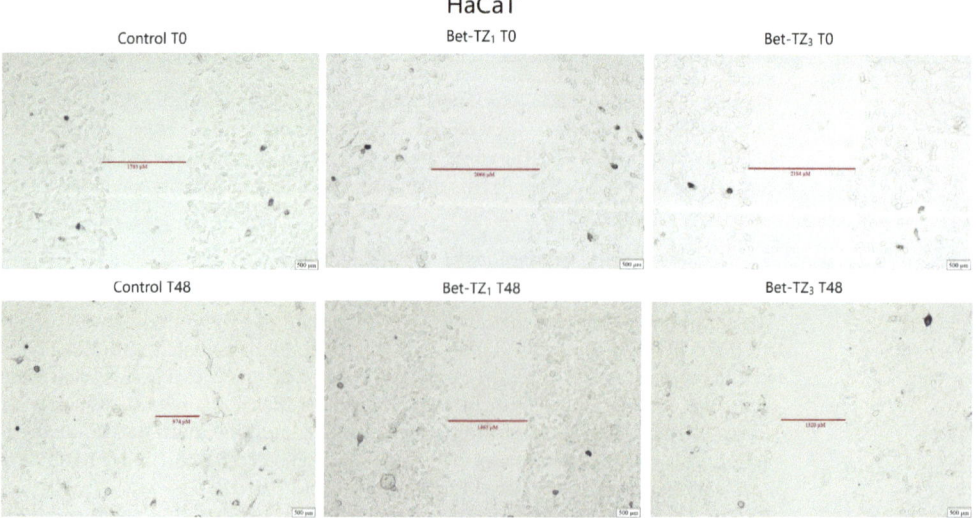

Figure 10. The effects of **Bet-TZ1** (10 µM) and **Bet-TZ3** (10 µM) on immortalized human keratinocytes' HaCaT migration capacity. Cell migration was measured at 0 h and 48 h after stimulation, indicating that the tested compounds reduced the scratch closure time when compared to untreated cells used (control).

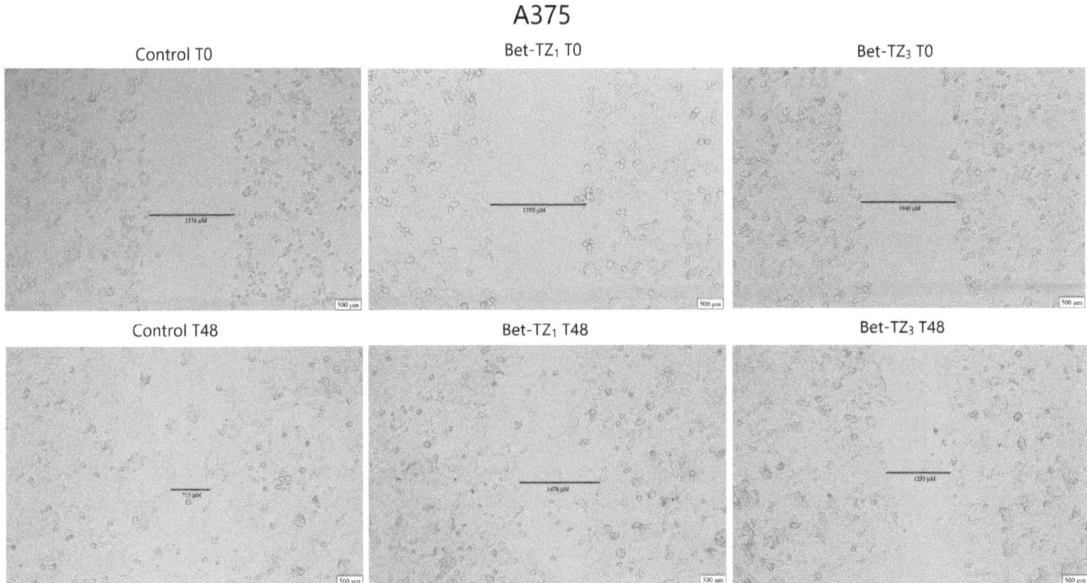

Figure 11. The effects of **Bet-TZ1** (10 µM) and **Bet-TZ3** (10 µM) on malignant melanoma cells' A375 migration capacity. Cell migration was measured at 0 h and 48 h after stimulation, indicating that the tested compounds reduced the scratch closure time when compared to untreated cells (control).

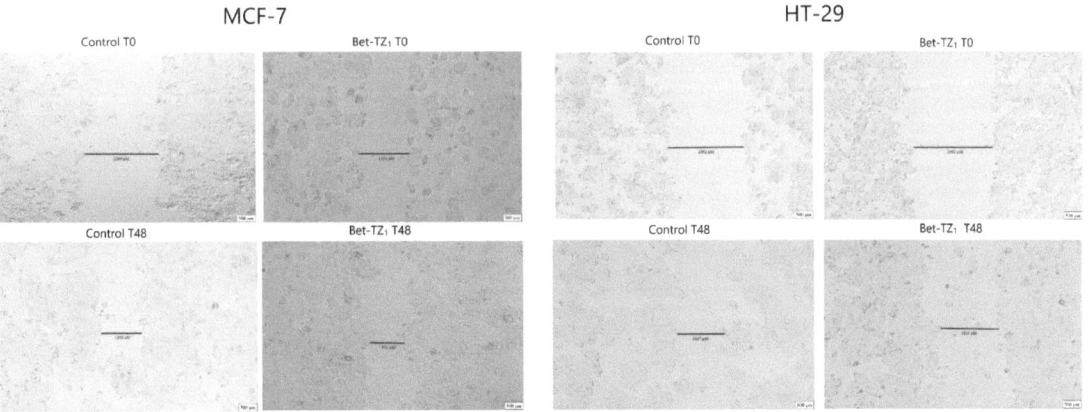

Figure 12. The effects of **Bet-TZ1** (10 µM) on breast cancer cells' MCF-7 and HT-29 migration capacity. Cell migration was measured at 0 h and 48 h after stimulation, indicating that the tested compounds reduced the scratch closure time when compared to untreated cells (controls).

Both **Bet-TZ1** and **Bet-TZ3** exhibited lower scratch closure rates for HaCaT and A375 cells (57.03% and 78.54%—HaCaT; 28.74% and 61.83%—A375) vs. control (100%), while **Bet-TZ1** expressed lower scratch closure rates compared to **Bet-TZ3** on both HaCaT and A375 cells (Figure 12). **Bet-TZ1** decreased the scratch closure area also on MCF-7 and HT-29 cells, as follows: 85.13% and 64.91% vs. control (100%) (Figure 12).

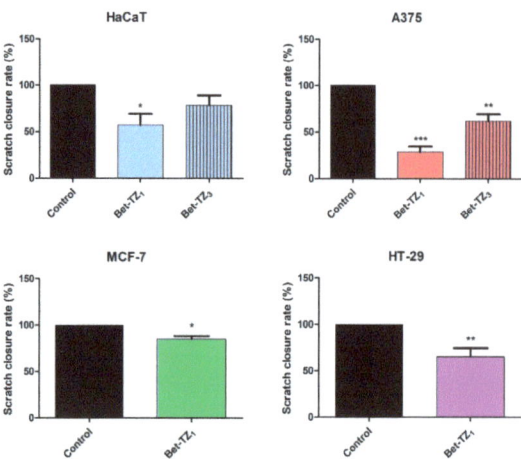

Figure 13. Scratch migration assay of **Bet-TZ1** (10 µM) on HaCaT, A375, MCF-7, and HT-29 cells and of **Bet-TZ3** (10 µM) on HaCaT and A375 cells. The presented values signify the remanent gap size 48 h post treatment and were calculated as a percentage of the initial gap size used as control (100%). Results are recorded as the mean values ± SD by one-way ANOVA test, followed by a Dunnett's post hoc test (for HaCaT and A375 cells) and with unpaired t-test (for MCF-7 and HT-29 cells). (*** $p < 0.001$, ** $p < 0.01$, and * $p < 0.05$).

2.6. HET−CAM Test

The HET−CAM test was used to assess the irritative potential of **Bet** and **Bet-TZ1-4**. By monitoring the effects induced 24 h after the application of 300 µL of each sample one can notice that **Bet** and **Bet-TZ2-4** did not produce any interference with the circulation process; by contrast, **Bet-TZ1** triggered some localized spotted hemorrhages, without influencing the embryo's viability (Figure 14).

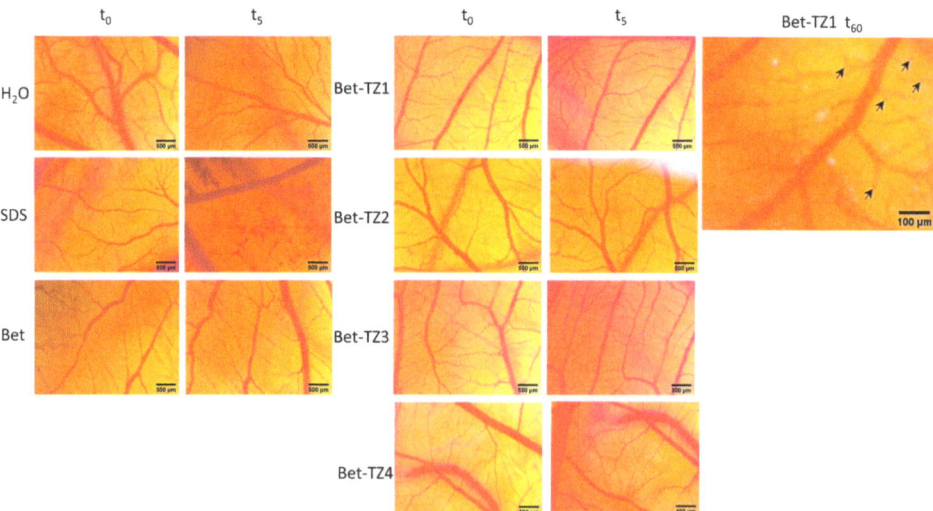

Figure 14. The HET−CAM method-based irritation test. Stereomicroscope images of the chorioallantoic membrane were captured before (T_0), 300 s (T_5) post treatment with 300 µL **Bet** and **Bet-TZ1-4**, respectively (tested at 100 µM), and after 24 h for **Bet-TZ1** indicating localized spotted hemorrhages (indicated by black arrows), without influencing the embryo's viability; distilled water and sodium dodecylsulfate (SDS) 0.5%, were used as negative and positive control, respectively. Scale bars were set at 500 µm.

The irritation potential of each compound was investigated by using the Luepke scale [29] which assigns scores ranging from 0 to 21 based on the degree of severity of the reaction of the chorioallantoic membrane. Non-irritant compounds are classified within the range of 0 to 0.9; slight irritation is indicated by scores between 1 and 4.9; moderate irritation is depicted by scores ranging from 5 to 8.9 and strongly irritant compounds are assigned scores between 9 and 21. According to the findings in Table 3, the compounds under investigation did not exhibit any signs of irritation, indicating that they are appropriate for both mucosal and cutaneous applications.

Table 3. The irritation factor for Bet and **Bet-TZ1-4**.

Samples	IF	Effect
H_2O	0	No irritation
SDS	16.29 ± 0.23	Severe irritation
Bet	0	No irritation
Bet-TZ1	0	No irritation
Bet-TZ2	0	No irritation
Bet-TZ3	0	No irritation
Bet-TZ4	0	No irritation

3. Discussion

Bet is the main triterpene isolated from the outer bark of *Betula* species, which possesses tremendous therapeutic potential [30]. Chemical modulation of key positions in betulin's molecule allowed the synthesis of various derivatives with improved pharmacological profile. The 1,2,4-triazole and its derivatives are common heterocycles found in the structure of various drugs due to their innate physicochemical properties such as dipole character, rigidity, and the capacity to form hydrogen bonds, which provide them with a suitable pharmacological profile [31,32]. The use of 1,2,4-triazoles as linkers [33] or pharmacophores [34–36] in the structure of various triterpenes has been previously reported in the literature; however, to the best of our knowledge, this study represents the first report regarding the introduction of 5-substituted-1,2,4-triazole-3-thiols to the C_{30} position of Bet. An interesting property of azoles is the annular tautomerism where the proton linked to a heteroatom can migrate to other heteroatoms within the heterocycle [37]; thus, the 1,2,4-triazoles can be found in three tautomeric forms, namely, 1H-, 2H-, and 4H-1,2,4-triazoles. Although, in general, the 1H tautomer was considered the only stable tautomer in solution, some derivatives, such as 3(5)-chloro-1,2,4-triazole and 3(5)-bromo-1,2,4-triazole, were identified as 4H tautomers in solution, contradicting the previous knowledge on the topic [38]. Currently, the effect of different tautomers on the biological effect is not clearly understood. The impact of one sole tautomer on the therapeutic properties of that compound is always dependent on the duration of the tautomeric equilibrium in relation to a given biological process. On one hand, the rapid interconversion of tautomers in relation to a certain biological process can lead to both forms being consumed. On the other hand, slow interconversion in a similar setting could end up in one tautomer being favored as the only active species [39]. Therefore they might induce a different impact on the biological effect, as some tautomers can be rapidly interchanged into the most favorable form to interact with the target while slow interconversion of others could result in the existence of a single active tautomer [40]. We established that all **Bet-TZ1-4** compounds exist in DMSO solutions in two stable forms in various percentages, as detected through ^{1}H NMR spectroscopy, with one major component (59% to 81%) that we hypothesize is responsible for the anticancer effect. However, because we have not identified a specific protein target for our compounds, we cannot determine which tautomer is responsible for the biological effect. To visualize the exact tautomer form in the binding site, a highly precise crystallographic analysis of the target–ligand complex would be required.

The **Bet-TZ1-4** cytotoxicity was assessed against HaCaT (human keratinocytes), A375 (melanoma), MCF-7 (breast cancer), and HT-29 (colorectal cancer) cell lines using the Alamar blue assay. The results in HaCaT cells showed that **Bet-TZ2-4** semisynthetic derivatives significantly inhibit cell viability even at the highest tested concentration (100 µM); however, when used in high concentrations (75 and 100 µM), **Bet-TZ1** significantly inhibited cell viability, compared to 5-FU used as a reference. These results indicate that **Bet-TZ2-4** does not cytotoxically affect non-malignant cells and can be administered in elevated doses without significant side effects; in contrast, **Bet-TZ1** exhibits clear cytotoxic effects against non-malignant keratinocytes. The selectivity index (SI) for **Bet-TZ1**, calculated as the IC_{50} HaCaT/IC_{50} cancer cell line, was less than 2 in all three cases (SI_{A375} 1.90, SI_{MCF-7} 1.27, and SI_{HT-29} 0.91), indicating non-selective cytotoxic activity. However, the use of only the selectivity index to assess the anticancer potential of a drug candidate has been shown to be a poor and insufficient predictor [41].

Shy et al. reported the synthesis of similar betulin derivatives only by using 1,2,3-triazole as a C30-substituent while maintaining the free C3-hydroxyl group; experimental results showed that all triazole derivatives exerted superior cytotoxic effects compared to the parent compound but the presence of large lipophilic aromatic side chains favored their bioactivity [42].

The cytotoxicity of **Bet-TZ1-4** against the melanoma cell line was similar or slightly enhanced compared to **Bet**. In particular, the effect of higher doses of **Bet-TZ1** (75 and 100 µM) against A375 was superior to **Bet** and even 5-FU; a dose-dependent cytotoxic effect was also recorded for **Bet-TZ3** after 48 h of exposure. In breast and colorectal cancer cells, the lowest dose of **Bet-TZ1** and **Bet-TZ3** (10 µM) and all samples of **Bet-TZ2** and **Bet-TZ4** showed inferior cytotoxicity compared with 5-FU and **Bet** alone; doses above 25 µM of **Bet-TZ1** and **Bet-TZ3** exhibited significantly stronger cytotoxic activity compared to Bet and 5-FU. In A375 cells, the IC_{50} values of **Bet-TZ1** and **Bet-TZ3** were 22.41 µM and 34.34 µM, compared to **Bet** alone (46.19 µM) and to 5-FU (1.06 µM). Intriguingly, despite a higher IC_{50} value on A375 cells, when compared to **Bet-TZ1**, **Bet-TZ3** can be viewed as a more effective agent due to the lack of cytotoxic effect on non-malignant HaCaT cells that reveals a selective cytotoxic effect against melanoma cells. In MCF-7 and HT-29 cells, **Bet-TZ3** was not active (IC_{50} > 100 µM) whereas **Bet-TZ1** had an IC_{50} of 33.52 µM and 46.92 µM, outperforming the parent-compound Bet (37.29 µM and 55.67 µM). Comparatively, the most active compounds were **Bet-TZ1**, in particular in higher concentrations, against all tested cell lines, and **Bet-TZ3** when used in A375 cells. While the unsubstituted triazole derivative was cytotoxic to both malignant and non-malignant cells, a substituted phenyl attached to the 5th position of the triazole ring reduced toxicity to non-malignant cells. **Bet-TZ3**, a p-chloro-phenyl triazole derivative of **Bet**, was more selective, being cytotoxic primarily to the A375 melanoma cell line. This case was previously encountered in a series of substituted 1,2,3-triazole derivatives of betulinic acid (linked to the triterpene in the same 28th position), with the p-fluoro-phenyl derivative being the most active compound [42]. It appears that p-halogeno-triazole groups linked at the allylic position of a lupane-type triterpene are beneficial for inducing in vitro cancer cell cytotoxicity. However, this hypothesis requires a larger compound series to be synthesized and tested in order to be validated. Considering these results, only these two compounds in concentrations equivalent to their IC_{50} values were further evaluated in terms of potential effect on cell morphology.

The induction of apoptosis is a well known cellular mechanism for Bet and other triterpenes [43], as well as their semisynthetic derivatives [44]. In the current study, a morphology assessment also showed that the newly synthesized betulin derivatives triggered apoptotic processes, identified as nuclei condensation and fragmentation which led to the formation of characteristic apoptotic bodies [45]. Apoptosis was also identified as the underlying mechanism for similar betulinic acid-triazole derivatives [34]; the authors established that large triazole substituents in the C30 position favorably influence the compound's cytotoxicity becoming an important element of the pharmacophore with the C3 substituent affecting its bioavailability. For betulinic acid derivatives, having two hydrophilic groups in C28 and C3 positions seemed to hinder cell membrane penetration, with acetylation of at least one such group being able to overcome this challenge. In this case, both hydroxylic groups in the C20 and C3 positions bear the lipophilic acetate moiety that apparently facilitates cell entrance. Our previous experiments on betulinic acid derivatives bearing 1,2,4-triazole scaffolds in the C30 position, together with acetylated C3-hydroxyl, supported such conclusions both in terms of the mechanism of action and the structure–activity relationships [46,47].

Betulin was also previously shown to trigger apoptosis in cancer cells via the intrinsic signaling pathway. However, unlike betulinic acid, **Bet** does not primarily affect the pro/anti-apoptotic protein (BAX, Bcl-2) normal ratio [48,49], but rather induces an upregulated/increased caspase activity [50,51]. Caspases 3 and 9 are key players in the onset of the intrinsic apoptotic pathway [52], and as stated above, are correlated with Bet pro-apoptotic activity. However, given the fact that MCF-7 is a caspase 3-deficient cell line [53], we proceeded to quantify the expression of caspase 9 in cell lines treated with Bet-TZ1 and **Bet-TZ3**, where a significant cytotoxic activity was recorded. As expected, Bet did increase the expression of caspase 9, but so did both **Bet** derivatives in each tested setting. There are currently no triazole-betulin derivatives tested for anti-apoptotic activity similar to the ones described in this study. However, previous studies reported that the synthesis of other types of betulin derivatives with various functional groups in positions 3, 28, or 30 has resulted in pro-apoptotic agents with increased caspase activity [54–56]. According to these findings, the increased expression of various caspases and the associated pro-apoptotic features appear to be more related to the triterpenic structural core than to the various functional groups present in their structure. As a result, future research focusing on additional **Bet** derivatizations may shed light on the big picture of betulin derivatives-induced apoptosis in cancer cells.

It has been shown that the migration of cancer cells is an important marker for tumor cell invasion and metastasis while inhibiting cell migration represents a strong and desirable quality for a potent anticancer agent [57]. The antimigratory effect of the leading compounds, **Bet-TZ1** and **Bet-TZ3**, was assessed in non-cancer and cancer cell lines; results revealed that although both compounds inhibit the migration of tested cells, the effect of **Bet-TZ1**, containing the unsubstituted 1,2,4-triazole, was superior to **Bet-TZ3**. The ability of the triterpene scaffold to prevent cancer cell migration was previously revealed for numerous betulin and betulinic acid derivatives displaying various chemical modulations in several cancer cell lines where the cytotoxic activity was clearly distinct from the anti-invasive capacity [58,59].

The HET–CAM assay represents a one of a kind model in biomedical testing since the chorioallantoic membrane provides a rich vascular network that enables a wide variety of non-invasive biological studies [60]. It is considered a better and more valid alternative to more invasive tests used to assess the local irritative potential of different substances, providing information regarding vascular events such as coagulation, hyperemia, and hemorrhage [61]. In our study, Bet, as well as its **Bet-TZ1-4** derivatives did not induce irritative phenomena thus predicting their safe use on skin and mucosae. These findings are in agreement with other studies supporting the non-irritative and wound-healing effect of triterpenes [62]; one such example is a randomized phase 3 trial developed by Frew et al. [63] in which a gel containing Bet accelerated the healing of superficial partial thickness burns.

These findings collectively show that Bet can be an ideal starting point for developing potent cytotoxic compounds for cancer cells. This is an important step because, unlike its acid counterpart (BA), Bet is more readily obtained and considerably less expensive. Future research could focus on expanding the synthesized series in order to assess precise structure–activity relationships and possibly pinpoint specific targets for the active compounds.

4. Materials and Methods

4.1. Chemistry

The reagents utilized for the chemical synthesis were commercially acquired from Merk (Darmstadt, Germany) and were subsequently used without any supplementary purification.

4.1.1. Instruments

The 1D (^{1}H and ^{13}C) and 2D NMR (H,H-COSY, H,C-HSQC, and H,C-HMBC) experiments were performed utilizing a Bruker Avance NEO Spectrometer 400 MHz (Bruker, Karlsruhe, Germany) that was equipped with a QNP direct detection probe (5 mm) and z-gradients. The spectra were recorded under standard conditions in either hexadeuterodimethyl sulfoxide (DMSO-d_6) or deuterochloroform (CDCl$_3$) and were referenced to the residual peak of the solvent (^{1}H: 2.51 ppm for DMSO-d_6 or 7.26 ppm for CDCl$_3$; ^{13}C: 39.5 ppm for DMSO-d_6 or 77.0 for CDCl$_3$). For **Bet-TZ1-4** derivatives, we first recorded the 1D and 2D NMR spectra in DMSO-d_6. Then, in each NMR tube containing the solutions of **Bet-TZ1-4**, a drop of trifluoroacetic acid (TFA) was added; the solutions were vortexed for 5 min at 500 rpm and then the 1D and 2D NMR experiments were recorded again. All the NMR experiments were recorded using standard parameter sets, as provided by Bruker. A Biobase melting point instrument (Biobase Group, Jinan, China) was utilized to record the melting points. Thin-layer chromatography was performed using 60 F254 silica gel-coated plates (Merck KGaA, Darmstadt, Germany). Fourier-transform infrared spectroscopy (FTIR) experiments were conducted with KBr pellets using a Shimadzu IR Affinity-1S apparatus (400–4000 cm^{-1} range and a 4 cm^{-1} resolution). Methanolic solutions were utilized to record LC/MS spectra in the negative ion mode, using an Agilent (Santa Clara, CA, USA) 6120 Quadrupole LC/MS system that was outfitted with an ESI ionization source, UV detector, and a SB–C18 Zorbax Rapid Resolution column. The samples were analyzed under the following conditions: 25 °C, 0.4 mL/min, and l = 250 nm. The mobile phase was composed of a 1 mM isocratic mixture comprising 15% ammonium formate and 85% methanol.

4.1.2. Synthesis Procedure for **Br-Bet**

The process of Bet acetylation was carried out using a modified version of a previously described method [64,65]. This involved the reaction of Bet (1 equivalent) with acetic anhydride (4 equivalents) in pyridine and dimethylaminopyridine (DMAP) (0.1 equivalent) at room temperature for a duration of 12 h. The reaction mixture underwent dilution with water and was subjected to triple extraction with CHCl$_3$. The organic phase was dehydrated using anhydrous MgSO$_4$, followed by solvent elimination through rotary evaporation. The freshly obtained 3-O, 28-O-diacetyl-betulin was subsequently used without undergoing supplementary purification. Subsequently, a solution of 2.5 g of acetylated Bet, approximately equivalent to 5 mmol, was prepared in 50 mL of CCl$_4$. Following this, 1.78 g of recently recrystallized NBS, equivalent to 10 mmol, was introduced into the solution. The reaction continued at room temperature for a duration of 48 h. Subsequently, the solution was subjected to filtration, followed by solvent evaporation. The resulting product was chromatographed over silica, utilizing a mixture of CHCl$_3$ and ethyl acetate in a volume ratio of 40:1.

3,28-O-diacetyl-betulin, white powder, m.p. 216–218 °C, yield 82%; ^{1}H NMR (CDCl$_3$, 400.13 MHz, δ, ppm): 4.68 (s, 1H, H29a), 4.58 (s, 1H, H29b), 4.46 (dd, J = 6.0 Hz, J = 10 Hz, 1H, H3), 4.24 (d, J = 10.9 Hz, 1H, H28a), 3.84 (d, J = 11.0 Hz, H28b), 2.44 (m, 1H, H19), 2.07 (s, 3H, H34), 2.04 (s, 3H, H32), 1.98.1.90 (m, 1H, H15a), 1.84 (d, J = 13.0 Hz, 1H, H21a), 1.76 (dd, J = 12.4 Hz, J = 8.4 Hz, 1H, H7a), 1.68–1.59 (m, 10H, H1a, H2a, H12a, H13, H18, H22, H30), 1.50–1.49 (m, 1H, H6a), 1.41–1.39 (m, 5H, H9, H11a, H15b, H16), 1.30–1.18 (m, 3H, H6b, H11b, H21b), 1.11–1.02 (m, 6H, H2b, H7b, H12b, H27), 0.96–0.93 (m, 4H, H1b, H26), 0.84–0.83 (m, H23–25), 0.78 (d, J = 9.0 Hz, 1H, H5). ^{13}C NMR (CDCl$_3$, 100.6 MHz, δ, ppm): 171.6 (C33), 171.0 (C31), 150.1 (C20), 109.9 (C29), 80.9 (C3), 62.8 (C28), 55.4 (C5), 50.3 (C9), 48.8 (C18), 47.7 (C19), 46.3 (C17), 42.7 (C14), 44.9 (C8), 38.4 (C1), 37.8 (C4), 37.5 (C13), 37.1 (C10), 34.5 (C7), 34.1 (C16), 29.7 (C21), 29.6 (C15), 27.9 (C23), 27.0 (C12), 25.1 (C2), 23.7 (C22), 21.3 (C32), 21.0 (C34), 20.8 (C11), 19.1 (C30), 18.2 (C6), 16.5 (C24), 16.1 (C27), 16.0 (C25), 14.7 (C26).

3,28-O-diacetyl-30-bromo-betulin (**Br-Bet**), white powder, m.p. 187–190 °C, yield 65%; ^{1}H NMR (CDCl$_3$, 400.13 MHz, δ, ppm): 5.13 (s, 1H, H29a), 5.02 (s, 1H, H29b), 4.45 (m, 1H, H3), 4.25 (m, 1H, H28a), 3.97 (s, 2H, H30), 3.84 (m, H28b), 2.44 (m, 1H, H19), 2.07 (s, 3H, H34), 2.03 (s, 3H, H32), 1.84–0.76 (m, betulinic protons). ^{13}C NMR (CDCl3, 100.6 MHz, δ, ppm)171.5 (C33), 171.0 (C31), 150.8 (C20), 113.3 (C29), 80.9 (C3), 62.5–14.6 (betulinic carbons). ESI-MS Rt = 4.74 min, m/z = 604 [M-H$^+$]$^-$.

4.1.3. Synthesis Procedure for **TZ1**

The procedure to synthesize 1,2,4-triazole-3-thiol (**TZ1**) was established based on the available methods in the literature [66,67] and was previously reported by our group along with the corresponding spectral data [46]. First, 0.5 moles of formic acid (90%, 20 mL) was stirred with 0.1 moles thiosemicarbazide for 30 min, when 1-formyl-3-thiosemicarbazide began to crystalize. Cold water was added and the emulsion was filtered and kept in an ice bath for the crystallization of 1H-1,2,4-triazole-3-thiol to occur. The crystals were filtered, dried, and utilized immediately without additional purification. For the following stage, 30 mmoles of NaOH, 20 mL H$_2$O, and 28.1 mmoles of 1-formyl-3-thiosemicarbazide were added into a 50 mL round-bottom flask and were refluxed for 1 h. After completion, the reaction was cooled and the final product was precipitated (concentrated HCl) and filtered.

4.1.4. Synthesis Procedure for **TZ2-4**

The procedure for synthesizing 5-substituted-1,2,4-triazole-3-thiol was carried out in accordance with established methodologies as previously reported [24]. A solution containing 20 mmol of thiosemicarbazide was prepared by dissolving it in 50 mL of DMF while being stirred magnetically. Then, 22 mmol of pyridine and 20 mmol of aroyl chloride were added to the solution. The process of magnetic stirring was sustained at room temperature for a duration of 30 min, following which the temperature was elevated to 50 °C and sustained for an approximate duration of 1 h. The endpoint of the reaction was verified by means of TLC. The aroyl-thiosemicarbazides that were obtained were subjected to precipitation using aqueous hydrochloric acid, followed by filtration and subsequent drying. Furthermore, the 5-substituted-1H-1,2,4-triazole-3-thiols (**TZ2-4**) were synthesized through the cyclization of 10 mmol of aroyl-thiosemicarbazide in ethanolic NaOH at reflux. The reaction was monitored using TLC until completion. The 5-substituted-1H-1,2,4-triazole-3-thiols were obtained through precipitation with HCl 4% and the further filtration of the resulting precipitate. Spectral data for **TZ2** and **TZ4** were previously reported [47]. Spectral data for TZ3 are listed below.

5-(4-chlorophenyl)-1H-1,2,4-triazole-3-thiol (**TZ3**); white powder, m.p. 296–298 °C (uncorrected), yield 65%; ^{1}H NMR (400.13 MHz, DMSO-d6, d, ppm): 13.93 (s, 1H), 13.75 (s, 1H), 7.93 (d, J = 8.6 Hz, 2H), 7.61 (d, J = 8.6 Hz, 2H). ^{13}C NMR (100.6 MHz, DMSO-d6, d, ppm): 167.1, 149.3, 135.2, 129.2, 127.4, 124.3. ESI−MS Rt = 0.5 min, m/z = 210 [M-H$^+$]$^-$.

4.1.5. Synthesis Procedure for **Bet-TZ1-4**

A quantity of 0.2 mmoles of 3,28-O-diacetyl-30-bromo-betulin (BetBr) and 0.3 mmoles of anhydrous K$_2$CO$_3$ were added in 5 mL of DMF and were stirred for 10 min at 25 °C. In the next stage, 0.2 mmoles of triazole derivative (**TZ1-4**) was added and the mixture was stirred for an additional 72 h at room temperature. In the following stage, the mixture was diluted with 50 mL H$_2$O and then extracted with CHCl$_3$ (4 × 15 mL). Anhydrous MgSO$_4$ was used to dry the organic phase and after solvent removal, the obtained product was chromatographed using a 2:1 ratio of CHCl$_3$ to ethyl acetate.

3,28-O-diacetyl-30-(1H-1,2,4-triazole-3-yl-sulfanyl)-betulin (**Bet-TZ1**), white powder, m.p. 113–119 °C (uncorrected), yield 38%; ^{1}H NMR (DMSO-d$_6$ + TFA, 400.13 MHz, δ, ppm): 8.49 (, s, 1H, H36), 4.95 (s, 1H, H29a), 4.91 (s, 1H, H29b), 4.36 (dd, J = 4.6 Hz, J = 10 Hz, 1H, H3), 4.23 (d, J = 10.8 Hz, 1H, H28a), 3.80 (s, 2H, H30) 3.72 (d, J = 10.9 Hz, H28b), 2.47 (m, 1H, H19),2.03 (m, 1H, H2a) 2.02 (s, 3H, H34), 1.99 (s, 3H, H32), 1.74–0.94 (betulinic protons), 0.80–0.78 (m, 10H, H5, H23–25). ^{13}C NMR (DMSO-d$_6$+ TFA, 400.13 MHz, δ, ppm): 170.9 (C33), 170.3 (C31), 156.4 (C35), 149.7 (C20), 146.3 (C36), 111.6 (C29), 80.1 (C3), 61.4 (C28), 54.7 (C5), 49.6 (C9), 49.2 (C18), 46.1 (C17), 44.6 (C19), 42.3 (C14), 40.5 (C8), 37.9 (C1), 37.5 (C4), 37.1 (C13), 36.7 (C10), 36.5 (C30), 33.9 (C7), 33.7 (C16), 30.9 (C21), 29.3 (C15), 27.6 (C23), 26.7 (C12), 26.2 (C2), 23.5 (C22), 21.1 (C32), 20.8 (C34), 20.6 (C11), 17.8 (C6), 16.5 (C24), 15.9 (C27),

15.7 (C25), 14.6 (C26). FTIR [KBr] (cm^{-1}) relevant peaks: 3117 (N-H stretch); 2945, 2872 (C-H stretch); 1735, 1244, 1030 (ester C=O, C-C-O, O-C-C stretch); ESI-MS Rt = 2.85 min, m/z = 625 [M-H$^+$]$^-$.

3,28-O-diacetyl-30-{5-[4-(dimethylamino)phenyl]-1H-1,2,4-triazole-3-yl-sulfanyl}-betulin (**Bet-TZ2**); white powder, m.p. 113–119 °C (uncorrected), yield 41%; ^{1}H NMR (DMSO-d$_6$ + TFA, 400.13 MHz, δ, ppm): 7.85 (d, J = 8.8 HZ, 2H, H38), 7.00 (d, J = 8.8 Hz, 2H, H39), 5.00 (s, 1H, H29a) 4.90 (s, 1H, H29b), 4.31 (dd, J = 4.8 Hz, J = 11.3 Hz, 1H, H3), 4.22 (d, J = 10.9 Hz, 1H, H28a), 3.90 (d, J = 14.4 Hz, 1H, H30a, AB spin system), 3.81 (d, J = 14.4 Hz, 1H, H30b, AB spin system), 3.73 (d, J = 10.9 Hz, H28b), 3.02 (s, 6H, H41), 2.47 (m, 1H, H19), 2.06 (m, 1H, H2a) 2.00 (s, 3H, H34), 1.97 (s, 3H, H32), 1.70–0.90 (betulinic protons), 0.75–0.72 (m, 10H, H5, H23–25). ^{13}C NMR (DMSO-d$_6$+ TFA, 400.13 MHz, δ, ppm): 171.0 (C33), 170.5 (C31), 160.6 (C40), 156.3 (C35), 155.8 (C35), 150.4 (C40) 149.6 (C20), 127.7 (C38), 116.1 (C37), 113.7 (C39), 111.5 (C29), 80.2 (C3), 61.7 (C28), 54.9 (C5), 49.7 (C9), 49.1 (C18), 46.2 (C17), 44.3 (C19), 42.4 (C14), 41.0 (C41), 40.6 (C8), 37.8 (C1), 37.5 (C4), 37.2 (C13), 36.7 (C10, C30), 34.0 (C7), 33.7 (C16), 31.0 (C21), 29.4 (C15), 27.8 (C23), 26.8 (C12), 26.4 (C2), 23.6 (C22), 21.1 (C32), 20.9 (C34), 20.7 (C11), 17.9 (C6), 16.6 (C24), 16.0 (C27), 15.8 (C25), 14.7 (C26). FTIR [KBr] (cm^{-1}) relevant peaks: 3232 (N-H stretch); 2945, 2873 (C-H stretch); 1735, 1244, 1029 (ester C=O, C-C-O, O-C-C stretch); ESI-MS Rt = 2.25 min, m/z = 744 [M-H$^+$]$^-$.

3,28-O-diacetyl-30-[5-(4-chlorophenyl)-1H-1,2,4-triazole-3-yl-sulfanyl]-betulin (**Bet-TZ3**); white powder, m.p. 128–135 °C (uncorrected), yield 32%; ^{1}H NMR (DMSO-d$_6$ + TFA, 400.13 MHz, δ, ppm): 7.97–7.95 (m, 2H, H38), 7.48 (d, J = 6.6 Hz, 2H, H39), 5.03 (s, 1H, H29a) 4.91 (s, 1H, H29b), 4.36 (dd, J = 4.5 Hz, J = 11.3 Hz, 1H, H3), 4.22 (d, J = 10.8 Hz, 1H, H28a), 3.93 (d, J = 14.5 Hz, 1H, H30a, AB spin system), 3.80 (d, J = 14.5 Hz, 1H, H30b, AB spin system) 3.73 (d, J = 10.9 Hz, H28b), 2.57 (m, 1H, H19), 2.06 (m, 1H, H2a) 2.00 (s, 3H, H34), 1.98 (s, 3H, H32), 1.72–0.91 (betulinic protons), 0.76–0.68 (m, 10H, H5, H23–25). ^{13}C NMR (DMSO-d$_6$+ TFA, 400.13 MHz, δ, ppm): 170.9 (C33), 170.3 (C31), 157.7 (C36), 156.0 (C35), 149.6 (C20), 130.0 (C40), 129.0 (C39), 128.5 (C37), 126.0 (C38), 114.5 (C29), 80.6 (C3), 61.6 (C28), 54.7 (C5), 49.6 (C9), 49.0 (C18), 46.1 (C17), 44.5 (C19), 42.3 (C14), 40.5 (C8), 37.9 (C1), 37.4 (C4), 37.1 (C13), 36.6 (C10, C30), 33.9 (C7), 33.7 (C16), 30.7 (C21), 29.4 (C15), 27.7 (C23), 26.7 (C12), 26.1 (C2), 23.4 (C22), 21.0 (C32), 20.8 (C34), 20.6 (C11), 17.8 (C6), 16.4 (C24), 15.9 (C27), 15.7 (C25), 14.6 (C26). FTIR [KBr] (cm^{-1}) relevant peaks: 3230 (N-H stretch); 2945, 2872 (C-H stretch); 1735, 1246, 1029 (ester C=O, C-C-O, O-C-C stretch); ESI-MS Rt = 3.05 min, m/z = 735 [M-H$^+$]$^-$.

3,28-O-diacetyl-30-[5-(4-methoxyphenyl)-1H-1,2,4-triazole-3-yl-sulfanyl]-betulin (**Bet-TZ4**); white powder, m.p. 132–138 °C (uncorrected), yield 35%; ^{1}H NMR (DMSO-d$_6$ + TFA, 400.13 MHz, δ, ppm): 7.88 (d, J = 8.8 HZ, 2H, H38), 7.04 (d, J = 8.8 Hz, 2H, H39), 5.00 (s, 1H, H29a) 4.90 (s, 1H, H29b), 4.36 (dd, J = 4.8 Hz, J = 11.1 Hz, 1H, H3), 4.22 (d, J = 10.9 Hz, 1H, H28a), 3.89 (d, J = 14.5 Hz, 1H, H30a, AB spin system), 3.81–3.79 (m, 4H, H30b, H41) 3.72 (d, J = 11.0 Hz, H28b), 2.47 (m, 1H, H19), 2.06 (m, 1H, H2a) 2.00 (s, 3H, H34), 1.97 (s, 3H, H32), 1.71–0.90 (betulinic protons), 0.76–0.69 (m, 10H, H5, H23–25). ^{13}C NMR (DMSO-d$_6$+ TFA, 400.13 MHz, δ, ppm): 170.7 (C33), 170.1 (C31), 160.6 (C40), 156.9 (C36), 156.4 (C35), 149.6 (C20), 127.5 (C38), 120.6 (C37), 114.3 (C39), 111.2 (C29), 79.9 (C3), 61.5 (C28), 55.3 (C41), 54.6 (C5), 49.5 (C9), 48.9 (C18), 46.0 (C17), 44.3 (C19), 42.2 (C14), 40.4 (C8), 37.6 (C1), 37.3 (C4), 37.0 (C13), 36.5 (C10), 36.4 (C30), 33.8 (C7), 33.6 (C16), 30.7 (C21), 29.2 (C15), 27.6 (C23), 26.6 (C12), 26.0 (C2), 23.3 (C22), 20.9 (C32), 20.7 (C34), 20.5 (C11), 17.7 (C6), 16.4 (C24), 15.7 (C27), 15.6 (C25), 14.5 (C26). FTIR [KBr] (cm^{-1}) relevant peaks: 3230 (N-H stretch); 2945, 2872 (C-H stretch); 1735, 1247, 1030 (ester C=O, C-C-O, O-C-C stretch); ESI-MS Rt = 2.14 min, m/z = 731 [M-H$^+$]$^-$.

4.2. Biological Assessment

4.2.1. Cell Culture

The selected cell lines for the study, namely, HaCat (immortalized human keratinocytes) were acquired from CLS Cell Lines Service GmbH (Eppelheim, Germany), whereas A375 (human malignant melanoma cells), HT-29 (human colorectal adenocarcinoma), and MCF7 (human breast adenocarcinoma) were purchased from American Type Culture Collection (ATCC, Lomianki, Poland). The aforementioned cells were obtained as frozen items and were subsequently stored in liquid nitrogen. Dulbecco's Modified Eagle Medium (DMEM) High Glucose added with 1% Penicillin/Streptomycin mixture (100 IU/mL) and with 10% fetal bovine serum (FBS) was used to culture HaCaT and A375 cells, while HT-29 cells were cultured using McCoy's 5A Medium, supplemented with the same 10% FBS and 1% antibiotic mixture. The MCF7 cells were propagated in Eagle's Minimum Essential Medium (EMEM), supplemented with 10% FBS, 1% antibiotic mixture, and 0.01 mg/mL human recombinant insulin. All cells were maintained in a humified incubator with 5% CO_2 at 37 °C. After reaching 80–90% confluence, cells were stimulated with the tested compounds (10, 25, 50, 75, and 100 µM) for 24 h and 48 h, respectively. The cell number was determined with Trypan Blue using a cell counting device (Thermo Fisher Scientific, Inc., Waltham, MA, USA).

4.2.2. Cell Viability Assessment

The Alamar blue colorimetric determination was used to assess the cell viability of HaCaT, A375, MCF7, and HT-29 cells, after stimulation with increasing concentrations (10, 25, 50, 75, and 100 µM) of four diacetylbetulin derivatives, betulin, and 5-fluorouracil as a positive control, at the same concentrations for 48 h. The cells (1×10^4) were seeded into 96-well plates and incubated (37 °C and 5% CO_2) until an 80–85% confluence was reached. The used medium was discarded using an aspiration station and swapped with fresh medium specific for each cell line, containing the compounds. The tested concentrations (10, 25, 50, 75, and 100 µM) were prepared from 20 mM compound stock solutions so that the final concentration of DMSO did not exceed 0.5%. After 48 h, 0.01% Alamar blue was used to counterstain all cells, after which the cells incubated for an additional 3 h. The absorbance measurements were carried out at 2 wavelengths (570 nm, and 600 nm) using a xMark™ Microplate Spectrophotometer, Bio-Rad (Hercules, CA, USA). The experiments were performed in triplicate.

4.2.3. Immunofluorescence Assay—Morphological Assessment of Apoptotic Cells

The assessment of nuclear localization and any signs of apoptosis (shrinkage, fragmentation) and cytoplasmatic alterations were determined using Hoechst staining, while the cytoplasmatic localization was assessed using beta-tubulin staining. HaCaT, A375, MCF-7, and HT-29 cells were seeded onto 12-well plates at 2×10^5 cells/well initial density. After reaching 80–90% confluence, the cells were stimulated with **Bet-TZ1** using its 48-h-treatment IC_{50} values obtained for each cell line and with **Bet-TZ3** at its 48-h-treatment IC_{50} value for the A375 cell line. Separately, some wells were stimulated with 5-fluorouracil using the concentration corresponding to its IC_{50} values for each cell line at 48 h. After 48 h, the old medium was removed and the cells were fixed with methanol for 15 min, permeabilized with Triton X 0.01% in phosphate buffer saline (PBS) for an additional 15 min, and finally blocked with Bovine serum albumin 3% (BSA) for 30 min at room temperature. Afterward, the cells were stained with beta-tubulin monoclonal antibody at a dilution of 1:2000 in BSA 3% for 1 h (room temperature) and subsequently incubated with Alexa Fluor 488 goat-anti mouse secondary antibody at a 1:5000 dilution in BSA 3% for 30 min in the dark. Finally, the Hoechst 33258 solution was added for 5 min. The nuclear and cytoplasmatic alterations were observed and recorded using the integrated DP74 digital camera of the inverted microscope, Olympus IX73 (Olympus, Tokyo, Japan).

4.2.4. Real-Time PCR Quantification of Apoptotic Markers

The total RNA was extracted using the peqGold RNAPureTM Package (Peqlab Biotechnology GmbH, Erlangen, Germany) following the manufacturer's instructions, and the total concentration of RNA was measured using a DS-11 spectrophotometer (DeNovix, Wilmington, DE, USA). Reverse transcription was achieved using the Maxima® First Strand cDNA Synthesis Kit (Thermo Fisher Scientific, Inc., Waltham, MA, USA). The Tadvanced

Biometra Product line (Analytik Jena AG, Göttingen, Germany) was used for sample incubation using the following thermal cycle: 10 min at 25 °C, 15 min at 50 °C, and 5 min at 85 °C. The Quant Studio 5 real-time PCR system (Thermo Fisher Scientific, Inc., Waltham, MA, USA) was used for quantitative real-time PCR determinations. The experiment was conducted using 20 µL aliquots containing Power SYBR-Green PCR Master Mix (Thermo Fisher Scientific, Inc., Waltham, MA, USA), pure water, the sense and antisense primer, and the sample cDNA. The primer pairs used for this method included 18 S (Thermo Fisher Scientific, Inc., Waltham, MA, USA), used as housekeeping gene (sense: 5′GTAACCCGTTGAACCCCATT 3′; antisense: 5′CCATCCAATCGGTAGTAGCG3′), and Caspase-9 (sense: 5′ATGGACGAAGCGGATCGGCGGCTCC3′; antisense: 5′GCACCACT-GGGGGTAAGGTTTTCTAG3′) (Eurogentec, Seraing, Belgium). Normalized, results were calculated using the comparative threshold cycle method ($2^{-\Delta\Delta Ct}$).

4.2.5. Scratch Assay

The regressive effect on the invasion capacity of **Bet-TZ1** (on A375, MCF7, and HT-29 cancer cells) and **Bet-TZ3** (on A375 cells) and their wound healing potential on HaCaT cells was determined using the scratch test. The cells were seeded onto 12-well plates at an initial density of 2×10^5 cells/well. After reaching 80–85% confluence, the old medium was removed and each well was washed with warm PBS, then treated with 5 µg/mL mitomycin C for 2 h at 37 °C. Mitomycin C is an antibiotic that inhibits DNA synthesis and cell proliferation used to determine the true anti-migratory effect of a substance. After mitomycin C treatment, the cells were again washed with PBS, scratched onto the diameter of the well with a sterile pipette tip, and then stimulated with 10 µM **Bet-TZ1** and **Bet-TZ3**. To establish the scratch closure rate (%), the wells were photographed at 0, 24, and 48 h using the Olympus IX73 inverted microscope (Olympus, Tokyo, Japan). The Sense Dimension software (version 1.8) was utilized for analyzing cell migration for each cell line.

4.2.6. Statistical Analysis

The statistical analysis was achieved by employing a *t*-test and one-way ANOVA followed by Dunnett's post hoc test using GraphPad Prism version 6.0.0 (GraphPad Software, San Diego, CA, USA). The IC_{50} values were calculated using the same software, according to the correlation between the log[concentration] and cell viability. The statistically significant threshold ($p < 0.05$) between groups was * $p < 0.05$, ** $p < 0.01$, and *** $p < 0.001$.

4.3. HET−CAM Assay

We used the HET−CAM in vivo protocol to evaluate the safety profile of a particular substance against a living tissue. The standard protocol involved the usage of a developing chorioallantoic membrane within an embryonated chicken (*Gallus domesticus*) egg. This method complied with the Interagency Coordinating Committee on the Validation of Alternative Methods recommendations [68], which were customized to suit the specific circumstances of the study. Based on an adapted approach to the established methodology [69], the eggs were subjected to incubation conditions of 37 °C and 50% relative humidity. On the third day of incubation, 5–6 mL of albumen was extracted, subsequently leading to the creation of an opening at the top of the eggs. In the context of the developing chorioallantoic membrane of the chick embryo, a volume of 300 µL of SLS (positive control), Bet, and **Bet-TZ1-4** were administered at a concentration of 100 µM. The alterations in CAM were observed through the use of stereomicroscopy, specifically, the Discovery 8 Stereomicroscope by Zeiss (Jena, Germany). The images were captured using the Zeiss Axio CAM 105 color camera, both before and 5 min after the application of the tested substances. During the five-minute duration, the impact on three specific parameters was observed (hemorrhage, lysis, and vascular plexus coagulability). Each determination was performed in triplicate. The obtained results were quantified as irritation factor (IF) values, which were determined using the provided formula. These values were then compared to a negative (distilled water) and a positive control (SLS 0.5%) with an IF of 16.29. The Luepke scale was used to interpret the IF values, where a range of 0–0.9 indicates non-irritation, 1–4.9 indicates weak irritation, 5–8.9 indicates moderate irritation, and 9–21 indicates strong irritation [70].

$$IF = 5 * \frac{301 - Sec\ H}{300} + 7 * \frac{301 - Sec\ L}{300} + 9 * \frac{301 - Sec\ C}{300};$$

where *IF* = irritation factor; *H* = hemorrhage; *L* = vascular lysis; *C* = coagulation; *Sec H* = start of hemorrhage reactions (s); *Sec L* = onset of vessel lysis on CAM (s); *Sec C* = onset of (s).

5. Conclusions

This study presented the synthesis, cytotoxicity assessment, and influence on angiogenesis of a series of diacetylbetulin derivatives containing 5-Substituted-1,2,4-triazoles at C_{30} (**Bet-TZ1-4**). While the synthesis protocol led to obtaining good yields of target compounds, the NMR analysis revealed that, in the DMSO solution, they exist in two tautomeric forms that could have an influence on the anticancer effect, the hypothesis that remains to be explored in further studies. The cytotoxicity assessment of **Bet-TZ1-4** against A375 (melanoma), MCF-7 (breast cancer), HT-29 (colorectal cancer), and HaCaT (human keratinocytes) revealed **Bet-TZ1** as the lead candidate of the series against all tested lines. However, the cytotoxicity of **Bet-TZ1** manifested also against the non-malignant HaCaT cell line, indicating a reduced selectivity of the derivative. Promising results were also obtained for **Bet-TZ3**, which exhibited a selective cytotoxic effect against melanoma cells, and along **Bet-TZ1**, which showed promising anti-migratory properties. A related cytotoxic correlated pro-apoptotic effect was observed for both compounds confirmed by morphological nuclear assessment and PCR results that showed an increase in the expression of caspase 9. The HET−CAM test revealed that **Bet-TZ1-4** does not have an irritative potential, supporting their safety application in local treatments. Although our study obtained modest results in terms of cytotoxicity, further investigation of betulin-triazole derivatives still remains a pathway that should be explored, focusing on the synthesis of more selective derivatives against cancer.

Supplementary Materials: The following supporting information can be downloaded at: https://www.mdpi.com/article/10.3390/pr12010024/s1, Figure S1. The three possible tautomeric forms of 3,5-disubstituted 1,2,4-triazoles; Figure S2. 1H NMR spectrum of 3-O,28-O-diacetyl-betulin (400 MHz, CDCl3); Figure S3. 13C NMR spectrum of 3-O,28-O-diacetyl-betulin (100 MHz, CDCl3); Figure S4. 1H NMR spectrum of 3-O, 28-O-diacetyl-30-bromo-betulin (400 MHz, CDCl3); Figure S5. 13C NMR spectrum of 3-O, 28-O-diacetyl-30-bromo-betulin (100 MHz, CDCl3); Figure S6. 1H NMR spectrum of **Bet-TZ1** in DMSO-d6 (bottom) and DMSO-d6 with one drop of TFA (up); Figure S7. 13C NMR spectrum of **Bet-TZ1** in DMSO-d6 (bottom) and DMSO-d6 with one drop of TFA; Figure S8. H,H-COSY NMR spectrum of **Bet-TZ1** in DMSO-d6 with one drop of TFA; Figure S9. H, C-HSQC NMR spectrum of **Bet-TZ1** in DMSO-d6 with one drop of TFA; Figure S10. H,C-HMBC NMR spectrum of **Bet-TZ1** in DMSO-d6 with one drop of TFA; Figure S11. 1H NMR spectrum of **Bet-TZ2** in DMSO-d6 (bottom) and DMSO-d6 with one drop of TFA (up); Figure S12. FTIR spectrum of **Bet-TZ2**; Figure S13. 13C NMR spectrum of **Bet-TZ2** in DMSO-d6 (bottom) and DMSO-d6 with one drop of TFA (up); Figure S14. H,H-COSY NMR spectrum of **Bet-TZ2** in DMSO-d6; Figure S15. H,C-HSQC NMR spectrum of **Bet-TZ2** in DMSO-d6 with one drop of TFA; Figure S16. H,C-HMBC NMR spectrum of **Bet-TZ2** in DMSO-d6 with one drop of TFA; Figure S17. FTIR spectrum of **Bet-TZ2**; Figure S18. 1H NMR spectrum of **Bet-TZ3** in DMSO-d6 (bottom) and DMSO-d6 with one drop of TFA (up); Figure S19. 13C NMR spectrum of **Bet-TZ3** in DMSO-d6 (bottom) and DMSO-d6 with one drop of TFA (up); Figure S20. H,H-COSY NMR spectrum of **Bet-TZ3** in DMSO-d6; Figure S21. H,C-HSQC NMR spectrum of **Bet-TZ3** in DMSO-d6 with one drop of TFA; Figure S22. H,C-HMBC NMR spectrum of **Bet-TZ3** in DMSO-d6 with one drop of TFA; Figure S23. FTIR spectrum of **Bet-TZ3** in DMSO-d6; Figure S24. 1H NMR spectrum of **Bet-TZ4** in DMSO-d6 (bottom) and DMSO-d6 with one drop of TFA (up); Figure S25. 13C NMR spectrum of **Bet-TZ4** in DMSO-d6 (bottom) and DMSO-d6 with one drop of TFA (up); Figure S26. H,H-COSY NMR spectrum of **Bet-TZ4** in DMSO-d6; Figure S27. H,C-HSQC NMR spectrum of **Bet-TZ4** in DMSO-d6 with one drop of TFA; Figure S28. H,C-HMBC NMR spectrum of **Bet-TZ4** in DMSO-d6 with one drop of TFA; Figure S29. FTIR spectrum of **Bet-TZ4**.

Author Contributions: Conceptualization, A.P., M.M. and C.Ș.; methodology, A.P., M.M., A.M. (Alexandra Mioc), M.B.-P., R.R., R.N.-G., A.M. (Andreea Milan), G.M., C.T., C.O., Ș.A., S.R., I.Ș. and C.Ș.; validation, A.P., A.M. (Alexandra Mioc) and M.M.; investigation, A.P., A.M. (Alexandra Mioc) and M.M.; writing—original draft preparation, A.P., M.M., A.M. (Alexandra Mioc), M.B.-P., A.M. (Andreea Milan), G.M., S.R., C.O., C.T. and I.Ș.; writing—review and editing A.P., A.M. (Alexandra Mioc), M.M. and C.Ș.; visualization, A.P., R.R. and R.N.-G.; supervision, M.M. and C.Ș.; project administration, M.M. and C.Ș.; funding acquisition, M.M. All authors have read and agreed to the published version of the manuscript.

Funding: This research was funded by the University of Medicine and Pharmacy "Victor Babes" Timisoara, grant number 26679/09.11.2022 (M.M.).

Informed Consent Statement: Not applicable.

Data Availability Statement: Data are contained within the article and Supplementary Materials.

Conflicts of Interest: The authors declare no conflict of interest.

References

1. Maitra, U.; Stephen, C.; Ciesla, L.M. Drug discovery from natural products—Old problems and novel solutions for the treatment of neurodegenerative diseases. *J. Pharm. Biomed. Anal.* **2022**, *210*, 114553. [CrossRef] [PubMed]
2. Choudhari, A.S.; Mandave, P.C.; Deshpande, M.; Ranjekar, P.; Prakash, O. Phytochemicals in Cancer Treatment: From Preclinical Studies to Clinical Practice. *Front. Pharmacol.* **2020**, *10*, 1614. [CrossRef] [PubMed]
3. Anand, U.; Dey, A.; Chandel, A.K.S.; Sanyal, R.; Mishra, A.; Pandey, D.K.; De Falco, V.; Upadhyay, A.; Kandimalla, R.; Chaudhary, A.; et al. Cancer chemotherapy and beyond: Current status, drug candidates, associated risks and progress in targeted therapeutics. *Genes Dis.* **2023**, *10*, 1367–1401. [CrossRef] [PubMed]
4. Ahmed, M.B.; Islam, S.U.; Alghamdi, A.A.A.; Kamran, M.; Ahsan, H.; Lee, Y.S. Phytochemicals as Chemo-Preventive Agents and Signaling Molecule Modulators: Current Role in Cancer Therapeutics and Inflammation. *Int. J. Mol. Sci.* **2022**, *23*, 15765. [CrossRef] [PubMed]
5. Andor, B.; Tischer, A.; Berceanu-Vaduva, D.; Lazureanu, V.; Cheveresan, A.; Poenaru, M. Antimicrobial activity and cytotoxic effect on gingival cells of silver nanoparticles obtained by biosynthesis. *Rev. Chim.* **2019**, *70*, 781–783. [CrossRef]
6. Dehelean, C.A.; Marcovici, I.; Soica, C.; Mioc, M.; Coricovac, D.; Iurciuc, S.; Cretu, O.M.; Pinzaru, I. Plant-Derived Anticancer Compounds as New Perspectives in Drug Discovery and Alternative Therapy. *Molecules* **2021**, *26*, 1109. [CrossRef] [PubMed]
7. Demets, O.V.; Takibayeva, A.T.; Kassenov, R.Z.; Aliyeva, M.R. Methods of Betulin Extraction from Birch Bark. *Molecules* **2022**, *27*, 3621. [CrossRef]
8. Özdemir, Z.; Rybková, M.; Vlk, M.; Šaman, D.; Rárová, L.; Wimmer, Z. Synthesis and Pharmacological Effects of Diosgenin–Betulinic Acid Conjugates. *Molecules* **2020**, *25*, 3546. [CrossRef]
9. Tuli, H.S.; Sak, K.; Gupta, D.S.; Kaur, G.; Aggarwal, D.; Chaturvedi Parashar, N.; Choudhary, R.; Yerer, M.B.; Kaur, J.; Kumar, M.; et al. Anti-Inflammatory and Anticancer Properties of Birch Bark-Derived Betulin: Recent Developments. *Plants* **2021**, *10*, 2663. [CrossRef]
10. John, R.; Dalal, B.; Shankarkumar, A.; Devarajan, P.V. Innovative Betulin Nanosuspension exhibits enhanced anticancer activity in a Triple Negative Breast Cancer Cell line and Zebrafish angiogenesis model. *Int. J. Pharm.* **2021**, *600*, 120511. [CrossRef]
11. Kadela-Tomanek, M.; Jastrzębska, M.; Chrobak, E.; Bębenek, E.; Boryczka, S. Chromatographic and Computational Screening of Lipophilicity and Pharmacokinetics of Newly Synthesized Betulin-1,4-quinone Hybrids. *Processes* **2021**, *9*, 376. [CrossRef]
12. Grymel, M.; Zawojak, M.; Adamek, J. Triphenylphosphonium Analogues of Betulin and Betulinic Acid with Biological Activity: A Comprehensive Review. *J. Nat. Prod.* **2019**, *82*, 1719–1730. [CrossRef] [PubMed]
13. Majhi, S.; Das, D. Chemical derivatization of natural products: Semisynthesis and pharmacological aspects—A decade update. *Tetrahedron* **2021**, *78*, 131801. [CrossRef]
14. Kuczynska, K.; Cmoch, P.; Rárová, L.; Oklešťková, J.; Korda, A.; Pakulski, Z.; Strnad, M. Influence of intramolecular hydrogen bonds on regioselectivity of glycosylation. Synthesis of lupane-type saponins bearing the OSW-1 saponin disaccharide unit and its isomers. *Carbohydr. Res.* **2016**, *423*, 49–69. [CrossRef] [PubMed]
15. Luginina, J.; Linden, M.; Bazulis, M.; Kumpiņš, V.; Mishnev, A.; Popov, S.A.; Golubeva, T.S.; Waldvogel, S.R.; Shults, E.E.; Turks, M. Electrosynthesis of Stable Betulin-Derived Nitrile Oxides and their Application in Synthesis of Cytostatic Lupane-Type Triterpenoid-Isoxazole Conjugates. *Eur. J. Org. Chem.* **2021**, *2021*, 2557–2577. [CrossRef]
16. Dubinin, M.V.; Semenova, A.A.; Ilzorkina, A.I.; Markelova, N.Y.; Penkov, N.V.; Shakurova, E.R.; Belosludtsev, K.N.; Parfenova, L.V. New quaternized pyridinium derivatives of betulin: Synthesis and evaluation of membranotropic properties on liposomes, pro- and eukaryotic cells, and isolated mitochondria. *Chem. Biol. Interact.* **2021**, *349*, 109678. [CrossRef]
17. Grishko, V.V.; Tolmacheva, I.A.; Nebogatikov, V.O.; Galaiko, N.V.; Nazarov, A.V.; Dmitriev, M.V.; Ivshina, I.B. Preparation of novel ring-A fused azole derivatives of betulin and evaluation of their cytotoxicity. *Eur. J. Med. Chem.* **2017**, *125*, 629–639. [CrossRef]
18. Heravi, M.M.; Zadsirjan, V. Prescribed drugs containing nitrogen heterocycles: An overview. *RSC Adv.* **2020**, *10*, 44247–44311. [CrossRef]

19. Strzelecka, M.; Świątek, P. 1,2,4-Triazoles as Important Antibacterial Agents. *Pharmaceuticals* **2021**, *14*, 224. [CrossRef]
20. Malik, M.S.; Ahmed, S.A.; Althagafi, I.I.; Ansari, M.A.; Kamal, A. Application of triazoles as bioisosteres and linkers in the development of microtubule targeting agents. *RSC Med. Chem.* **2020**, *11*, 327–348. [CrossRef]
21. Lengerli, D.; Ibis, K.; Nural, Y.; Banoglu, E. The 1,2,3-triazole 'all-in-one' ring system in drug discovery: A good bioisostere, a good pharmacophore, a good linker, and a versatile synthetic tool. *Expert Opin. Drug Discov.* **2022**, *17*, 1209–1236. [CrossRef] [PubMed]
22. Matin, M.M.; Matin, P.; Rahman, M.R.; Ben Hadda, T.; Almalki, F.A.; Mahmud, S.; Ghoneim, M.M.; Alruwaily, M.; Alshehri, S. Triazoles and Their Derivatives: Chemistry, Synthesis, and Therapeutic Applications. *Front. Mol. Biosci.* **2022**, *9*, 864286. [CrossRef] [PubMed]
23. Bębenek, E.; Jastrzębska, M.; Kadela-Tomanek, M.; Chrobak, E.; Orzechowska, B.; Zwolińska, K.; Latocha, M.; Mertas, A.; Czuba, Z.; Boryczka, S. Novel Triazole Hybrids of Betulin: Synthesis and Biological Activity Profile. *Molecules* **2017**, *22*, 1876. [CrossRef] [PubMed]
24. Mioc, M.; Soica, C.; Bercean, V.; Avram, S.; Balan-Porcarasu, M.; Coricovac, D.; Ghiulai, R.; Muntean, D.; Andrica, F.; Dehelean, C.; et al. Design, synthesis and pharmaco-toxicological assessment of 5-mercapto-1,2,4-triazole derivatives with antibacterial and antiproliferative activity. *Int. J. Oncol.* **2017**, *50*, 1175–1183. [CrossRef] [PubMed]
25. Gonçalves, S.M.C.; Silva, G.N.; da Rocha Pitta, I.; Melo Rêgo, M.J.B.; Gnoato, S.C.B.; da Rocha Pitta, M.G. Novel betulin derivatives inhibit IFN-γ and modulates COX-2 expression. *Nat. Prod. Res.* **2020**, *34*, 1702–1711. [CrossRef] [PubMed]
26. Bodrikov, I.V.; Kurskii, Y.A.; Chiyanov, A.A.; Subbotin, A.Y. Electrophilic Substitution of Hydrogen in Betulin and Diacetylbetulin. *Russ. J. Org. Chem.* **2018**, *54*, 131–138. [CrossRef]
27. Phalgune, U.D.; Vanka, K.; Rajamohanan, P.R. GIAO/DFT studies on 1,2,4-triazole-5-thiones and their propargyl derivatives. *Magn. Reson. Chem.* **2013**, *51*, 767–774. [CrossRef]
28. Chaudhary, P.M.; Chavan, S.R.; Kavitha, M.; Maybhate, S.P.; Deshpande, S.R.; Likhite, A.P.; Rajamohanan, P.R. Structural elucidation of propargylated products of 3-substituted-1,2,4-triazole-5-thiols by NMR techniques. *Magn. Reson. Chem.* **2008**, *46*, 1168–1174. [CrossRef]
29. Luepke, N.P.; Kemper, F.H. The HET-CAM test: An alternative to the draize eye test. *Food Chem. Toxicol.* **1986**, *24*, 495–496. [CrossRef]
30. Szoka, Ł.; Isidorov, V.; Nazaruk, J.; Stocki, M.; Siergiejczyk, L. Cytotoxicity of Triterpene Seco-Acids from Betula pubescens Buds. *Molecules* **2019**, *24*, 4060. [CrossRef]
31. Aggarwal, R.; Sumran, G. An insight on medicinal attributes of 1,2,4-triazoles. *Eur. J. Med. Chem.* **2020**, *205*, 112652. [CrossRef] [PubMed]
32. Patel, K.R.; Brahmbhatt, J.G.; Pandya, P.A.; Daraji, D.G.; Patel, H.D.; Rawal, R.M.; Baran, S.K. Design, synthesis and biological evaluation of novel 5-(4-chlorophenyl)-4-phenyl-4H-1,2,4-triazole-3-thiols as an anticancer agent. *J. Mol. Struct.* **2021**, *1231*, 130000. [CrossRef]
33. Kadela-Tomanek, M.; Jastrzębska, M.; Marciniec, K.; Chrobak, E.; Bębenek, E.; Boryczka, S. Lipophilicity, Pharmacokinetic Properties, and Molecular Docking Study on SARS-CoV-2 Target for Betulin Triazole Derivatives with Attached 1,4-Quinone. *Pharmaceutics* **2021**, *13*, 781. [CrossRef] [PubMed]
34. Sidova, V.; Zoufaly, P.; Pokorny, J.; Dzubak, P.; Hajduch, M.; Popa, I.; Urban, M. Cytotoxic conjugates of betulinic acid and substituted triazoles prepared by Huisgen Cycloaddition from 30-azidoderivatives. *PLoS ONE* **2017**, *12*, e0171621. [CrossRef] [PubMed]
35. Dangroo, N.A.; Singh, J.; Rath, S.K.; Gupta, N.; Qayum, A.; Singh, S.; Sangwan, P.L. A convergent synthesis of novel alkyne–azide cycloaddition congeners of betulinic acid as potent cytotoxic agent. *Steroids* **2017**, *123*, 1–12. [CrossRef] [PubMed]
36. Kuczynska, K.; Bończak, B.; Rárová, L.; Kvasnicová, M.; Strnad, M.; Pakulski, Z.; Cmoch, P.; Fiałkowski, M. Synthesis and cytotoxic activity of 1,2,3-triazoles derived from 2,3-seco-dihydrobetulin via a click chemistry approach. *J. Mol. Struct.* **2022**, *1250*, 131751. [CrossRef]
37. Alkorta, I.; Elguero, J.; Liebman, J.F. The annular tautomerism of imidazoles and pyrazoles: The possible existence of nonaromatic forms. *Struct. Chem.* **2006**, *17*, 439–444. [CrossRef]
38. Claramunt, R.M.; López, C.; Angeles García, M.; Dolores Otero, M.; Rosario Torres, M.; Pinilla, E.; Alarcón, S.H.; Alkorta, I.; Elguero, J. The structure of halogeno-1,2,4-triazoles in the solid state and in solution. *New J. Chem.* **2001**, *25*, 1061–1068. [CrossRef]
39. Katritzky, A.R.; Hall, C.D.; El-Gendy, B.E.-D.M.; Draghici, B. Tautomerism in drug discovery. *J. Comput. Aided. Mol. Des.* **2010**, *24*, 475–484. [CrossRef]
40. Larina, L.I. Tautomerism and Structure of Azoles. *Adv. Heterocycl. Chem.* **2018**, *124*, 233–321.
41. Indrayanto, G.; Putra, G.S.; Suhud, F. Validation of in-vitro bioassay methods: Application in herbal drug research. *Profiles Drug Subst. Excip. Relat. Methodol.* **2021**, *46*, 273–307. [PubMed]
42. Shi, W.; Tang, N.; Yan, W.-D. Synthesis and cytotoxicity of triterpenoids derived from betulin and betulinic acid via click chemistry. *J. Asian Nat. Prod. Res.* **2015**, *17*, 159–169. [CrossRef] [PubMed]
43. Zhang, Q.; Chen, W.; Zhang, B.; Li, C.; Zhang, X.; Wang, Q.; Wang, Y.; Zhou, Q.; Li, X.; Shen, X.L. Central role of TRAP1 in the ameliorative effect of oleanolic acid on the mitochondrial-mediated and endoplasmic reticulum stress-excitated apoptosis induced by ochratoxin A. *Toxicology* **2021**, *450*, 152681. [CrossRef] [PubMed]

44. Chakraborty, B.; Dutta, D.; Mukherjee, S.; Das, S.; Maiti, N.C.; Das, P.; Chowdhury, C. Synthesis and biological evaluation of a novel betulinic acid derivative as an inducer of apoptosis in human colon carcinoma cells (HT-29). *Eur. J. Med. Chem.* **2015**, *102*, 93–105. [CrossRef] [PubMed]
45. Eidet, J.R.; Pasovic, L.; Maria, R.; Jackson, C.J.; Utheim, T.P. Objective assessment of changes in nuclear morphology and cell distribution following induction of apoptosis. *Diagn. Pathol.* **2014**, *9*, 92. [CrossRef] [PubMed]
46. Nistor, G.; Mioc, M.; Mioc, A.; Balan-Porcarasu, M.; Raoviceanu, R.; Prodea, A.; Milan, A.; Ghiulai, R.; Semenescu, A.; Dehelean, C.; et al. The C30-Modulation of Betulinic Acid Using 1,2,4-Triazole: A Promising Strategy for Increasing Its Antimelanoma Cytotoxic Potential. *Molecules* **2022**, *27*, 7807. [CrossRef] [PubMed]
47. Nistor, G.; Mioc, A.; Mioc, M.; Balan-Porcarasu, M.; Ghiulai, R.; Racoviceanu, R.; Avram, Ș.; Prodea, A.; Semenescu, A.; Milan, A.; et al. Novel Semisynthetic Betulinic Acid–Triazole Hybrids with In Vitro Antiproliferative Potential. *Processes* **2022**, *11*, 101. [CrossRef]
48. Rzeski, W.; Stepulak, A.; Szymański, M.; Juszczak, M.; Grabarska, A.; Sifringer, M.; Kaczor, J.; Kandefer-Szerszeń, M. Betulin Elicits Anti-Cancer Effects in Tumour Primary Cultures and Cell Lines In Vitro. *Basic Clin. Pharmacol. Toxicol.* **2009**, *105*, 425–432. [CrossRef]
49. Pfarr, K.; Danciu, C.; Arlt, O.; Neske, C.; Dehelean, C.; Pfeilschifter, J.M.; Radeke, H.H. Simultaneous and Dose Dependent Melanoma Cytotoxic and Immune Stimulatory Activity of Betulin. *PLoS ONE* **2015**, *10*, e0118802. [CrossRef]
50. Zehra, B.; Ahmed, A.; Sarwar, R.; Khan, A.; Farooq, U.; Abid Ali, S.; Al-Harrasi, A. Apoptotic and antimetastatic activities of betulin isolated from Quercus incana against non-small cell lung cancer cells. *Cancer Manag. Res.* **2019**, *11*, 1667–1683. [CrossRef]
51. Li, Y.; He, K.; Huang, Y.; Zheng, D.; Gao, C.; Cui, L.; Jin, Y. Betulin induces mitochondrial cytochrome c release associated apoptosis in human cancer cells. *Mol. Carcinog.* **2010**, *49*, 630–640. [CrossRef] [PubMed]
52. Slee, E.A.; Harte, M.T.; Kluck, R.M.; Wolf, B.B.; Casiano, C.A.; Newmeyer, D.D.; Wang, H.-G.; Reed, J.C.; Nicholson, D.W.; Alnemri, E.S.; et al. Ordering the Cytochrome c–initiated Caspase Cascade: Hierarchical Activation of Caspases-2, -3, -6, -7, -8, and -10 in a Caspase-9–dependent Manner. *J. Cell Biol.* **1999**, *144*, 281–292. [CrossRef] [PubMed]
53. Tian, T. MCF-7 cells lack the expression of Caspase-3. *Int. J. Biol. Macromol.* **2023**, *231*, 123310. [CrossRef] [PubMed]
54. Orchel, A.; Chodurek, E.; Jaworska-Kik, M.; Paduszyński, P.; Kaps, A.; Chrobak, E.; Bębenek, E.; Boryczka, S.; Borkowska, P.; Kasperczyk, J. Anticancer Activity of the Acetylenic Derivative of Betulin Phosphate Involves Induction of Necrotic-Like Death in Breast Cancer Cells In Vitro. *Molecules* **2021**, *26*, 615. [CrossRef] [PubMed]
55. Pęcak, P.; Świtalska, M.; Chrobak, E.; Boryczka, G.; Bębenek, E. Betulin Acid Ester Derivatives Inhibit Cancer Cell Growth by Inducing Apoptosis through Caspase Cascade Activation: A Comprehensive In Vitro and In Silico Study. *Int. J. Mol. Sci.* **2022**, *24*, 196. [CrossRef] [PubMed]
56. Zhuo, Z.; Xiao, M.; Lin, H.; Luo, J.; Wang, T. Novel betulin derivative induces anti-proliferative activity by G2/M phase cell cycle arrest and apoptosis in Huh7 cells. *Oncol. Lett.* **2018**, *15*, 2097–2104. [CrossRef] [PubMed]
57. Entschladen, F.; Drell, T.L.; Lang, K.; Joseph, J.; Zaenker, K.S. Tumour-cell migration, invasion, and metastasis: Navigation by neurotransmitters. *Lancet Oncol.* **2004**, *5*, 254–258. [CrossRef] [PubMed]
58. Härmä, V.; Haavikko, R.; Virtanen, J.; Ahonen, I.; Schukov, H.-P.; Alakurtti, S.; Purev, E.; Rischer, H.; Yli-Kauhaluoma, J.; Moreira, V.M.; et al. Optimization of Invasion-Specific Effects of Betulin Derivatives on Prostate Cancer Cells through Lead Development. *PLoS ONE* **2015**, *10*, e0126111. [CrossRef]
59. Bache, M.; Bernhardt, S.; Passin, S.; Wichmann, H.; Hein, A.; Zschornak, M.P.; Kappler, M.; Taubert, H.; Paschke, R.; Vordermark, D. Betulinic Acid Derivatives NVX-207 and B10 for Treatment of Glioblastoma—An in Vitro Study of Cytotoxicity and Radiosensitization. *Int. J. Mol. Sci.* **2014**, *15*, 19777–19790. [CrossRef]
60. Winter, G.; Koch, A.B.F.; Löffler, J.; Jelezko, F.; Lindén, M.; Li, H.; Abaei, A.; Zuo, Z.; Beer, A.J.; Rasche, V. In vivo PET/MRI Imaging of the Chorioallantoic Membrane. *Front. Phys.* **2020**, *8*, 151. [CrossRef]
61. de Araujo Lowndes Viera, L.M.; Silva, R.S.; da Silva, C.C.; Presgrave, O.A.F.; Boas, M.H.S.V. Comparison of the different protocols of the Hen's Egg Test-Chorioallantoic Membrane (HET-CAM) by evaluating the eye irritation potential of surfactants. *Toxicol. Vitr.* **2022**, *78*, 105255. [CrossRef] [PubMed]
62. Ghiulai, R.; Roșca, O.J.; Antal, D.S.; Mioc, M.; Mioc, A.; Racoviceanu, R.; Macașoi, I.; Olariu, T.; Dehelean, C.; Crețu, O.M.; et al. Tetracyclic and Pentacyclic Triterpenes with High Therapeutic Efficiency in Wound Healing Approaches. *Molecules* **2020**, *25*, 5557. [CrossRef] [PubMed]
63. Frew, Q.; Rennekampff, H.-O.; Dziewulski, P.; Moiemen, N.; Zahn, T.; Hartmann, B. Betulin wound gel accelerated healing of superficial partial thickness burns: Results of a randomized, intra-individually controlled, phase III trial with 12-months follow-up. *Burns* **2019**, *45*, 876–890. [CrossRef] [PubMed]
64. Tolmacheva, I.A.; Shelepen'kina, L.N.; Vikharev, Y.B.; Anikina, L.V.; Grishko, V.V.; Tolstikov, A.G. Synthesis and biological activity of S-containing betulin derivatives. *Chem. Nat. Compd.* **2005**, *41*, 701–705. [CrossRef]
65. Uzenkova, N.V.; Petrenko, N.I.; Shakirov, M.M.; Shul'ts, E.E.; Tolstikov, G.A. Synthesis of 30-amino derivatives of lupane triterpenoids. *Chem. Nat. Compd.* **2005**, *41*, 692–700. [CrossRef]
66. Hu, J.; Wang, Y.; Wei, X.; Wu, X.; Chen, G.; Cao, G.; Shen, X.; Zhang, X.; Tang, Q.; Liang, G.; et al. Synthesis and biological evaluation of novel thiazolidinone derivatives as potential anti-inflammatory agents. *Eur. J. Med. Chem.* **2013**, *64*, 292–301. [CrossRef]
67. Ainsworth, C. 1,2,4-TRIAZOLE. *Org. Synth.* **1960**, *40*, 99. [CrossRef]

68. Interagency Coordinating Committee on the Validation of Alternative Methods (ICCVAM). *ICCVAM-Recommended Test Method Protocol: Hen's Egg Test—Chorioallantoic Membrane (HET-CAM) Test Method*; National Institute of Environmental Health Sciences: Research Triangle Park, NC, USA, 2010.
69. Maghiari, A.L.; Coricovac, D.; Pinzaru, I.A.; Macașoi, I.G.; Marcovici, I.; Simu, S.; Navolan, D.; Dehelean, C. High Concentrations of Aspartame Induce Pro-Angiogenic Effects in Ovo and Cytotoxic Effects in HT-29 Human Colorectal Carcinoma Cells. *Nutrients* **2020**, *12*, 3600. [CrossRef]
70. Guercio, B.J.; Zhang, S.; Niedzwiecki, D.; Li, Y.; Babic, A.; Morales-Oyarvide, V.; Saltz, L.B.; Mayer, R.J.; Mowat, R.B.; Whittom, R.; et al. Associations of artificially sweetened beverage intake with disease recurrence and mortality in stage III colon cancer: Results from CALGB 89803 (Alliance). *PLoS ONE* **2018**, *13*, e0199244. [CrossRef]

Disclaimer/Publisher's Note: The statements, opinions and data contained in all publications are solely those of the individual author(s) and contributor(s) and not of MDPI and/or the editor(s). MDPI and/or the editor(s) disclaim responsibility for any injury to people or property resulting from any ideas, methods, instructions or products referred to in the content.

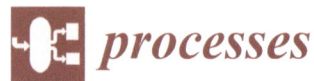

Article

Exploring the Antimelanoma Potential of Betulinic Acid Esters and Their Liposomal Nanoformulations

Andreea Milan [1,2], Marius Mioc [1,2], Alexandra Mioc [2,3,*], Narcisa Marangoci [4], Roxana Racoviceanu [1,2], Gabriel Mardale [2,3], Mihaela Bălan-Porcărașu [4], Slavița Rotunjanu [2], Irina Șoica [5] and Codruța Șoica [2,3]

[1] Department of Pharmaceutical Chemistry, Faculty of Pharmacy, Victor Babes University of Medicine and Pharmacy, Eftimie Murgu Square, No. 2, 300041 Timișoara, Romania; andreea.milan@umft.ro (A.M.); marius.mioc@umft.ro (M.M.); babuta.roxana@umft.ro (R.R.)
[2] Research Centre for Pharmaco-Toxicological Evaluation, Victor Babes University of Medicine and Pharmacy, Eftimie Murgu Square, No. 2, 300041 Timișoara, Romania; mardale.gabriel@umft.ro (G.M.); slavita.rotunjanu@umft.ro (S.R.); codrutasoica@umft.ro (C.Ș.)
[3] Department of Pharmacology-Pharmacotherapy, Faculty of Pharmacy, Victor Babes University of Medicine and Pharmacy, Eftimie Murgu Square, No. 2, 300041 Timișoara, Romania
[4] Institute of Macromolecular Chemistry 'Petru Poni', 700487 Iasi, Romania; nmarangoci@icmpp.ro (N.M.); mihaela.balan@icmpp.ro (M.B.-P.)
[5] University College London Medical School, 74 Huntley St., London WC1E 6DE, UK; irina.soica.20@ucl.ac.uk
* Correspondence: alexandra.mioc@umft.ro

Abstract: Betulinic acid is a naturally occurring pentacyclic triterpene belonging to the lupane-group that exhibits a wide range of pharmacological activities. BA derivatives are continuously being researched due to their improved anticancer efficacy and bioavailability. The current research was conducted in order to determine the antiproliferative potential of three synthesized BA fatty esters using palmitic, stearic and butyric acids and their liposomal nanoformulations. The cytotoxic potential of BA fatty esters (Pal-BA, St-BA, But-BA) and their respective liposomal formulations (Pal-BA-Lip, St-BA-Lip, But-BA-Lip) has been assessed on HaCaT immortalized human keratinocytes and A375 human melanoma cells. Both the esters and their liposomes acted as cytotoxic agents against melanoma cells in a time- and dose-dependent manner. The butyryl ester But-BA outperformed BA in terms of cytotoxicity (IC$_{50}$ 60.77 µM) while the nanoformulations St-BA-Lip, But-BA-Lip and BA-Lip also displayed IC$_{50}$ values (60.11, 50.71 and 59.01 µM) lower compared to BA (IC$_{50}$ 65.9 µM). The morphological evaluation revealed that the A375 cells underwent morphological changes consistent with apoptosis following 48 h treatment with the tested compounds, while the HaCaT cells' morphology remained unaltered. Both the esters and their liposomal formulations were able to inhibit the migration of the melanoma cells, suggesting a significant antimetastatic effect. The quantitative real-time PCR revealed that all tested samples were able to significantly increase the expression of the pro-apoptotic Bax and inhibit the anti-apoptotic Bcl-2 proteins. This effect was more potent in the case of liposomal nanoformulations versus non-encapsulated compounds, and overall, But-BA and its formulation exhibited the best results in this regard.

Keywords: betulinic acid; betulinic acid derivatives; liposomal formulation; cytotoxicity; melanoma

Citation: Milan, A.; Mioc, M.; Mioc, A.; Marangoci, N.; Racoviceanu, R.; Mardale, G.; Bălan-Porcărașu, M.; Rotunjanu, S.; Șoica, I.; Șoica, C. Exploring the Antimelanoma Potential of Betulinic Acid Esters and Their Liposomal Nanoformulations. *Processes* **2024**, *12*, 416. https://doi.org/10.3390/pr12020416

Academic Editors: Alina Bora and Luminita Crisan

Received: 12 December 2023
Revised: 15 February 2024
Accepted: 16 February 2024
Published: 19 February 2024

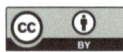

Copyright: © 2024 by the authors. Licensee MDPI, Basel, Switzerland. This article is an open access article distributed under the terms and conditions of the Creative Commons Attribution (CC BY) license (https://creativecommons.org/licenses/by/4.0/).

1. Introduction

Natural products have long been a major focus in finding treatments for a wide range of maladies. Their enormous pharmacological potential and formulation versatility have designated them as an interesting starting point in the development of different drugs [1]. Several breakthroughs in organic chemistry have been inspired by natural compounds, leading to significantly improved semisynthetic analogues that retain the main scaffold of the natural compound but exert enhanced pharmacological properties [2].

Betulinic acid (BA, 3β-hydroxy-lup-20(29)-en-28-oic acid) is a pentacyclic triterpene, belonging to the lupane group and widely distributed throughout the plant kingdom, but mainly found in the birch tree bark (*Betula* sp., Betulaceae) [3]. Due to Pisha's discovery that betulinic acid (BA) exhibits specific cytotoxic effects against human melanoma, the pentacyclic triterpene has been analyzed and further developed for its various biological properties [4]. BA exerts significant in vitro cytotoxic effects against a plethora of tumor cell lines, its properties being demonstrated against colon, breast, prostate, hepatocellular, bladder, neck, pancreatic, lung, ovarian and human melanoma [5]. Moreover, several researches have been conducted to confirm and identify BA's mechanism of action as an anticancer, anti-inflammatory, antioxidant, antidiabetic, antiviral, cardioprotective, neuroprotective agent [6–8]. Despite its high pharmacological potential, its current use in therapy is limited particularly by its low in vivo bioavailability [9], a challenge that was tackled both technically through cyclodextrin complexation [10] and liposomal nanoformulations [11,12], and by chemical modulation [13]. Amongst different chemical derivatizations, the esterification with fatty acids has emerged as a promising method for the synthesis of active compounds with improved biological activities. Fatty acids have been identified as cell apoptosis inducers as well as inhibitors of cancer cell proliferation [14]. Al-Hwaiti et al. have demonstrated that palmitic acid and stearic acid, alongside oleic and linoleic acids exerted anticancer effects against colorectal cancer Caco-2 and HCT-116 cells [15]; furthermore, ω-hydroxypalmitic acid and ω-hydroxystearic acid were able to induce cell apoptosis against G361 melanoma cells [16]. It was also reported that butyric acid could facilitate the chemoprevention in colorectal carcinogenesis; Chodurek et al. have tested its chemopreventive effect against A375 melanoma cells while also revealing that sodium butyrate was able to inhibit cell proliferation [17]. Long-chain BA and betulin fatty esters have been previously synthesized by Pinzaru et al. who assessed their anticancer activity, revealing improved pharmacological potential compared to the parent active compound [18]. Furthermore, the evaluation of other pentacyclic triterpenes fatty esters has been performed by Mallavadhani et al. who had synthesized 3-O-fatty ester chains (C_{12}-C_{18}) of amyrins and ursolic acid, the dodecanoate derivatives showing potent antimicrobial activity against the Gram—*P. syringae*, significantly higher compared to the reference tetracycline [19]. Pentacyclic triterpenes' antiproteolytic effectiveness of the anti-inflammatory potential has been evaluated by Hodges et al.; the authors have obtained two fatty acid esters analogues of lupeol using palmitic and linoleic acids and demonstrated their selective trypsin inhibition properties [20]. Similarly, the synthesis of fatty acids ester derivatives of lupeol by Fotie et al. proved that the introduction of the long side chain has a positive effect on the antimalarial activity against drug-resistant clones of *Plasmodium falciparum* W-2 and D-6 [21].

To address the bioavailability issue associated with the highly lipophilic nature of BA fatty esters, their inclusion in liposomal formulations has been regarded as a potentially viable solution. Due to their unique chemical and physical features such as their amphiphilic characteristics, resemblance to human cells and the possibility of being extensively surface-modified, liposomes provide a myriad of advantages over other nanoparticles, including great preparation versatility, the capacity to encapsulate a large number of distinct compounds, and targeted delivery resulting in high patient tolerance [22]. However, conventional liposomes are easily unstable in the plasma due to their chemical composition and their interaction with lipoproteins [23]; sterically stabilized through surface modifications (stealth) liposomes are able to prevent drug leakage prior to delivery [24].

The current study proposes the synthesis of BA fatty esters using stearic, palmitic and butyric acids, which are reported to possess individually unique pharmacological effects [25–27] followed by their encapsulation in surface-modified liposomal nanoformulations bearing polyethylene glycol fragments in order to prolong their lifespan. The resulting formulations were assessed as anticancer agents against human malignant melanoma (A375) cells.

2. Results

2.1. Chemistry

2.1.1. Synthesis and Characterization of Fatty Acid Esters of BA

The reaction conditions for obtaining fatty BA esters are depicted in Figure 1. All three compounds were obtained in high yields (>65%). The ^{1}H NMR spectra of the esters' derivatives show the peaks for the two H30 protons from the BA backbone as two singlets at 4.74 and 4.61 ppm, H3 resonates at 4.47 ppm, H19 is found at 3.00 ppm and the CH_2 protons adjacent to the ester group of the fatty acid residue resonate at 2.30 and 2.27 ppm, overlapped with one of the H15 protons from the BA. The integral values of the peaks from the ^{1}H NMR spectra are in accordance with the proposed structures (Figures S1, S7 and S13, Supplementary Materials). The ^{13}C NMR spectra show the peak for the COOH group from BA at around 182 ppm, the COO carbon of the ester group at about 173 ppm and the peaks for the rest of the carbon atoms at the appropriate chemical shift values (Figures S2, S8 and S14, Supplementary Materials). The peak for the ester carbon from 173 ppm gives long range correlation peaks in the H,C-HMBC spectra (Figures S6, S12 and S18, Supplementary Materials) with both H3 from BA and with CH_2 from the fatty acid chain, thus demonstrating the covalent bonding between BA and the fatty acids. Ester formation is also supported by FTIR spectroscopy, which shows an adjacent C=O signal belonging to the ester function at 1730 cm^{-1} in the spectra of each compound. Furthermore, the strong OH signal from the BA spectra at 3349 cm^{-1} is no longer present in the FTIR spectra of the obtained esters (Figure S19, Supplementary Materials). The most relevant physicochemical properties of each newly synthetized BA derivative are presented in Table 1.

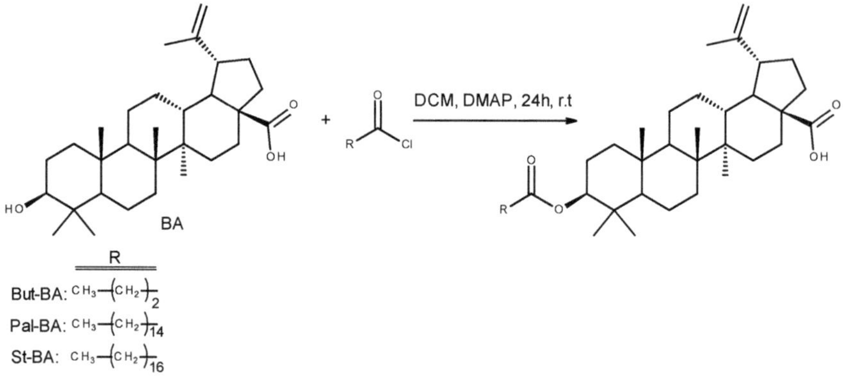

Figure 1. Synthesis of BA fatty acid ester derivatives; BA: betulinic acid, But-BA: 3-O-butiryl-betulinic acid, Pal-BA: 3-O-palmitoyl-betulinic acid, St-BA: 3-O-stearoyl-betulinic acid; DCM: dichloromethane, DMAP: 4-Dimethylaminopyridine.

Table 1. Physicochemical properties of synthetized BA derivatives.

Compound	Melting Point	Yield	Appearance	m/z [M-H+]$^-$
But-BA	265–280 °C	74%	white powder	525
Pal-BA	160–170 °C	70%	translucent crystals	693
St-BA	150–162 °C	65%	translucent crystals	721

2.1.2. Synthesis and Characterization of BA-Fatty Acid Ester Liposomal Formulation

The lipid film hydration method, which has previously been shown to be suitable for our current purpose [28], was used to obtain bare liposomes as well as liposomal formulations loaded with BA and its newly synthesized esters. Transmission electron microscopy (TEM), scanning electron microscopy (SEM), and dynamic light scattering (DLS) were used to examine the liposomes. Results are depicted in Figures 2–4. The TEM and SEM images revealed stable spherical liposomes of various sizes. The diameters of the bare liposomes were rarely larger than 100 nm, whereas the addition of triterpenes increased their diameter. The liposomal formulations containing the palmitoyl and stearoyl esters of BA displayed the largest particles, with sizes occasionally exceeding 200 nm (Figures 2 and 3). While the microscopy-recorded diameters and the mean hydrodynamic size of the particles slightly differ, DLS measurements were within the expected range (Figure 4). The measured polydispersity index was roughly related to the measured liposome diameters; bare liposomes had the lowest dispersity (PI 0.1955), BA-Lip and But-BA-Lip had PI values in the around 0.2, while the large ester formulations exhibited PI values in the 0.4–0.5 range (Figure 4). DLS measurements were repeated daily for one week; no significant changes in the recorded PI values and hydrodynamic size occurred, indicating that these formulations were stable within the tested time period. The determined ζ potential values for empty liposomes, BA-Lip, But-BA-Lip, Pal-BA-Lip and St-BA-Lip were −22.1 mV, −19.4 mV, −18.7 mV, −18.2 mV and −17.8 mV, respectively. Drug loading efficiency (DLE) ranged from 78 to 85% for all liposomal formulations; DLE values for BA-Lip, But-BA-Lip, Pal-BA-Lip and St-BA-Lip were 78%, 85%, 82% and 80%, respectively. Furthermore, liposome stability related to drug loading efficiency was assessed over a 15-day period at two different temperatures. As depicted in Table 2, minor changes in drug encapsulation efficiency were observed during the stability study at 4 °C, but there was a significant decrease in stability when the formulations were stored at 25 °C. As indicated by the percentage difference between day 1 and day 15, liposomes containing BA were the most stable formulation, while But-BA-Lip was the least stable.

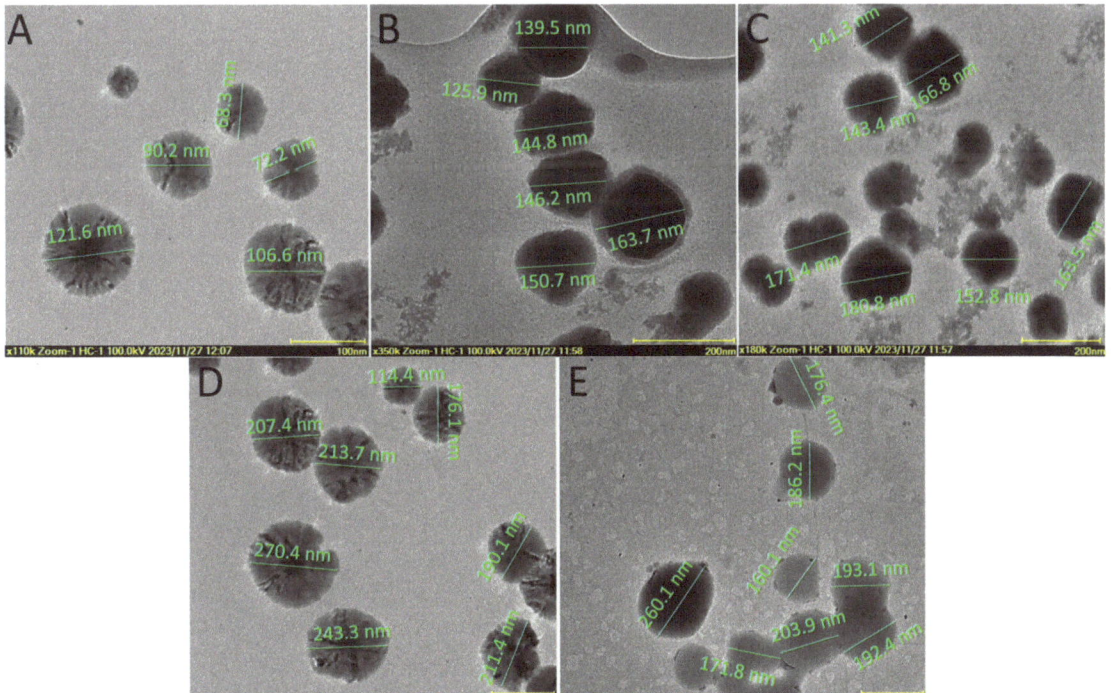

Figure 2. TEM images of (**A**) bare liposome (scale bar 100 nm), (**B**) BA-Lip (scale bar 200 nm), (**C**) But-BA-Lip (scale bar 200 nm), (**D**) Pal-BA-Lip (scale bar 200 nm) and (**E**) St-BA-Lip (scale bar 200 nm).

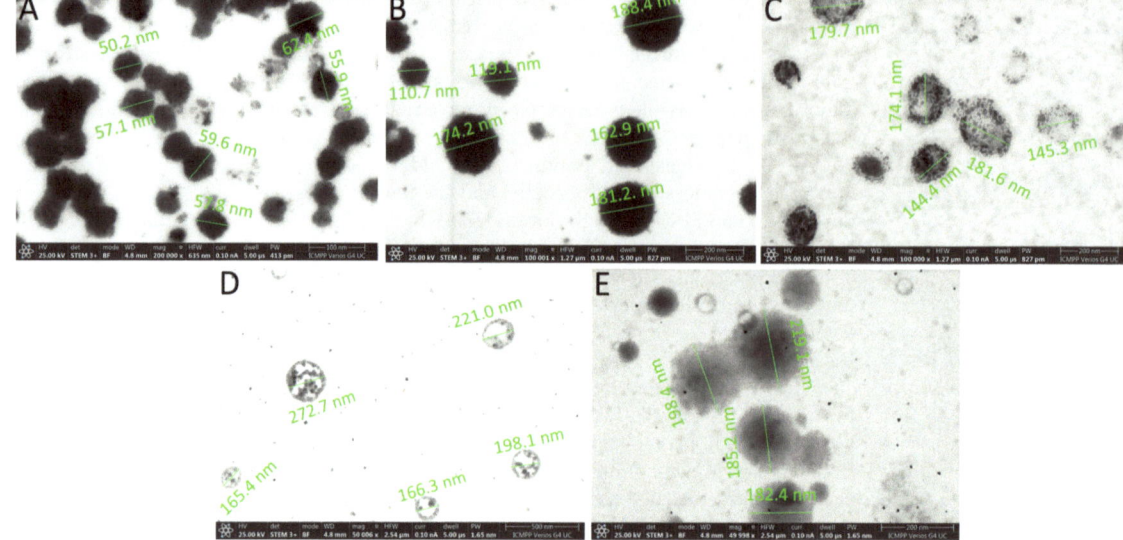

Figure 3. SEM images of (**A**) bare liposome (scale bar 100 nm), (**B**) BA-Lip (scale bar 200 nm), (**C**) But-BA-Lip (scale bar 200 nm), (**D**) Pal-BA-Lip (scale bar 500 nm) and (**E**) St-BA-Lip (scale bar 200 nm).

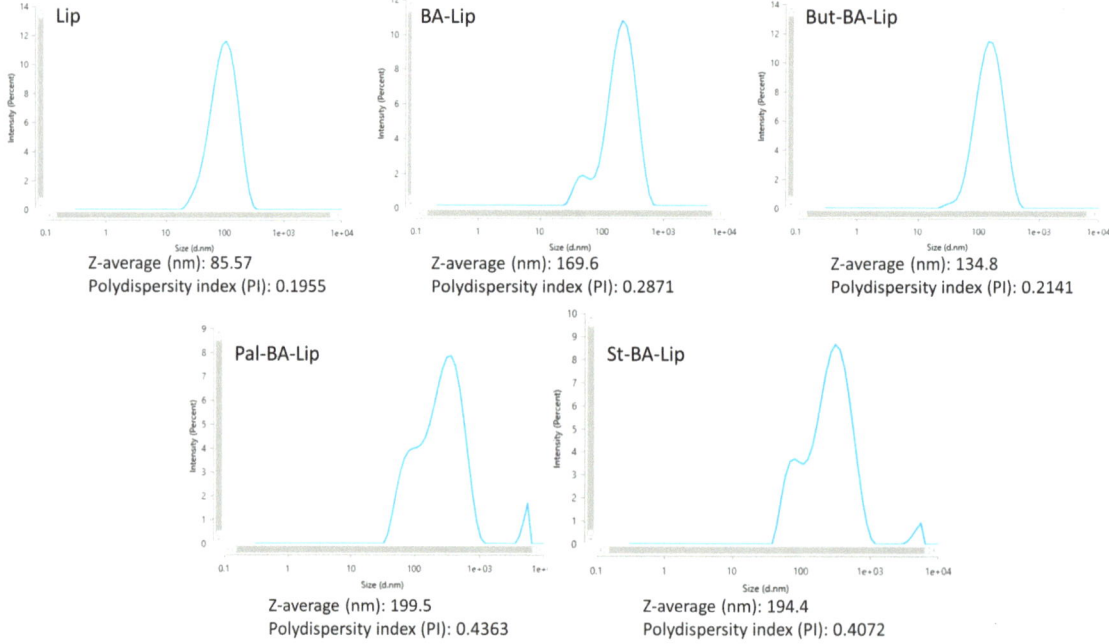

Figure 4. Measured hydrodynamic size and polydispersity index of the obtained liposomal formulations.

Table 2. Drug loading efficiency of liposomal formulations determined at 4 °C and 25 °C, for 15 days.

| | Drug Loading Efficiency (DLE %) | | | | | | | |
| | BA-Lip | | But-BA-Lip | | Pal-BA-Lip | | St-BA-Lip | |
	4 °C	25 °C	4 °C	25 °C	4 °C	25 °C	4 °C	25 °C
Day 1	78.12	78.12	85.22	85.22	82.06	82.06	80.18	80.18
Day 3	78.08	77.66	84.91	84.51	81.65	81.42	79.72	79.71
Day 5	77.65	77.13	84.58	83.72	81.17	80.68	79.16	78.88
Day 7	76.87	76.35	83.96	82.82	80.58	79.81	78.44	77.85
Day 9	76.11	75.38	83.15	80.91	79.83	78.87	77.53	76.71
Day 11	75.76	74.4	82.21	78.82	78.95	77.72	76.49	75.46
Day 13	74.58	73.17	81.03	76.51	78.01	76.25	75.35	73.89
Day 15	73.89	71.11	78.84	73.64	76.63	74.56	74.07	72.14
Day 1–15 difference	4.23	7.01	6.38	11.58	5.43	7.5	6.11	8.04

2.2. Evaluation of Betulinic Acid Fatty Esters and Liposomes Cytotoxic Effect

The viability of nonmalignant human keratinocytes—HaCaT and human malignant melanoma—A375 cells was evaluated at 24 h and 48 h post-treatment with the newly synthesized compounds (10, 25, 50, 75 and 100 µM) using the Alamar blue assay. The incubation of nonmalignant HaCaT cells for 24 and 48 h revealed that, except for But-BA and But-BA-Lip, the tested compounds did not exhibit cytotoxic effects against HaCaT cells even at the highest tested concentrations (75 and 100 µM). However, the slightly cytotoxic effects of But-BA and But-BA-Lip were only recorded at the highest tested concentration with cell viability (%) decreasing at 73.15 ± 3.9 (48 h), 75.24 ± 2.57 (24 h) for But-BA and 84.12 ± 1.5 (48 h), 84.92 ± 0.06 (24 h) for But-BA-Lip; neither effect was comparable to 5-FU (5-Fluorouracil) where cell viabilities dropped to 30.61 ± 3.54 (48 h), 35.58 ± 2.87 (24 h) when the same concentration (100 µM) was applied (Figure 5).

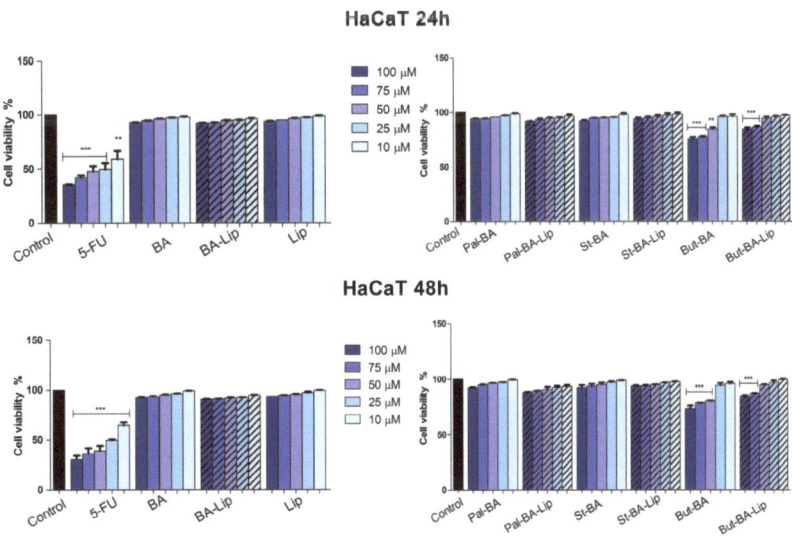

Figure 5. Cell viability after 24 and 48 h treatment with 5-FU, BA, BA-Lip, Pal-BA, Pal-BA-Lip, St-BA, St-BA-Lip, But-BA and But-BA-Lip (10, 25, 50, 75 and 100 µM) on HaCaT cells. The results are expressed as viability percentages compared to the control group, considered 100% (** $p < 0.01$ and *** $p < 0.001$ vs. control cells). The slash bars are represented by the liposomal nanoformulations of BA's esters. The data represents the mean values ± SD of three independent experiments performed in triplicate.

In terms of antimelanoma effects, the results revealed that among the synthetized esters, only But-BA decreased cell viability more aggressively than BA alone subsequently displaying lower IC$_{50}$ value after 48 h incubation (60.77 µM vs. 65.9 µM) (Table 3); the other esters (Pal-BA and St-BA) significantly decreased cell viability (%) vs. control (100%) but displayed a similar cytotoxic profile with pure BA when the highest concentrations were applied for 48 h (47.29 ± 1.39 for Pal-BA and 45.54 ± 2.8 for St-BA vs. 40.24 ± 0.89 for BA). Moreover, the results showed that the inclusion of BA or its fatty esters in liposomes induced stronger cytotoxic effects compared to the fatty esters and pure BA, respectively; however, neither compound was able to match the antiproliferative activity of 5-FU, as follows: 37.34 ± 2.74 (Pal-BA-Lip 100 µM–48 h), 46.73 ± 4.96 (Pal-BA-Lip 100 µM–24 h), 44.52 ± 0.52 (St-BA-Lip 100 µM–48 h), 45.43 ± 1.68 (St-BA-Lip 100 µM–24 h), 33.42 ± 0.03 (But-BA-Lip 100 µM–48 h), 42.94 ± 4.87 (But-BA-Lip 100 µM–24 h), 40.24 ± 0.89 (BA 100 µM–48 h) and 52.47 ± 1.01 (BA 100 µM–24 h) compared to 20.23 ± 2.24 (5-FU 100 µM, 48 h) and 26.45 ± 7.53 (5-FU 100 µM–24 h). Empty liposomes did not exert cytotoxic effects in either HaCaT human keratinocytes or melanoma A375 cells (Figure 6).

Table 3. The calculated IC$_{50}$ values (µM) of 5-FU, BA, BA-Lip, Pal-BA, Pal-BA-Lip, St-BA, St-BA-Lip, But-BA and But-BA-Lip on HaCaT and A375 cell lines 48 h post-stimulation.

Compounds	HaCaT	A375
5-FU	40.14 ± 1.2	26.61 ± 0.82
BA	>100	65.9 ± 1.07
BA-LIP	>100	59.01 ± 0.45
PAL-BA	>100	85.58 ± 1.32
PAL-BA-LIP	>100	67.59 ± 0.33
ST-BA	>100	75.75 ± 0.75
ST-BA-LIP	>100	60.11 ± 1.56
BUT-BA	>100	60.77 ± 0.29
BUT-BA-LIP	>100	50.71 ± 0.67

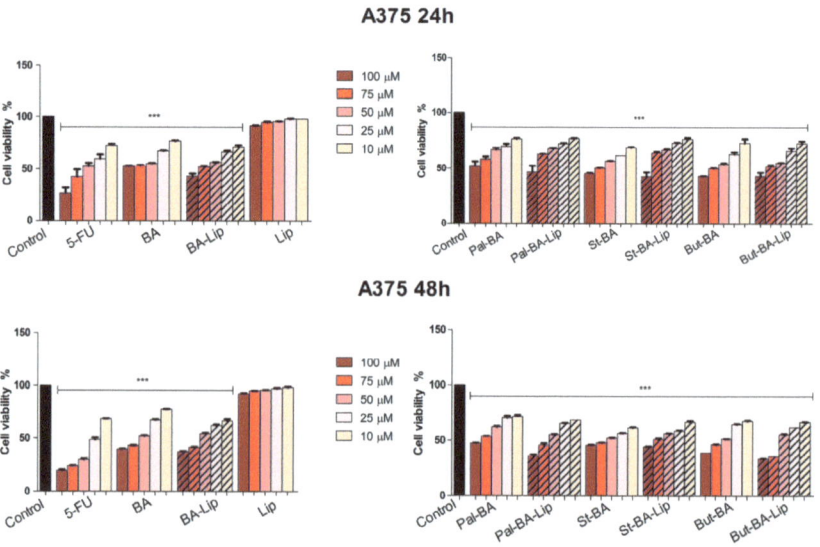

Figure 6. Cell viability after 24 and 48 h treatment with 5-FU, BA, BA-Lip, Pal-BA, Pal-BA-Lip, St-BA, St-BA-Lip, But-BA and But-BA-Lip (10, 25, 50, 75 and 100 µM) on A375 cells. The results are expressed as viability percentages compared to the control group, considered 100% (*** $p < 0.001$ vs. control cells). The slash bars represent viability data for liposomal nanoformulations of BA's esters. The data represents the mean values ± SD of three independent experiments performed in triplicate.

2.3. Fatty Ester Derivatives Effects on Cell Morphology

In nonmalignant HaCaT cells, no significant differences have been observed in terms of cell morphology and confluence between treated and untreated (control) cells after 48 h. But-BA (100 µM) and But-BA-Lip (100 µM) only slightly altered cellular morphology, some of the cells becoming rounder and on the verge of detaching (Figure S20A–C, Supplementary Materials). The positive control, 5-FU, decreased the number and altered HaCaT morphology and confluence, making them round and detached (Figure S20A).

In A375 melanoma cells, treatment with 5-FU, the highest concentration of esters (Pal-BA, St-BA and But-BA) and their liposomes (Pal-BA-Lip, St-BA-Lip and But-BA-Lip) induced several morphological changes such as round and detached cells, changes that occurred simultaneously with a reduced number of cells, thus correlating to viability results (Figure S21A–C, Supplementary Materials).

No significant changes in HaCaT cell morphology were detected in terms of cell cytoskeleton architecture and nuclei upon treatment with BA, esters or their liposomal formulations (BA, Ba-Lip, But-BA, But-Ba-Lip, Pal-BA, Pal-BA-Lip, St-BA and St-BA-Lip) in the highest tested concentration (100 µM) for 48 h (Figure 7A,B).

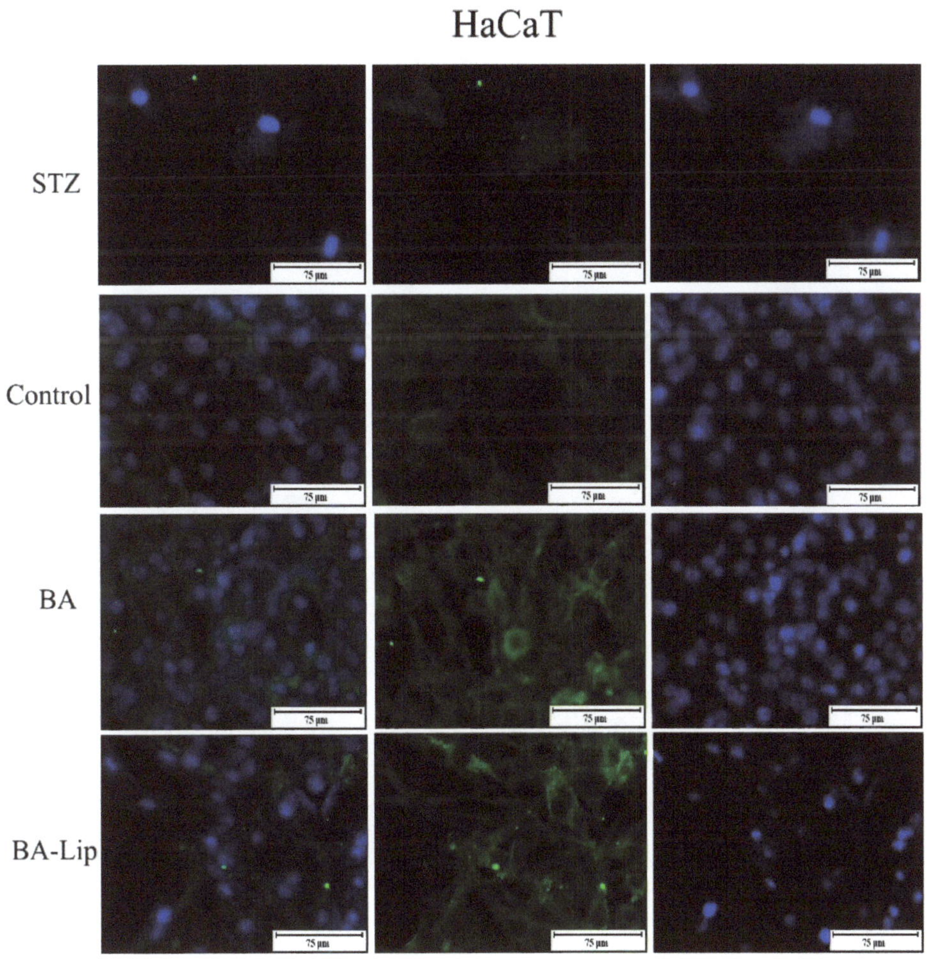

Figure 7. *Cont.*

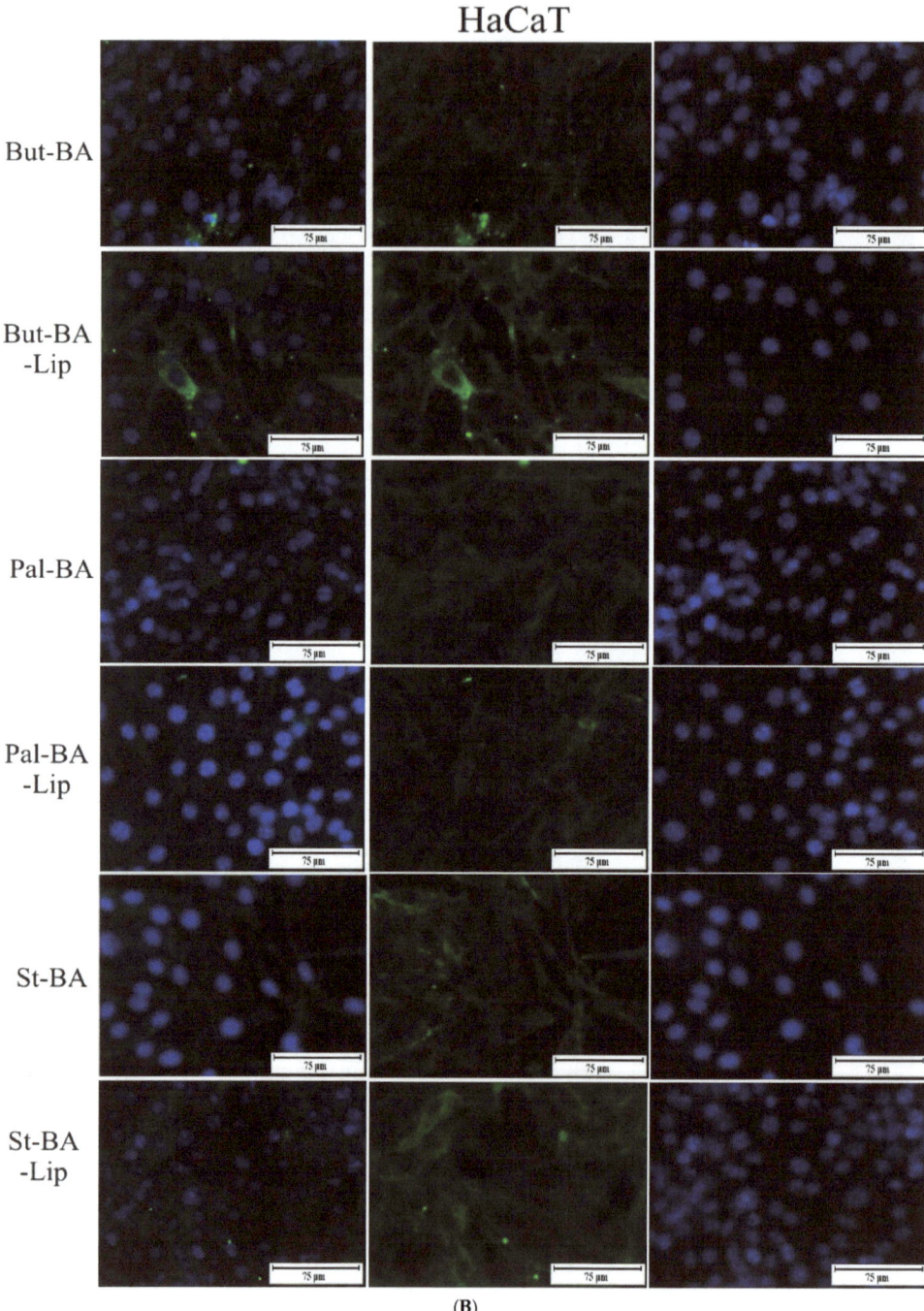

Figure 7. The impact of 48 h treatment with BA, Ba-Lip (100 μM) (**A**) and But-BA, But-Ba-Lip, Pal-BA, Pal-BA-Lip, St-BA and St-BA-Lip (100 μM) (**B**) on HaCaT cells nuclei (blue–Hoechst staining–third column), cytoskeleton (beta-actin–green staining–second column) and the merged picture (first column). Staurosporine (STZ, 5 μM) was used as a positive control for necrotic cell death. The scale bar was 150 μm.

The 48 h treatment of A375 melanoma cells with BA, fatty acid esters and their liposomal formulation (Ba-Lip, But-BA, But-Ba-Lip, Pal-BA, Pal-BA-Lip, St-BA and St-BA-Lip) using their IC$_{50}$ values induced various morphological changes that are consistent with apoptosis (Figure 8A,B). In particular, the treated cells underwent observable cytoskeletal rearrangement accompanied by the alteration of cell shape and loss of structural integrity; other morphological changes can be observed at nuclear level, such as: chromatin condensation (the nucleus appears highly compacted), nuclear shrinkage and fragmentation and the formation of apoptotic bodies that can be seen as widely spread small condensed chromatin fragments with various sizes.

Quantitative real-time PCR was used to determine gene expression variations of anti-apoptotic Bcl-2 and pro-apoptotic Bax in order to further investigate the pro-apoptotic effect of BA, BA-fatty acid esters, and their liposomal formulations against melanoma cells. After a 24-h incubation period, measurements were carried out on A375 cells treated with test compounds at a sub-cytotoxic concentration of 10 µM. The results show that all compounds and formulations increase the expression of the pro-apoptotic Bax gene while decreasing the expression of the anti-apoptotic Bcl-2 gene (Figure 9). BA induced a two-fold reduction in the relative fold expression of Bcl-2. In this case, BA was outperformed by its liposomal formulations Pal-BA and Pal-BA-Lip. This trend could be observed in the case of BAX, where the 2.5 increase in relative fold expression induced by BA was surpassed by the same BA-Lip, Pal-BA, and Pal-BA-Lip. It is also worth noting that the liposomal formulation outperformed the unencapsulated compound in each case.

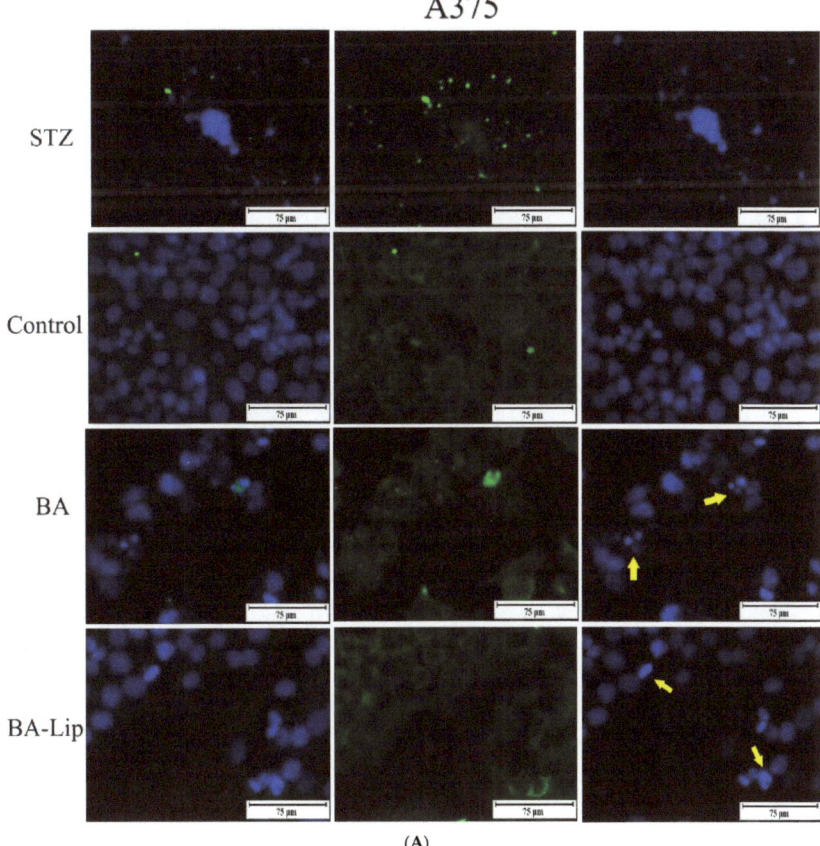

(A)

Figure 8. Cont.

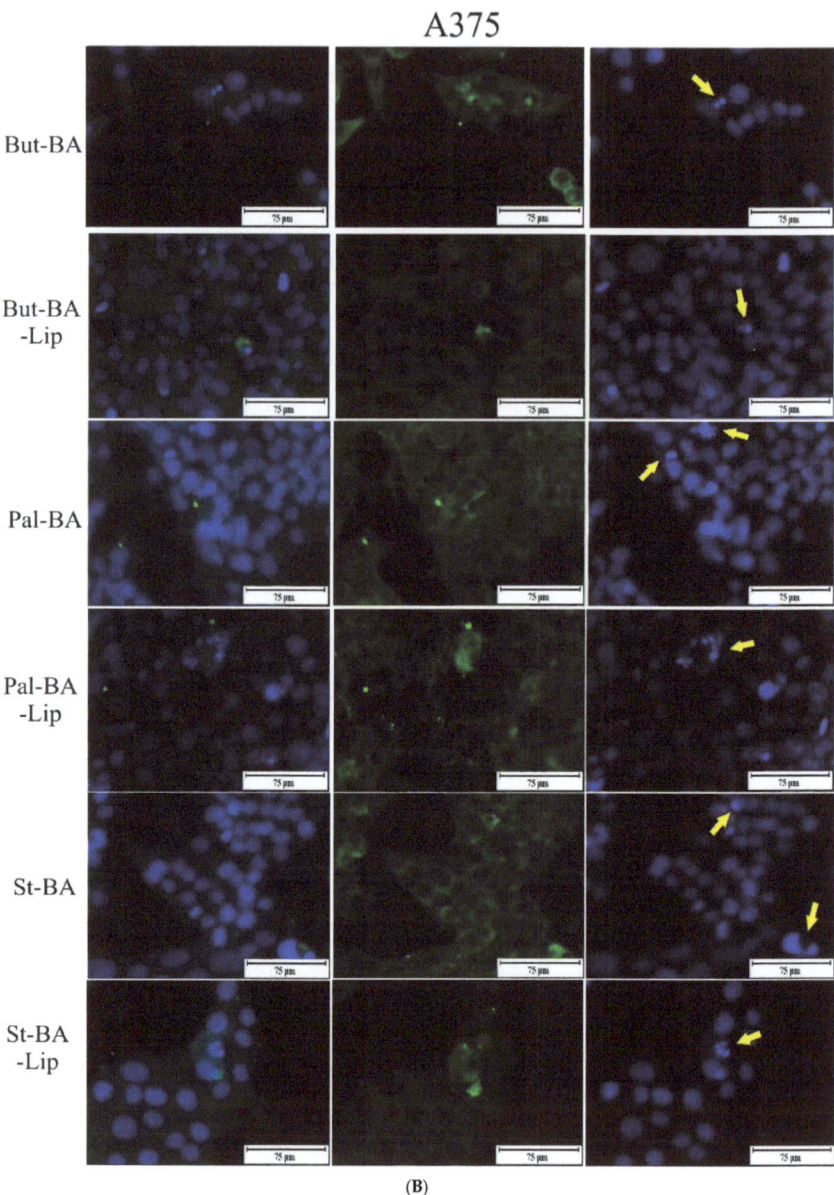

Figure 8. The impact of 48 h treatment with BA, Ba-Lip (IC$_{50}$) (**A**) and But-BA, But-Ba-Lip, Pal-BA, Pal-BA-Lip, St-BA and St-BA-Lip (IC$_{50}$) (**B**) on A375 cells nuclei (blue—Hoechst staining—third column), cytoskeleton (beta-actin—green staining—second column) and the merged picture (first column). Staurosporine (STZ, 5 μM) was used as a positive control for necrotic cell death. The yellow arrows indicate signs of apoptotic cell death. The scale bar was 150 μm.

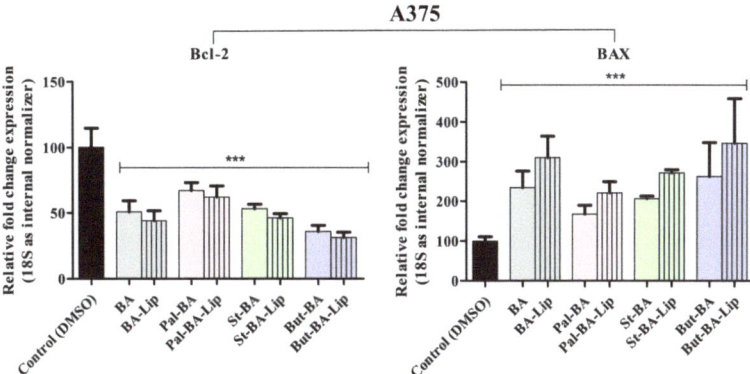

Figure 9. Relative fold change expression in mRNA of Bcl-2 and BAX in A375 cells after stimulation with BA, BA-Lip, But-BA, But-Ba-Lip, Pal-BA, Pal-BA-Lip, St-BA and St-BA-Lip at 10 μM. The expressions were normalized to 18S and DMSO was used as control. Data represents the mean values ± SD of three independent experiments. One-way ANOVA with Dunnett's post-test was applied to determine the statistical differences in rapport with DMSO stimulated cells (*** $p < 0.001$ vs. control cells).

2.4. Scratch Assay

In order to determine the anti-migratory effects of BA, BA fatty acid esters and their liposomal formulations, a scratch assay technique was performed. Stimulation of A375 melanoma cells with BA esters and their respective liposomes revealed an efficient anti-migratory effect for the tested concentration (10 μM) both 24 h and 48 h post-treatment (Figures 10 and 11A–C). All compounds exhibited scratch closure rates below 30% compared to control with a scratch closure rate of 70% after 24 h and 81.49% after 48 h. BA esters (Pal-BA, St-BA and But-BA) inhibited the scratch closure rate to 14.5%, 23.31% and 19.98%, respectively. The most impressive anti-migratory effects were exhibited by But-BA-Lip, with a scratch closure rate of 8.23%, and Pal-BA-Lip, with a scratch closure rate of 8.61%, values that were slightly lower compared to those of BA at 16.48% and BA-Lip at 9.62%. St-BA-Lip decreased the scratch closure rate to 22.36%. Furthermore, at this concentration, cells with round shape and detached cells could be observed, thus clearly showing the cytotoxic effects of these compounds against melanoma cells.

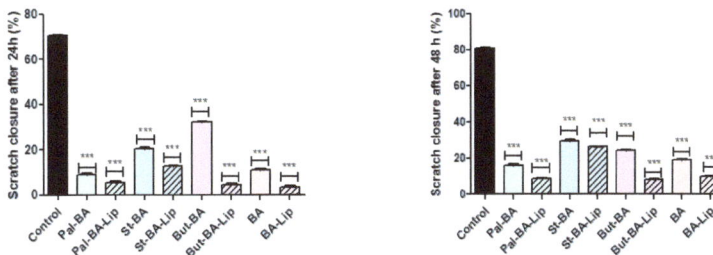

Figure 10. Scratch migration assay of Pal-BA, Pal-BA-Lip, St-BA, St-BA-Lip, But-BA, But-BA-Lip, BA and BA-Lip (10 μM) on A375 cells. The percentage signifies the remnant gap size 24 h and 48 h after conducting the scratches compared to the initial gap size. Values were expressed as mean ± SD and the asterisk values show significant results of the tested compounds compared to the control group using the one-way ANOVA's test followed by Dunnett's post-test.

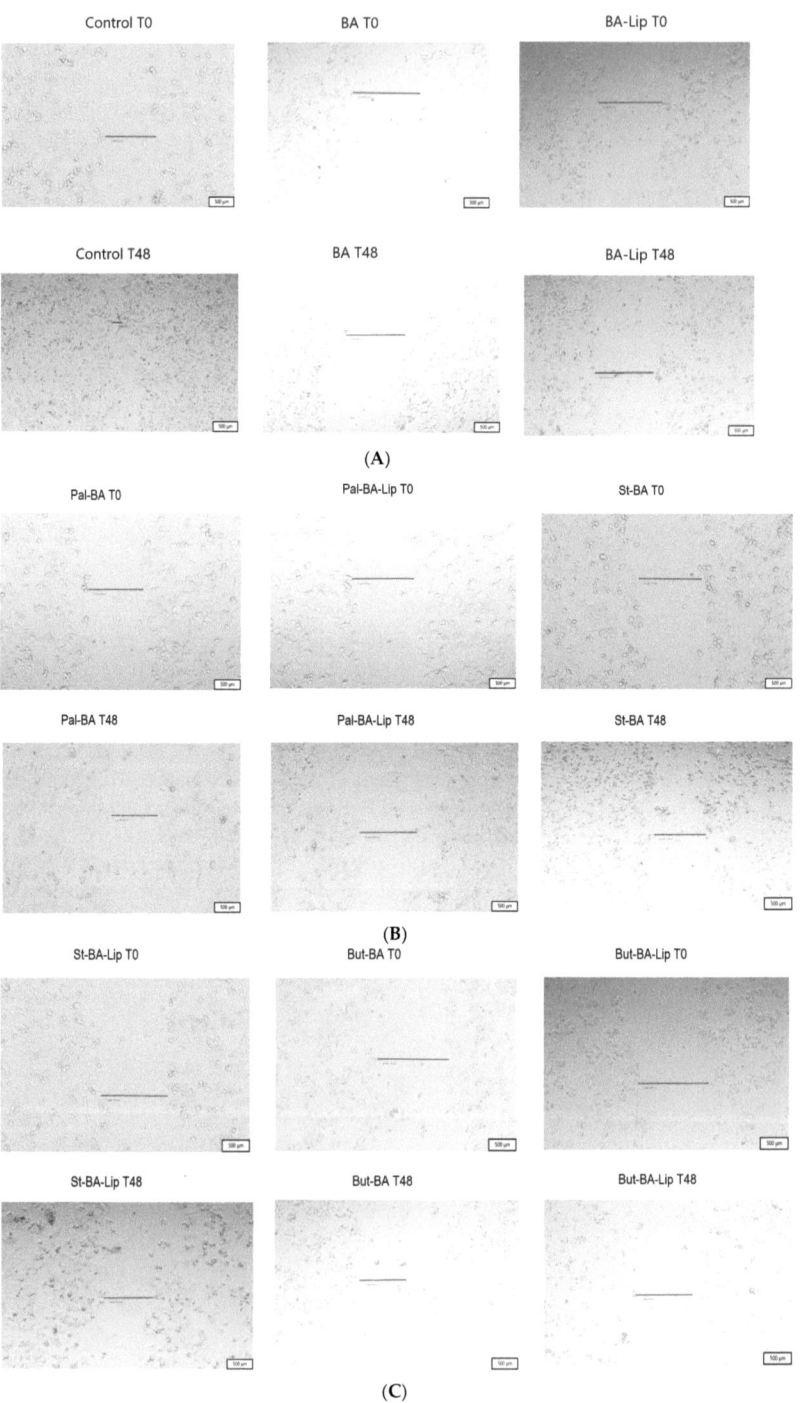

Figure 11. The effects of BA and BA-Lip (**A**), Pal-BA, Pal-BA-Lip, St-BA (**B**), St-BA-Lip, But-BA and But-BA-Lip (**C**) (10 μM) on malignant melanoma cells A375 migration capacity. The images were taken by light microscopy at 10× magnification. The cell migration was measured both at 0 h and at 48 h after stimulation. The red line represents the measured width of the scratched/wounded area.

2.5. Betulinic Acid Esters Effect on BAX and Bcl-2 Protein Levels

In order to determine whether the treatment with BA, BA-Lip, Pal-BA, Pal-BA-Lip, St-BA, St-BA-Lip, But-BA and But-BA-Lip induce apoptotic cell death in A375 cancer cells, the pro-apoptotic BAX and anti-apoptotic Bcl-2 levels were quantitatively measured using an in vitro Enzyme-Linked Immunosorbent assay (ELISA). The results indicate that all compounds were able to increase the pro-apoptotic BAX protein level, while decreasing the anti-apoptotic Bcl-2 protein level (Figure 12).

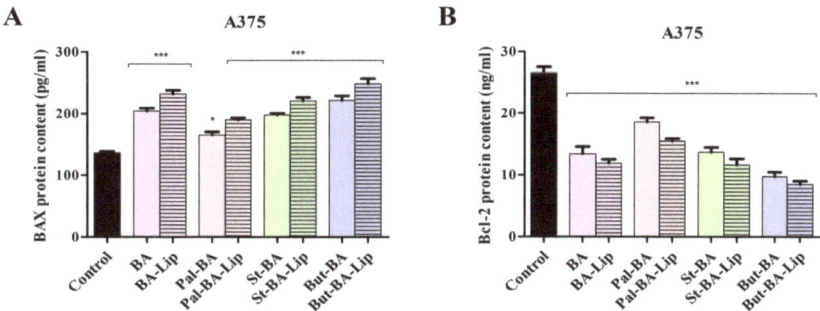

Figure 12. Effect of BA, BA-Lip, Pal-BA, Pal-BA-Lip, St-BA, St-BA-Lip, But-BA and But-BA-Lip, (IC50) on BAX (**A**) and Bcl-2 (**B**) protein levels in A375 cell lines after 48 h treatment. The results were reported as mean values ± SD with $p < 0.05$ (*) and $p < 0.001$ (***), when compared to control. All experiments were performed in triplicate.

3. Discussion

When comparing natural compounds versus synthetic ones as treatments against malignant diseases, nature wins points by presenting certain advantages such as superior efficacy and safety, lower costs and chemical diversity; moreover, natural compounds have the ability to modulate multiple oncogenic signaling pathways while conventional chemotherapeutic drugs usually aim at only one particular target [29]. Betulinic acid, which can be found in many tree and plant species, shows a wide range of biologic activities [30] including selective anticancer effects against numerous types of cancer cells [31]; its ability to directly target mitochondria and trigger cancer death provides the possibility of alternative anticancer treatment when conventional therapy fails [32]. Despite its promising anticarcinogenic effects, BA's low bioavailability has impelled many researchers to synthesize new analogues that exhibit improved pharmacokinetic and pharmacodynamic profiles [33]. The chemical modulation of betulinic acid may lead to the synthesis of hybrid molecules that occupy a special place in the development of effective anticancer agents, since they provide the possibility to enhance and enlarge the biological effects of the parent molecule while circumventing drug resistance [34]. Some researchers reported that the biological activities of several pentacyclic triterpenes such as amyrin, oleanolic acid, lupeol and ursolic acid might be improved through esterification with fatty acids [19,35]. Despite general knowledge that saturated fatty acids are associated with increased risks of cardiovascular events, they are also involved in important physiological regulatory mechanisms in protein activation and subcellular trafficking as well as gene transcription; moreover, saturated fatty acids may induce apoptosis through several pathways [36]. To the best of our knowledge, fatty acid conjugates of anticancer agents are rather poorly explored although several studied revealed that both saturated and unsaturated fatty acids have the ability to improve the anticancer efficacy and selectivity of conjugated drugs [37]. Betulinic acid is currently regarded as unsuitable for therapeutic use due to its low solubility and bioavailability; the introduction of a hydrophobic fragment in the molecule's scaffold causes an increase in lipophilicity that may induce an increased uptake of the compound through the cell membrane, thus optimizing its bioavailability [38].

Triterpene esterification can be accomplished using a variety of reagents such as free acids, anhydrides or acyl chlorides; since BA contains a single hydroxyl group that can be acylated, the more reactive acyl chlorides were chosen as reaction partners. One previous study used anhydrides to synthesize various 3-O-BA esters [39], including 3-O-butiryl-BA; however, the resulting compound was obtained in lower yields compared to the current study. BA esters were subsequently incorporated in liposomes which are able to prolong circulation time and facilitate intracellular absorption; in addition, liposome entrapment may delay ester hydrolysis, thus providing in vivo controlled drug release [40].

Several previous studies reported BA-containing liposomes with similar characteristics which were also prepared by using the film hydration method employed in the current study, thus making it highly reproducible. As an example, Farcas et al. described a BA formulation containing magnetic nanoparticles entrapped in PEGylated liposomes [28] where, similar to our case, the addition of BA resulted in an increase in hydrodynamic size and PI values; the authors also reported comparable DLE values. Liu Y et al. prepared BA PEGylated liposomes with a mean diameter of 142 nm and DLE of up to 95% [12]; Mullauer et al. used the film hydration method to obtain BA-liposomes with sizes ranging from 100 to 200 nm [41]. Even when the liposomal formulation contains a mixture of BA with other active compounds, it appears that the DLE reported for BA is maintained; Jin et al. developed a PEGylated liposomal formulation that included BA, parthenolide, honokiol and ginsenoside Rh2 that exhibited 89.5% DLE related to BA alone. To the best of our knowledge, this is the first report on liposomes containing BA esters with fatty acids; their diameters are clearly larger than those recorded for BA formulations presumably due to their higher molecular weight, while their DLE reached similar values (around 80%). For But-BA-Lip, the particle size fell within the range of 100–200 nm, while for the other two liposomal formulations the diameter exceeded 200 nm; however, the tumor neo-angiogenesis process induces the occurrence of gaps between endothelial cells of up to 2 μm that allow a preferential access to tumor sites compared to normal cells that display a tighter structure with 5–10 nm pores [40]. Liposomes remained unchanged in size and PDI values for 7 days. However, when all formulations were tested for 15 days for drug loading fluctuations, we discovered that when stored at room temperature (25 °C), drug loading efficiency decreased significantly, with the But-BA-Lip formulation being the least stable. When the samples were refrigerated (4 °C), the reductions in drug loading efficiency were minor. This phenomenon, in which the drug content of liposomal formulations degrades at higher temperatures during storage, is common in PEGylated liposomes, including those containing pentacyclic triterpenes [12,42]. The observed reduction in ζ potentials (-22.1 mV, -19.4 mV, -18.7 mV, -18.2 mV, and -17.8 mV) across the five formulations (Lip, Ba-Lip, But-Ba-Lip, Pal-Ba-Lip and St-Ba-Lip) indicates an apparent correlation with the loaded drug's mass. The ζ potential values slightly decrease as the loaded drug's mass increases. This phenomenon can be caused by the interaction of drug molecules with the liposomes' surface charge. The accumulation of drug molecules towards the liposome's surface may shield the charges, lowering the absolute value of the overall zeta potential. Such fluctuations in zeta potential indicate changes in the electrostatic stability of liposomal formulations [43]. Given that stable liposomes typically have zeta potential values that fall outside of the -30 mV to 30 mV range [44], the observed decrease in zeta potential is not that concerning given that these values fall in the same range (-20 mV–-10 mV) as similar liposomes that were previously reported [28,45,46].

The fatty acids esters (Pal-BA, St-BA, But-BA) as well as their liposomal formulations (Pal-BA-Lip, St-BA-Lip, But-BA-Lip) were assessed against immortalized human keratinocytes HaCaT and human melanoma A375 cells in terms of cell viability using the Alamar blue assay. HaCaT is a non-cancerous monoclonal cell line derived from adult human keratinocytes that can support long-term growth without supplemented growth factors; it displays all morphological features, surface markers and functions of normal keratinocytes and has been used in numerous cell viability studies as model of non-malignant cells for anticancer selectivity assessments [47]. The experimental results revealed that except for But-BA and But-BA-Lip none of the tested compounds exerted cytotoxic effects against HaCaT keratinocytes, regardless of concentration; these findings indicate that Pal-BA and St-BA, as well as their liposomal formulations, Pal-BA-Lip and St-BA-Lip, may selectively act against cancer cells without affecting healthy cells even when used in high dosages.

Regarding the But-BA and But-BA-Lip effect in HaCaT cells, only the highest tested concentration exhibited cytotoxic effects, yet these were significantly lower compared to 5-FU employed as positive control. Since butyric acid is not toxic against skin cells and is also able to modulate cutaneous immune and inflammatory reactions [48], one may only assume that the slightly cytotoxic effect in HaCaT cells is attributable to the ester itself; however, following inclusion in liposomes, the cytotoxic effect is clearly attenuated.

The tested compounds acted as cytotoxic agents in A375 melanoma cells in a dose- and time-dependent manner; the results revealed a calculated IC_{50} value of 65.9 µM for BA. While these values may seem high compared to other studies, this variability can be attributed, in part, to differences in the experimental methodologies employed, particularly regarding the concentration of DMSO used in the assays and the method of compound dilution. A similar case was reported by Suresh et al. where IC_{50} values for betulinic acid, of 154 µM and 112 µM for A375 and MCF-7 cell line, respectively. [49]. The authors attribute the high IC_{50} value obtained for BA on the low DMSO concentration that was used, namely 0.1% final concentration, as compared to other studies that vary this concentration from 0.5% to 2%. This low concentration led to the precipitation of BA, but the authors stated that testing BA in this suspended state mimics the in vivo scenario better in terms of drug release [49].

Out of the three tested esters, only But-BA exhibited a lower IC_{50} value than BA alone, thus revealing higher cytotoxic efficacy. A similar decrease of viability in A375 melanoma cells was recorded for BA ester with myristic acid; the study demonstrated that although both BA and its ester induced cytotoxic effects, the strongest inhibition was recorded for the esterified triterpenic acid [18]. The higher IC_{50} values for Pal-BA and St-BA may be correlated with the fact that when the stock solutions were diluted, at lower concentrations, the compounds formed precipitates, thus there being less available dissolved active substance at the cell site. This occurrence was previously mentioned for BA, as well, when the authors tried to obtain final BA dilution samples with a DMSO maximum concentration of 0.1% [49]. Following liposomal inclusion, an enhanced anticancer activity was recorded compared to both BA alone as well as its fatty acid esters; however, only BA-Lip, St-BA-Lip and But-BA-Lip display lower IC_{50} values than the one recorded for pure BA. In agreement to the current results, numerous studies demonstrated that the inclusion of BA in surface-modified nanoformulations will result in an enhancement of their anticancer potential, as revealed in several types of cancer cells: hepatocellular carcinoma HepG2 cells (IC_{50} value of 63.07 µg/mL–BA folate-functionalized liposomes) [46], cervical cancer HeLa cells (84.31% inhibition rates 48 h post-stimulation with PEGylated BA liposomes 125 µg/mL) [12], lung cancer A549 cells (IC_{50} > 15 µg/mL for BA liposomes, after stimulation with a cocktail of BA, parthenolide, honokiol and ginsenoside) [45].

Although its anti-melanoma mechanisms are yet to be fully elucidated, it is known that BA acts as proapoptotic inducer in various human cancer cell lines through multiple mitochondrial-dependent mechanisms [50]; in addition, the anticancer mechanism of BA relies on the excessive production of reactive oxygen species (ROS), the regulation of the cell cycle and the inhibition of angiogenesis [51]. Apoptosis can be described as regulated cell death, typically characterized by cell shrinkage, nuclei fragmentation and dynamic membrane blebbing [52]; BA can induce cell apoptosis through several signaling pathways, being able to modulate the Bax/Bcl-2 ratio and to activate caspases-3, -7, as well as MAPK/ERK pathway [8,53]. One may assume that BA hybrid molecules such as the fatty acid esters will trigger cell death through similar apoptotic mechanisms as the parent compound; taking into consideration the effective antiproliferative activities recorded for the tested compounds, the IC_{50} concentrations were selected for further examination of the underlying molecular mechanisms of action of the hybrid compounds and their liposomal formulations as well through Hoechst (nuclei) and beta-actin (cytoskeleton) staining. Non-cancerous HaCaT cells were examined by means of the same techniques after treatment with the highest concentration previously used (100 µM) that induced cytotoxic effects. The morphological assessment in melanoma cells showed several signs of apoptosis, such as nuclei shrinkage and condensation and nuclear fragmentation, as well as disrupted cytoskeletons in melanoma cells; the proapoptotic anticancer mechanism is shared by both BA alone and the fatty acids used as esterification partners. In addition to being a source of energy and a player in the membrane structure and functions, palmitic acid exerts antitumor effects through apoptosis induction, the inhibition of tumor cell proliferation and metastasis and immunostimulation; moreover, its derivatives are able to exert additional cytoprotective effects [14]. Stearate conjugates are able to cause significant growth inhibition in cancer cells through apoptosis induction in a concentration-dependent manner while also limiting cell migration [54]. Butyric acid is among the main short-chain fatty acids secreted by the gut bacteria and may be accountable for 70% of the energy available for epithelial intestinal cells [55]; it shows strong dose-dependent anti-inflammatory and cytotoxic effects based on apoptosis induction. In particular, butyrate derivatives were revealed as antimelanoma agents acting as pro-drugs of butyric acid [56]. The delivery and release of butyric acid in cancer cell can be optimized through its inclusion in liposomes [57]. The fact that the esters synthesized in the current study adopt a proapoptotic anticancer mechanism comes as a natural consequence of the individual mechanisms of action of the conjugated molecules; also, their liposomal formulations may facilitate their delivery inside cancer cells.

Keratinocytes evaluation could not reveal any pro-apoptotic signs regardless of the tested compound. This level of anticancer selectivity is characteristic for BA alone and has long been reported starting with Pisha et al. in 1995 [58]; it is therefore to be expected that BA hybrid molecules will show similar behavior. Indeed, BA esters with palmitic and stearic acids, respectively, did not cause morphological changes in HaCaT cells which correlates well with their lack of cytotoxicity in the same cell line during cell viability studies; despite exerting slightly cytotoxic effects against HaCaT cells when used in high dosage, But-BA and But-BA-Lip did not induce any of the morphological signs associated with cell apoptosis.

Internal cellular stress initiates the mitochondrial apoptotic pathway, which involves the coordinated actions of pro-apoptotic (BAX, Bak) and anti-apoptotic (BCL-2, BCL-X, BCL-w, MCL-1, BFL-1/A1) proteins. BA was found to increase BAX expression while decreasing Bcl-2 expression, triggering apoptosis in PANC-1, SW1990, A549, HT-29, T47D, FTC 238, C6, SKNAS, TE671, Jurkat E6.1 and RPMI 8226 cells [59,60]. BA exhibited the same previously reported effect correlated with BCL2/BAX gene modulation on A375 melanoma cells, with quantitative results similar to other studies where PCR was used to determine BCL-2/BAX relative fold gene expression [60]. This pattern extends to other BA derivatives that were designed by chemical modulations of various positions (3-OH, 28-COOH or 30-allyl) [61–63] that in some cases led to a slight modification of the triterpene core as well [64]. This collectively suggests that the hydrophobic triterpene scaffold is essential for the alteration of the Bcl-2/BAX normal ratio. Considering this information, the PCR results, together with the quantitative measurements of Bax and Bcl-2 protein level, obtained for the three fatty acid esters, fell in the expected range since no significant chemical alterations were carried out on the core structure of BA. There have been a few reports in the literature related to 3-O-BA esters that show an increased pro-apoptotic activity against cancer cells when compared to BA alone by altering the expression of Bcl-2 protein family members. Saha et al. reported the biological evaluation of 3-O-dichloroacetyl-BA, which showed increased cytotoxicity and pro-apoptotic activity compared to BA by decreasing Bcl-XL levels and increasing BAX expression in MCF7 cells [65]. Drag-Zalesinska et al. showed that an increase in pro-apoptotic activity in EPP85-181P was recorded for the 3-O-lysine ester of BA, which outperformed the parent compound [66]. While this data suggests that

3-O esters of BA can have a greater pro-apoptotic effect in cancer cells than the parent compound, more research is needed to determine why But-BA was the only compound that outperformed BA.

The scratch assay is an in vitro method used to evaluate the effects of active compounds as well as their involvement in cell migration [67]. Since aberrant cell migration is a feature of cancer cells, the anti-migratory effect that would stop tumor cell invasion represents a desirable effect for any potent anticancer agent [68,69]. The antimigratory effect of our newly synthesized compounds was tested in vitro in A375 melanoma cells by using lower concentrations than cytotoxic ones; the most promising results were recorded for Pal-BA-Lip and But-BA-Lip that significantly inhibited the migration of the cancer cells in a time-dependent manner, thus revealing their potential for preventing cancer metastasis. The anti-migratory effect of BA in various cancer cells has already been described [70,71]; however, to the best of our knowledge, this is the first report on the antimigratory activity of betulinic acid esters with fatty acids which not only succeeded in inhibiting cell migration with a potency comparable to betulinic acid but in some cases even surpassing it.

Collectively, the biological data reported a significant antiproliferative and antimigratory activity for all hybrid compounds, with the butyric derivative exhibiting the strongest anticancer potential against melanoma cells. Such C-3 fatty esters of pentacyclic triterpenes also occur in plants [72] and have been under investigation for their biological effects; their natural origin indicates them as less toxic in healthy cells than synthetic drugs, a [73] fact that was verified in HaCaT keratinocytes in the current study for the similar, newly synthesized esters. Fatty acid esters may provide an additional advantage of acting as pro-drugs for the active triterpene, betulinic acid, whose release and delivery to the cancer cell can be thus influenced [74]; also, the fatty acids released as a result of ester cleavage are able to induce intrinsic cytotoxic effects through complementary pro-apoptotic activity thus adding to the overall therapeutic benefit. The inclusion of the active compounds in liposomes increased their anticancer effects in all cases, with the liposomal formulation of But-BA achieving lower IC_{50} values and therefore stronger cytotoxic effects than the similar formulation of pure BA. Future research should focus on the study of the pharmacokinetic profile of these BA fatty acid prodrugs, whose delivery to the cancer cell may be controlled in order to provide prolonged anticancer activity; further in vivo studies are necessary for the complete characterization of the biological effects and toxicity of these compounds and their liposomal formulations.

4. Materials and Methods

4.1. Chemistry

4.1.1. Instruments and Reagents

Betulinic acid (BA), butyryl chloride, palmitoyl chloride, stearoyl chloride, 4-dimethylaminopyrindine and and all other necessary solvents were commercially available products (Merck KGaA, Darmstadt, Germany) and were further used without any additional purification.

The 1D (^{1}H and ^{13}C) and 2D (H,H-COSY, H,C-HSQC and H,C-HMBC) NMR experiments were performed utilizing a Bruker Avance NEO 400 MHz Spectrometer (Bruker, Billerica, MA, USA) that was equipped with a 5 mm QNP direct detection probe and z−gradients. The spectra were recorded under standard conditions in either DMSO-d_6 or CDCl$_3$ and were referenced on the residual peak of the solvent (^{1}H: 2.51 ppm for DMSO-d_6 or 7.26 ppm for CDCl$_3$; ^{13}C: 39.5 ppm for DMSO-d_6 or 77.0 for CDCl$_3$).

The Biobase melting point instrument (Biobase Group in Shandong, Jinan, China), was utilized to record the melting points. Thin-layer chromatography was performed using 60 F254 silica gel-coated plates obtained from Merck KGaA in Darmstadt, Germany.

FTIR spectra were generated using KBr pellets on a Shimadzu IR Affinity-1S spectrophotometer with a 400–4000 cm^{-1} range and a 4 cm^{-1} resolution.

Methanolic solutions were utilized to record LC/MS spectra on an Agilent 6120 Quadrupole LC/MS system (Santa Clara, CA, USA) that was equipped with a UV detector, an ESI ionization source, and a Zorbax Eclipse Plus C18 column (3.0 mm × 100 mm × 3.5 µm) at 40 °C in the negative ion mode. The samples were analyzed under the following conditions: 0.4 mL/min, 25 °C, and λ = 200 nm. The mobile phase was composed of a 1 mM isocratic mixture comprising 85% methanol and 15% ammonium formate. This procedure was also employed for the determination of BA content in each liposomal formulation in order to calculate the drug loading efficiency (DLE). Liposomal formulations were previously subjected to NaOH degradation and ester hydrolysis to free esterified BA. After 24 h, the aqueous solutions containing hydrolyzed BA were neutralized, extracted with ethyl acetate, evaporated and the residue was redispersed in methanol. Methanolic solutions were analyzed by the above-mentioned technique where the quantity of liposome encapsulated BA was determined using a 7-point plot calibration curve, obtained in the 50–2000 ng·mL^{-1} range (R^2 > 0.999 linearity). DLE for each sample was calculated as the percentage ratio between the encapsulated and total amount of used BA.

The particle morphology of the synthesized samples was analyzed in STEM Mode with a Verios G4 UC Scanning electron microscope (Thermo Scientific, Brno, Czech Republic) equipped with Energy Dispersive X-ray spectroscopy analyzer (Octane Elect Super SDD detector, Gatan, Pleasanton, CA, USA). The STEM studies were performed using the STEM 3+ detector (Bright-Field Mode) at accelerating voltage of 25 kV. For STEM analysis the samples were dispersed in water and then they were placed on carbon-coated copper grids with 300-mesh size and dried until the solvent was removed. Hydrodynamic diameters of the liposomes (BA-Lip, But-BA-Lip, Pal-BA-Lip, St-BA-Lip) were determined by DLS with a Zetasizer Pro (Malvern Panalytical, Malvern, UK). Each sample was measured at a dilution of 1:10 in deionized water and measurements were performed in triplicate. The following parameters were used for these measurements: general purpose as analysis model, automatic for size display limit mode, automatic for size threshold mode, equilibration time of 120 s and a temperature of 25 °C.

4.1.2. Synthesis Procedure for BA Fatty Acid Esters

A quantity of 1 mmol BA was dispersed in 20 mL of dichloromethane (DCM) and stirred for 15 min before being followed by 2 mmoles of 4-dimethylaminopyridine (DMAP). Following that, 2 mmoles of acyl chloride were added dropwise. The reaction was stirred at room temperature for 24 h. Thin-layer chromatography using chloroform as the eluent confirmed the completion of the reaction. Following water extraction, the organic phase was dried over anhydrous MgSO4 and removed by rotary evaporation. The crude product was chromatographed over silica using chloroform as the mobile phase.

3-O-butiryl-betulinic acid (But-BA); translucent crystals, m.p. 265–280 °C, yield 74%; ^{1}H NMR (CDCl$_3$, 400 MHz, δ, ppm): 11.09 (s, 1H, COOH), 4.74 (s, 1H, H29a), 4.61 (s, 1H, H29b), 4.47 (dd, J = 4 Hz, J = 8 Hz, 1H, H3), 3.00 (m, 1H, H19), 2.29–2.26 (m, 3H, -CH_2-COO-; H15a), 2.21–0.78 (m, 42H from betulinic acid backbone, 5H from butyric acid chain). ^{13}C NMR (CDCl$_3$, 100 MHz, δ, ppm): 182.2 (COOH), 173.6 (-COO-), 150.4 (C20), 109.7 (C29), 80.6 (C3), 56.4, 55.4, 50.4, 49.2, 46.9, 42.4, 40.7, 38.4, 38.4, 37.8, 37.1, 37.0, 36.8, 34.2, 32.1, 30.6, 29.7, 27.9, 25.4, 23.7, 20.8, 19.3, 18.6, 18.1, 16.5, 16.1, 16.0, 14.7, 13.7. FTIR [KBr] (cm^{-1}) relevant peaks: 2941, 2874 (C-H stretch); 1730, 1254, 1010 (ester C=O, C-C-O, O-C-C stretch); ESI-MS, m/z = 525 [M-H$^+$]$^-$.

3-O-palmitoyl-betulinic acid (Pal-BA); white powder, m.p. 160–170 °C, yield 70%; ^{1}H NMR (CDCl$_3$, 400 MHz, δ, ppm): 11.15 (s, 1H, COOH), 4.74 (s, 1H, H29a), 4.61 (s, 1H, H29b), 4.47 (dd, J = 4 Hz, J = 8 Hz, 1H, H3), 3.00 (m, 1H, H19), 2.30–2.27 (m, 3H, -CH_2-COO-; H15a), 2.21–0.86 (m, 42H from betulinic acid backbone, 29H from palmitic acid chain). ^{13}C NMR (CDCl$_3$, 100 MHz, δ, ppm): 182.3 (COOH), 173.8 (-COO-), 150.4 (C20), 109.7 (C29), 80.6 (C3), 56.4, 55.4, 50.4, 49.2, 46.9, 42.4, 40.7, 38.4, 38.4, 37.8, 37.1, 37.0, 34.8, 34.2, 32.1, 31.9, 30.6, 29.7, 29.6, 29.6, 29.5, 29.4, 29.2, 29.2, 28.0, 25.4, 25.2, 23.7, 22.7, 20.8, 19.3, 18.1, 16.5, 16.1, 16.0, 14.7, 13.7. FTIR [KBr] (cm^{-1}) relevant peaks: 2930, 2859 (C-H stretch); 1730, 1242, 1010 (ester C=O, C-C-O, O-C-C stretch); ESI-MS, m/z = 693 [M-H$^+$]$^-$.

3-O-stearoyl-betulinic acid (St-BA); white powder, m.p. 150–162 °C, yield 65%; ^{1}H NMR (CDCl$_3$, 400 MHz, δ, ppm): 10.85 (s, 1H, COOH), 4.74 (s, 1H, H29a), 4.61 (s, 1H, H29b), 4.47 (dd, J = 4 Hz, J = 8 Hz, 1H, H3), 3.00 (m, 1H, H19), 2.30–2.27 (m, 3H, -CH$_2$-COO-; H15a), 2.21–0.88 (m, 41H from betulinic acid backbone, 31H from stearic acid chain). ^{13}C NMR (CDCl$_3$, 100 MHz, δ, ppm): 182.0 (COOH), 173.8 (-COO-), 150.4 (C20), 109.7 (C29), 80.6 (C3), 56.4, 55.4, 50.4, 49.3, 46.9, 42.4, 40.7, 38.4, 38.4, 37.8, 37.1, 37.1, 34.9, 34.2, 32.2, 31.9, 30.6, 29.7, 29.6, 29.6, 29.5, 29.4, 29.3, 29.2, 28.0, 25.4, 25.2, 23.7, 22.7, 20.8, 19.3, 18.2, 16.5, 16.2, 16.0, 14.7, 13.7. FTIR [KBr] (cm^{-1}) relevant peaks: 2924, 2853 (C-H stretch); 1730, 1242, 1010 (ester C=O, C-C-O, O-C-C stretch); ESI-MS, m/z = 721 [M-H$^+$]$^-$.

4.1.3. Synthesis Procedure for BA Fatty Acid Esters Liposomal Formulations

The liposomes were made using the thin-layer hydration method using a slightly modified, previously published procedure [28]. A quantity of 100 mg of L-α- phosphatidylcholine followed by 0.03 mmols of cholesterol, 0.004 mmols of DSPE-PEG2000, and 0.02 mmols of triterpene were dissolved in chloroform and stirred until a clear solution was obtained. The solvent was then removed with a rotary evaporator, and the resulting lipid film was hydrated with 10 mL of phosphate buffer saline (PBS). The mixture was allowed to hydrate for 24 h before being redispersed for 30 min using sonication. To remove unencapsulated BA, the emulsion was centrifuged at 3000 rpm for 10 min, 3 times, the supernatant was collected and was stored at 4 °C.

4.2. In Vitro Assessment

4.2.1. Cell Culture

The cell lines selected for our study were noncancerous human keratinocytes—HaCaT, acquired from CLS Cell Lines Service GmbH (Eppelheim, Germany), and human malignant melanoma—A375, purchased from American Type Culture Collection (ATTC, Lomianki, Poland). The cells were acquired as frozen items and were stored in liquid nitrogen. Both HaCaT and A375 were cultured and propagated in Dulbecco's Modified Eagle Medium (DMEM) high glucose, supplemented with 10% fetal bovine serum (FBS) and 1% antibiotic mixture of Penicillin/Streptomycin (100 IU/mL). The cells were maintained in a humified incubator with 5% CO$_2$ at 37 °C.

4.2.2. Cell Viability Assessment

Alamar blue assay. The Alamar blue staining method was used to determine the cell viability of HaCaT and A375 cells, post stimulation with increasing concentrations (10, 25, 50, 75 and 100 µM) of BA and its fatty esters Pal-BA, St-BA and But-BA, and the PEGylated liposomes Pal-BA-Lip, St-BA-Lip, But-BA-Lip, BA-Lip, the liposome in a free form (Lip) and using 5-fluorouracil as positive control, for 24 h and 48 h. The tested concentrations for the liposomal formulations were obtained considering previously recorded DLE values. The cells (1 × 10^4 cells/well) were seeded onto 96-well plates and incubated 37 °C and 5% CO$_2$ until reaching 80–85% confluence. The cell number was determined with Trypan blue coloring using an automated cell counting device (Thermo Fisher Scientific, Inc., Waltham, MA, USA). The used medium was removed using an aspiration station and replaced with fresh medium containing the tested compounds. The tested concentrations (10, 25, 50, 75 and 100 µM) were prepared using stock solutions of 20 mM and the final concentration of DMSO did not exceed 0.5%. After 24 h, and 48 h, respectively, the cells were stained with Alamar blue 0.01% by adding to each well 20 µL Alamar blue 0.01%, obtaining a finale volume of 220 µL/well and then incubated for another 3 h in a humified incubator with 5% CO$_2$ at 37 °C. The absorbance was measured at two wavelengths, 570 nm, and 600 nm using xMark™ Microplate Spectrophotometer, Bio-Rad (Hercules, CA, USA).

4.2.3. Fatty Ester Derivatives Effects on Cell Morphology

The A375 melanoma cells and the human keratinocytes HaCaT cells were seeded onto 12-well plates at initial density of 2 × 10^5 cells/well until reaching 80–85% confluence.

Afterwards, the cells were stimulated with the tested compounds for 48 h at the highest tested concentration (100 µM) for HaCaT cells and the corresponding IC_{50} values for A375. All the cells were stimulated with 5-FU as positive control. After 48 h, the morphology of the cells was evaluated using the EVOS™ M5000 Imaging System equipped with a highly sensitive CMOS camera (Thermo Fisher Scientific, Inc., Waltham, MA, USA).

4.2.4. Immunofluorescence Assay—Morphological Assessment of Apoptotic Cells

Hoechst staining was used to assess the nuclear localization and determine signs of apoptosis (fragmentation, shrinkage), while beta-actin staining was utilized to determine the cytoplasmatic localization. HaCaT and A375 cells were seeded onto 12-well plates at initial density of 2×10^5 cells/well. After reaching 80–85% confluence, the cells were stimulated for 48 h with the tested compounds at their IC_{50} values for A375 cells and at 100 µM—the highest concentration for HaCaT cells. Separately, some wells were treated with staurosporine 5 µM as positive control. After 48 h the old medium was removed and the cells were fixed with methanol for 15 min, permeabilized with Triton X 0.01% in PBS for 15 min and blocked with 3% BSA for 30 min at room temperature. Later on, the cells were stained with beta actin monoclonal antibody using a 1:2000 dilution (Thermo Fisher Scientific, Inc., Waltham, MA, USA) in BSA 3% for 1 h at room temperature and then were incubated with Alexa fluor 488 goat-anti mouse secondary antibody (Thermo Fisher Scientific, Inc., Waltham, MA, USA) at a dilution of 1:5000 in BSA 3% for 30 min in the dark, at room temperature. Finally, for nuclear staining the Hoechst 33258 solution was added for 5 min. The nuclear and cytoplasmatic modifications were analyzed using the EVOS™ M5000 Imaging System equipped with a highly sensitive CMOS camera (Thermo Fisher Scientific, Inc., Waltham, MA, USA).

4.2.5. Real-Time PCR Quantification of Apoptotic Markers

The total RNA content was extracted using the peqGold RNAPureTM Package (Peqlab Biotechnology GmbH, Erlangen, Germany) following the manufacturer's instructions, and the total concentration of RNA was measured using a DS-11 spectrophotometer (DeNovix, Wilmington, DE, USA). The Maxima® First Strand cDNA Synthesis Kit (Thermo Fisher Scientific, Inc., Waltham, MA, USA) was used for reverse transcription, and the samples were incubated in the Tadvanced Biometra Product line (Analytik Jena AG, Göttingen, Germany) using the following thermal cycle: 10 min at 25 °C, 15 min at 50 °C, and 5 min at 85 °C. Quantitative real-time PCR was conducted employing a Quant Studio 5 real-time PCR system (Thermo Fisher Scientific, Inc., Waltham, MA, USA). The analysis was performed using 20 µL aliquots containing Power SYBR-Green PCR Master Mix (Thermo Fisher Scientific, Inc., Waltham, MA, USA), sample cDNA, the sense and antisense primer and pure water. The primer pairs used for this method included 18S, used as housekeeping gene (sense: 5′ GTAACCCGTTGAACCCCATT 3′; antisense: 5′ CCATCCAATCGGTAGTAGCG 3′), Bax (sense: 5′ GCCGGGTTGTCGCCCTTTT 3′; antisense: 5′CCGCTCCCGGAGGAAGTCCA 3′) and Bcl-2 (sense: 5′CGGGAGATGTCGCCCCTGGT 3′; antisense: 5′GCATGCTGGGGCCGTACAGT 3′) (Thermo Fisher Scientific, Inc., Waltham, MA, USA). Normalized, relative expression results were calculated using the comparative threshold cycle method ($2^{-\Delta\Delta Ct}$).

4.2.6. Scratch Assay

The scratch test was performed in order to assess the regressive effect of Pal-BA, St-BA, But-BA, Pal-BA-Lip, St-BA-Lip, But-BA-Lip, compared to the parent compound BA and BA-Lip on the invasion capacity of malignant melanoma A375 cells. The cells (2×10^5/well) were seeded onto 12-well plates until reaching 80–85% confluence. Then, the old medium was removed and the attached cells were scratched onto the diameter of the well using a sterile pipette tip. After washing the cells with warm PBS, the cells were stimulated with each tested compound at 10 µM. To establish the growing rate of the stimulated cells compared to control, the wells were photographed at 0, 24 and 48 h using the Olympus

IX73 inverted microscope (Olympus, Tokyo, Japan). The cells Sense Dimension software (version 1.8) was utilized for analyzing cell migration for each cell line.

The following formula was used in order to calculate the scratch closure rate [75]:

$$\text{Scratch closure rate} = \left[\frac{At_0 - At}{At_0}\right] \times 100$$

where At_0 is the scratch at time 0 h and At is the scratch area at 24 h or 48 h.

4.3. BAX and Bcl-2 Detection

The apoptotic protein markers, Bcl-2 and BAX, were determined in A375 melanoma cells 48 h post-treatment with BA fatty esters (Pal-BA, St-BA, But-BA) and their liposomes (Pal-BA-Lip, St-BA-Lip, But-BA-Lip) as well as with the parent compound BA and its liposome BA-Lip using their respective IC50 values. Bcl-2 (ab119506) and BAX (ab199080) concentrations in cell lysates were assessed using the Elisa kits purchased from Abcam, according to the manufacturers' protocols [76]. To conduct the assay, samples or standards are added to the wells, followed by the antibody mix. After incubation, unbound material is washed away. TMB substrate is added, and in the presence of HRP, it catalyzes a reaction producing a blue color. This color reaction is halted by adding Stop Solution, resulting in a color change from blue to yellow. Optical densities were read using a microplate reader (xMark™ Microplate Spectrophotometer, Biorad, Hercules, CA, USA) at 450 nm.

4.4. Statistical Analysis

The statistical tests were carried out using one-way ANOVA followed by Dunnett's post-test (GraphPad Prism version 6.0.0, GraphPad Software, San Diego, CA, USA). The differences between the groups were considered statistically significant if $p < 0.05$, as follows: * $p < 0.05$, ** $p < 0.01$ and *** $p < 0.001$. The IC_{50} values presented in Table 3 were calculated using GraphPad Prism version 6.0.0 (GraphPad Software, San Diego, CA, USA).

5. Conclusions

Our study described the synthesis and cytotoxic evaluation of a series of BA derivatives obtained through the esterification with fatty acids such as palmitic, stearic and butyric acid, as well as their surface-modified liposomal nanoformulations. The synthesis protocol elicited good yields for each BA fatty ester, which were further incorporated in PEGylated liposomes. Both fatty esters as well as their liposomal nanoformulations exhibited significant cytotoxic effects in A375 human melanoma cells, comparable and, for some compounds, stronger than those recorded for parent compound BA and its liposomal formulation, BA-Lip. A related cytotoxic corelated pro-apoptotic effect was observed for all compounds and their subsequent formulations. Similar to the cytotoxicity results, the tested derivatives and formulations decreased the expression of the antiapoptotic marker Bcl-2 and increased the expression of the proapoptotic marker BAX. The cytotoxicity assessment against HaCaT cells revealed only slight cytotoxic effects for But-BA and its respective liposomal formulation, such effects lacking for palmitic and stearic BA conjugates. In all cases, the inclusion in liposomes enhanced the anticancer potential of the active compound. Our findings suggest that the further optimization of these compounds, particularly focusing on improving their solubility and formulation dynamics, could lead to significant advancements in cancer therapy. Future studies should prioritize pharmacokinetic evaluations and in vivo assessments to better understand the therapeutic potential of these compounds. Ultimately, our study provides new avenues for effective cancer treatment strategies, describing the successful development of BA derivatives and their liposomal formulations that may offer novel additions to the development of similar compounds with increased and selective cytotoxic effect.

Supplementary Materials: The following supporting information can be downloaded at: https://www.mdpi.com/article/10.3390/pr12020416/s1, Figure S1. 1H NMR spectrum of 3-O-butyryl-betulinic acid

(But-BA); Figure S2. 13C NMR spectrum of 3-O-butyryl-betulinic acid (But-BA); Figure S3. 13C DEPT NMR spectrum of 3-O-butyryl-betulinic acid (But-BA); Figure S4. H,H-COSY NMR spectrum of of 3-O-butyryl-betulinic acid (But-BA); Figure S5. H,C-HSQC NMR spectrum of 3-O-butyryl-betulinic acid (But-BA); Figure S6. H,C-HMBC NMR spectrum of 3-O-butyryl-betulinic acid (But-BA); Figure S7. 1H NMR spectrum of 3-O-palmitoyl-betulinic acid (Pal-BA); Figure S8. 13C NMR spectrum of 3-O-palmitoyl-betulinic acid (Pal-BA); Figure S9. 13C DEPT NMR spectrum of 3-O-palmitoyl-betulinic acid (Pal-BA); Figure S10. H,H-COSY NMR spectrum of 3-O-palmitoyl-betulinic acid (Pal-BA); Figure S11. H,C-HSQC NMR spectrum of 3-O-palmitoyl-betulinic acid (Pal-BA); Figure S12. H,C-HMBC NMR spectrum of 3-O-palmitoyl-betulinic acid (Pal-BA); Figure S13. 1H NMR spectrum of 3-O-stearoyl-betulinic acid (St-BA); Figure S14. 13C NMR spectrum of 3-O-stearoyl-betulinic acid (St-BA); Figure S15. 13C DEPT NMR spectrum of 3-O-stearoyl-betulinic acid (St-BA); Figure S16. H,H-COSY NMR spectrum of 3-O-stearoyl-betulinic acid (St-BA); Figure S17. H,C-HSQC NMR spectrum of 3-O-stearoyl-betulinic acid (St-BA); Figure S18. H,C-HMBC NMR spectrum of 3-O-stearoyl-betulinic acid (St-BA); Figure S19. FTIR spectra of BA, But-BA, Pal-BA and St-BA; Figure S20. The evaluation of morphological changes of HaCaT cells 48 h treatment with BA, BA-Lip, 5-FU (A), Pal-BA, Pal-BA-Lip, St-BA (B), St-BA-Lip, But-BA and But-BA-Lip (C); Figure S21. The evaluation of morphological changes of A375 cells after 0 h and 48 h treatment with BA, BA-Lip, 5-FU (A), Pal-BA, Pal-BA-Lip, St-BA (B), St-BA-Lip, But-BA and But-BA-Lip (C).

Author Contributions: Conceptualization, A.M. (Andreea Milan), M.M. and C.Ș.; methodology, A.M. (Andreea Milan), M.M., A.M. (Alexandra Mioc), M.B.-P., R.R., G.M., S.R., N.M. and C.Ș.; formal analysis, M.B.-P., G.M. and S.R.; validation, A.M. (Andreea Milan), A.M. (Alexandra Mioc) and M.M.; investigation, A.M. (Andreea Milan), A.M. (Alexandra Mioc) and M.M.; software, A.M. (Andreea Milan), A.M. (Alexandra Mioc), M.B.-P., R.R., S.R. and I.Ș.; writing—original draft preparation, A.M. (Andreea Milan); writing—review and editing A.M. (Andreea Milan), A.M. (Alexandra Mioc), M.M. and C.Ș.; visualization, R.R., I.Ș. and C.Ș.; supervision, A.M. (Alexandra Mioc), M.M. and C.Ș.; project administration, M.M. and C.Ș.; funding acquisition, M.M. All authors have read and agreed to the published version of the manuscript.

Funding: This research was funded by the University of Medicine and Pharmacy "Victor Babes" Timisoara, grant number 26679/09.11.2022 (M.M.).

Data Availability Statement: The original contributions presented in the study are included in the article/Supplementary Material, further inquiries can be directed to the corresponding author/s.

Conflicts of Interest: The authors declare no conflicts of interest.

References

1. Majolo, F.; de Oliveira Becker Delwing, L.K.; Marmitt, D.J.; Bustamante-Filho, I.C.; Goettert, M.I. Medicinal Plants and Bioactive Natural Compounds for Cancer Treatment: Important Advances for Drug Discovery. *Phytochem. Lett.* **2019**, *31*, 196–207. [CrossRef]
2. Harvey, A. Natural Products in Drug Discovery. *Drug Discov. Today* **2008**, *13*, 894–901. [CrossRef] [PubMed]
3. Ríos, J.; Máñez, S. New Pharmacological Opportunities for Betulinic Acid. *Planta Med.* **2018**, *84*, 8–19. [CrossRef] [PubMed]
4. Mioc, M.; Milan, A.; Malița, D.; Mioc, A.; Prodea, A.; Racoviceanu, R.; Ghiulai, R.; Cristea, A.; Căruntu, F.; Șoica, C. Recent Advances Regarding the Molecular Mechanisms of Triterpenic Acids: A Review (Part I). *Int. J. Mol. Sci.* **2022**, *23*, 7740. [CrossRef] [PubMed]
5. Seca, A.; Pinto, D. Plant Secondary Metabolites as Anticancer Agents: Successes in Clinical Trials and Therapeutic Application. *Int. J. Mol. Sci.* **2018**, *19*, 263. [CrossRef] [PubMed]
6. Ghiulai, R.; Roșca, O.J.; Antal, D.S.; Mioc, M.; Mioc, A.; Racoviceanu, R.; Macașoi, I.; Olariu, T.; Dehelean, C.; Crețu, O.M.; et al. Tetracyclic and Pentacyclic Triterpenes with High Therapeutic Efficiency in Wound Healing Approaches. *Molecules* **2020**, *25*, 5557. [CrossRef] [PubMed]
7. Paduch, R.; Kandefer-Szerszen, M. Antitumor and Antiviral Activity of Pentacyclic Triterpenes. *Mini. Rev. Org. Chem.* **2014**, *11*, 262–268. [CrossRef]
8. Mioc, M.; Prodea, A.; Racoviceanu, R.; Mioc, A.; Ghiulai, R.; Milan, A.; Voicu, M.; Mardale, G.; Șoica, C. Recent Advances Regarding the Molecular Mechanisms of Triterpenic Acids: A Review (Part II). *Int. J. Mol. Sci.* **2022**, *23*, 8896. [CrossRef]
9. Furtado, N.A.J.C.; Pirson, L.; Edelberg, H.; Miranda, M.L.; Loira-Pastoriza, C.; Preat, V.; Larondelle, Y.; André, C. Pentacyclic Triterpene Bioavailability: An Overview of In Vitro and In Vivo Studies. *Molecules* **2017**, *22*, 400. [CrossRef]
10. Prodea, A.; Mioc, A.; Banciu, C.; Trandafirescu, C.; Milan, A.; Racoviceanu, R.; Ghiulai, R.; Mioc, M.; Soica, C. The Role of Cyclodextrins in the Design and Development of Triterpene-Based Therapeutic Agents. *Int. J. Mol. Sci.* **2022**, *23*, 736. [CrossRef]

11. Valdés, K.; Morales, J.; Rodríguez, L.; Günther, G. Potential Use of Nanocarriers with Pentacyclic Triterpenes in Cancer Treatments. *Nanomedicine* **2016**, *11*, 3139–3156. [CrossRef]
12. Liu, Y.; Gao, D.; Zhang, X.; Liu, Z.; Dai, K.; Ji, B.; Wang, Q.; Luo, L. Antitumor Drug Effect of Betulinic Acid Mediated by Polyethylene Glycol Modified Liposomes. *Mater. Sci. Eng. C* **2016**, *64*, 124–132. [CrossRef] [PubMed]
13. Nistor, G.; Trandafirescu, C.; Prodea, A.; Milan, A.; Cristea, A.; Ghiulai, R.; Racoviceanu, R.; Mioc, A.; Mioc, M.; Ivan, V.; et al. Semisynthetic Derivatives of Pentacyclic Triterpenes Bearing Heterocyclic Moieties with Therapeutic Potential. *Molecules* **2022**, *27*, 6552. [CrossRef] [PubMed]
14. Wang, X.; Zhang, C.; Bao, N. Molecular Mechanism of Palmitic Acid and Its Derivatives in Tumor Progression. *Front. Oncol.* **2023**, *13*, 1224125. [CrossRef] [PubMed]
15. Al-Hwaiti, M.S.; Alsbou, E.M.; Abu Sheikha, G.; Bakchiche, B.; Pham, T.H.; Thomas, R.H.; Bardaweel, S.K. Evaluation of the Anticancer Activity and Fatty Acids Composition of "Handal" (*Citrullus Colocynthis* L.) Seed Oil, a Desert Plant from South Jordan. *Food Sci. Nutr.* **2021**, *9*, 282–289. [CrossRef] [PubMed]
16. Abe, A.; Sugiyama, K. Growth Inhibition and Apoptosis Induction of Human Melanoma Cells by ω-Hydroxy Fatty Acids. *Anticancer. Drugs* **2005**, *16*, 543–549. [CrossRef] [PubMed]
17. Chodurek, E.; Orchel, A.; Gawlik, N.; Kulczycka, A.; Gruchlik, A.; Dzierzewicz, Z. Proliferation and Cellular Death of A375 Cell Line in the Presence of HDACs Inhibitors. *Acta Pol. Pharm.—Drug Res.* **2010**, *67*, 686–689.
18. Pinzaru, I.; Trandafirescu, C.; Szabadai, Z.; Mioc, M.; Ledeti, I.; Coricovac, D.; Ciurlea, S.; Ghiulai, R.M.; Crainiceanu, Z.; Simu, G. Synthesis and Biological Evaluation of Some Pentacyclic Lupane Triterpenoid Esters. *Rev. Chim.* **2014**, *65*, 848–851.
19. Mallavadhani, U.V.; Mahapatra, A.; Jamil, K.; Reddy, P.S. Antimicrobial Activity of Some Pentacyclic Triterpenes and Their Synthesized 3-O-Lipophilic Chains. *Biol. Pharm. Bull.* **2004**, *27*, 1576–1579. [CrossRef]
20. Hodges, L.D.; Kweifio-Okai, G.; Macrides, T.A. Antiprotease Effect of Anti-Inflammatory Lupeol Esters. *Mol. Cell. Biochem.* **2003**, *252*, 97–101. [CrossRef]
21. Fotie, J.; Bohle, D.S.; Leimanis, M.L.; Georges, E.; Rukunga, G.; Nkengfack, A.E. Lupeol Long-Chain Fatty Acid Esters with Antimalarial Activity from Holarrhena f Loribunda. *J. Nat. Prod.* **2006**, *69*, 62–67. [CrossRef] [PubMed]
22. Gregory, G. Engineering Liposomes for Drug Delivery: Progress and Problems. *Trends Biotechnol.* **1995**, *13*, 527–537.
23. Sofou, S. Surface-Active Liposomes for Targeted Cancer Therapy. *Nanomedicine* **2007**, *2*, 711–724. [CrossRef] [PubMed]
24. Mineart, K.P.; Venkataraman, S.; Yang, Y.Y.; Hedrick, J.L.; Prabhu, V.M. Fabrication and Characterization of Hybrid Stealth Liposomes. *Macromolecules* **2018**, *51*, 3184–3192. [CrossRef] [PubMed]
25. Habib, N.; Wood, C.; Apostolov, K.; Barker, W.; Hershman, M.; Aslam, M.; Heinemann, D.; Fermor, B.; Williamson, R.; Jenkins, W. Stearic Acid and Carcinogenesis. *Br. J. Cancer* **1987**, *56*, 455–458. [CrossRef] [PubMed]
26. Zhu, S.; Jiao, W.; Xu, Y.; Hou, L.; Li, H.; Shao, J.; Zhang, X.; Wang, R.; Kong, D. Palmitic Acid Inhibits Prostate Cancer Cell Proliferation and Metastasis by Suppressing the PI3K/Akt Pathway. *Life Sci.* **2021**, *286*, 120046. [CrossRef] [PubMed]
27. Zafaryab, M.; Fakhri, K.K.; Hajela, K.; Moshahid, M.; Rizvi, A.; Moshahid, A.; Rizvi, M. In Vitro Assessment of Cytotoxic and Apoptotic Potential of Palmitic Acid for Breast Cancer Treatment. *J. Life Sci. Res.* **2019**, *7*, 166–174. [CrossRef]
28. Farcas, C.G.; Dehelean, C.; Pinzaru, I.A.; Mioc, M.; Socoliuc, V.; Moaca, E.-A.; Avram, S.; Ghiulai, R.; Coricovac, D.; Pavel, I.; et al. Thermosensitive Betulinic Acid-Loaded Magnetoliposomes: A Promising Antitumor Potential for Highly Aggressive Human Breast Adenocarcinoma Cells Under Hyperthermic Conditions. *Int. J. Nanomed.* **2020**, *15*, 8175–8200. [CrossRef]
29. Naeem, A.; Hu, P.; Yang, M.; Zhang, J.; Liu, Y.; Zhu, W.; Zheng, Q. Natural Products as Anticancer Agents: Current Status and Future Perspectives. *Molecules* **2022**, *27*, 8367. [CrossRef]
30. Hordyjewska, A.; Ostapiuk, A.; Horecka, A.; Kurzepa, J. Betulin and Betulinic Acid: Triterpenoids Derivatives with a Powerful Biological Potential. *Phytochem. Rev.* **2019**, *18*, 929–951. [CrossRef]
31. Zhang, X.; Hu, J.; Chen, Y. Betulinic Acid and the Pharmacological Effects of Tumor Suppression. *Mol. Med. Rep.* **2016**, *14*, 4489–4495. [CrossRef] [PubMed]
32. Ali-Seyed, M.; Jantan, I.; Vijayaraghavan, K.; Bukhari, S.N.A. Betulinic Acid: Recent Advances in Chemical Modifications, Effective Delivery, and Molecular Mechanisms of a Promising Anticancer Therapy. *Chem. Biol. Drug Des.* **2016**, *87*, 517–536. [CrossRef] [PubMed]
33. Fulda, S. Betulinic Acid for Cancer Treatment and Prevention. *Int. J. Mol. Sci.* **2008**, *9*, 1096–1107. [CrossRef] [PubMed]
34. Wang, J.; Shi, Y.-m. Recent Updates on Anticancer Activity of Betulin and Betulinic Acid Hybrids (A Review). *Russ. J. Gen. Chem.* **2023**, *93*, 610–627. [CrossRef]
35. Wang, K.-W. A New Fatty Acid Ester of Triterpenoid from *Celastrus rosthornianus* with Anti-Tumor Activities. *Nat. Prod. Res.* **2007**, *21*, 669–674. [CrossRef]
36. Legrand, P.; Rioux, V. The Complex and Important Cellular and Metabolic Functions of Saturated Fatty Acids. *Lipids* **2010**, *45*, 941–946. [CrossRef] [PubMed]
37. Jóźwiak, M.; Filipowska, A.; Fiorino, F.; Struga, M. Anticancer Activities of Fatty Acids and Their Heterocyclic Derivatives. *Eur. J. Pharmacol.* **2020**, *871*, 172937. [CrossRef]
38. Jóźwiak, M.; Struga, M.; Roszkowski, P.; Filipek, A.; Nowicka, G.; Olejarz, W. Anticancer Effects of Alloxanthoxyletin and Fatty Acids Esters—In Vitro Study on Cancer HTB-140 and A549 Cells. *Biomed. Pharmacother.* **2019**, *110*, 618–630. [CrossRef]
39. Ahmad, F.B.H.; Ghafari, M.; Basri, M.; Abdul, M.B. Anticancer Activity of 3-O-Acylated Betulinic Acid Derivatives Obtained by Enzymatic Synthesis. *Biosci. Biotechnol. Biochem.* **2010**, *74*, 1025–1029. [CrossRef]

40. Abbasi, H.; Kouchak, M.; Mirveis, Z.; Hajipour, F.; Khodarahmi, M.; Rahbar, N.; Handali, S. What We Need to Know about Liposomes as Drug Nanocarriers: An Updated Review. *Adv. Pharm. Bull.* **2022**, *13*, 7. [CrossRef]
41. Mullauer, F.B.; Van Bloois, L.; Daalhuisen, J.B.; Ten Brink, M.S.; Storm, G.; Medema, J.P.; Schiffelers, R.M.; Kessler, J.H. Betulinic Acid Delivered in Liposomes Reduces Growth of Human Lung and Colon Cancers in Mice without Causing Systemic Toxicity. *Anticancer. Drugs* **2011**, *22*, 223–233. [CrossRef] [PubMed]
42. Gao, D.; Tang, S.; Tong, Q. Acid Liposomes with Polyethylene Glycol Modification: Promising Antitumor Drug Delivery. *Int. J. Nanomed.* **2012**, *7*, 3517–3526. [CrossRef] [PubMed]
43. Németh, Z.; Csóka, I.; Semnani Jazani, R.; Sipos, B.; Haspel, H.; Kozma, G.; Kónya, Z.; Dobó, D.G. Quality by Design-Driven Zeta Potential Optimisation Study of Liposomes with Charge Imparting Membrane Additives. *Pharmaceutics* **2022**, *14*, 1798. [CrossRef] [PubMed]
44. Berbel Manaia, E.; Paiva Abuçafy, M.; Chiari-Andréo, B.G.; Lallo Silva, B.; Oshiro-Júnior, J.A.; Chiavacci, L. Physicochemical Characterization of Drug Nanocarriers. *Int. J. Nanomed.* **2017**, *12*, 4991–5011. [CrossRef] [PubMed]
45. Jin, X.; Yang, Q.; Cai, N.; Zhang, Z. A Cocktail of Betulinic Acid, Parthenolide, Honokiol and Ginsenoside Rh2 in Liposome Systems for Lung Cancer Treatment. *Nanomedicine* **2020**, *15*, 41–54. [CrossRef] [PubMed]
46. Guo, B.; Xu, D.; Liu, X.; Yi, J. Enzymatic Synthesis and in Vitro Evaluation of Folate-Functionalized Liposomes. *Drug Des. Devel. Ther.* **2017**, *11*, 1839–1847. [CrossRef]
47. Colombo, I.; Sangiovanni, E.; Maggio, R.; Mattozzi, C.; Zava, S.; Corbett, Y.; Fumagalli, M.; Carlino, C.; Corsetto, P.A.; Scaccabarozzi, D.; et al. HaCaT Cells as a Reliable In Vitro Differentiation Model to Dissect the Inflammatory/Repair Response of Human Keratinocytes. *Mediators Inflamm.* **2017**, *2017*, 7435621. [CrossRef]
48. Keshari, S.; Balasubramaniam, A.; Myagmardoloonjin, B.; Herr, D.R.; Negari, I.P.; Huang, C.-M. Butyric Acid from Probiotic Staphylococcus Epidermidis in the Skin Microbiome Down-Regulates the Ultraviolet-Induced Pro-Inflammatory IL-6 Cytokine via Short-Chain Fatty Acid Receptor. *Int. J. Mol. Sci.* **2019**, *20*, 4477. [CrossRef]
49. Suresh, C.; Zhao, H.; Gumbs, A.; Chetty, C.S.; Bose, H.S. New Ionic Derivatives of Betulinic Acid as Highly Potent Anti-Cancer Agents. *Bioorg. Med. Chem. Lett.* **2012**, *22*, 1734–1738. [CrossRef]
50. Coricovac, D.; Dehelean, C.A.; Pinzaru, I.; Mioc, A.; Aburel, O.-M.; Macasoi, I.; Draghici, G.A.; Petean, C.; Soica, C.; Boruga, M.; et al. Assessment of Betulinic Acid Cytotoxicity and Mitochondrial Metabolism Impairment in a Human Melanoma Cell Line. *Int. J. Mol. Sci.* **2021**, *22*, 4870. [CrossRef]
51. Jiang, W.; Li, X.; Dong, S.; Zhou, W. Betulinic Acid in the Treatment of Tumour Diseases: Application and Research Progress. *Biomed. Pharmacother.* **2021**, *142*, 111990. [CrossRef] [PubMed]
52. Jan, R.; Chaudhry, G.-E.-S. Understanding Apoptosis and Apoptotic Pathways Targeted Cancer Therapeutics. *Adv. Pharm. Bull.* **2019**, *9*, 205–218. [CrossRef] [PubMed]
53. Shen, M.; Hu, Y.; Yang, Y.; Wang, L.; Yang, X.; Wang, B.; Huang, M. Betulinic Acid Induces ROS-Dependent Apoptosis and S-Phase Arrest by Inhibiting the NF-κB Pathway in Human Multiple Myeloma. *Oxid. Med. Cell. Longev.* **2019**, *2019*, 5083158. [CrossRef] [PubMed]
54. Khan, A.A.; Alanazi, A.M.; Jabeen, M.; Chauhan, A.; Abdelhameed, A.S. Design, Synthesis and in Vitro Anticancer Evaluation of a Stearic Acid-Based Ester Conjugate. *Anticancer Res.* **2013**, *33*, 2517–2524. [PubMed]
55. Nakkarach, A.; Foo, H.L.; Song, A.A.-L.; Mutalib, N.E.A.; Nitisinprasert, S.; Withayagiat, U. Anti-Cancer and Anti-Inflammatory Effects Elicited by Short Chain Fatty Acids Produced by Escherichia Coli Isolated from Healthy Human Gut Microbiota. *Microb. Cell Fact.* **2021**, *20*, 36. [CrossRef] [PubMed]
56. Salomone, B.; Ponti, R.; Gasco, M.R.; Ugazio, E.; Quaglino, P.; Osella-Abate, S.; Bernengo, M.G. In Vitro Effects of Cholesteryl Butyrate Solid Lipid Nanospheres as a Butyric Acid Pro-Drug on Melanoma Cells: Evaluation of Antiproliferative Activity and Apoptosis Induction. *Clin. Exp. Metastasis* **2000**, *18*, 663–673. [CrossRef] [PubMed]
57. Quagliariello, V.; Masarone, M.; Armenia, E.; Giudice, A.; Barbarisi, M.; Caraglia, M.; Barbarisi, A.; Persico, M. Chitosan-Coated Liposomes Loaded with Butyric Acid Demonstrate Anticancer and Anti-Inflammatory Activity in Human Hepatoma HepG2 Cells. *Oncol. Rep.* **2019**, *41*, 1476–1486. [CrossRef] [PubMed]
58. Pisha, E.; Chai, H.; Lee, I.-S.; Chagwedera, T.E.; Farnsworth, N.R.; Cordell, G.A.; Beecher, C.W.W.; Fong, H.H.S.; Kinghorn, A.D.; Brown, D.M.; et al. Discovery of Betulinic Acid as a Selective Inhibitor of Human Melanoma That Functions by Induction of Apoptosis. *Nat. Med.* **1995**, *1*, 1046–1051. [CrossRef]
59. Guo, Y.; Zhu, H.; Weng, M.; Wang, C.; Sun, L. Chemopreventive Effect of Betulinic Acid via MTOR -Caspases/Bcl2/Bax Apoptotic Signaling in Pancreatic Cancer. *BMC Complement. Med. Ther.* **2020**, *20*, 178. [CrossRef]
60. Rzeski, W.; Stepulak, A.; Szymański, M.; Sifringer, M.; Kaczor, J.; Wejksza, K.; Zdzisińska, B.; Kandefer-Szerszeń, M. Betulinic Acid Decreases Expression of Bcl-2 and Cyclin D1, Inhibits Proliferation, Migration and Induces Apoptosis in Cancer Cells. *Naunyn. Schmiedebergs. Arch. Pharmacol.* **2006**, *374*, 11–20. [CrossRef]
61. Khan, I.; Guru, S.K.; Rath, S.K.; Chinthakindi, P.K.; Singh, B.; Koul, S.; Bhushan, S.; Sangwan, P.L. A Novel Triazole Derivative of Betulinic Acid Induces Extrinsic and Intrinsic Apoptosis in Human Leukemia HL-60 Cells. *Eur. J. Med. Chem.* **2016**, *108*, 104–116. [CrossRef] [PubMed]
62. Mioc, M.; Mioc, A.; Racoviceanu, R.; Ghiulai, R.; Prodea, A.; Milan, A.; Barbu Tudoran, L.; Oprean, C.; Ivan, V.; Șoica, C. The Antimelanoma Biological Assessment of Triterpenic Acid Functionalized Gold Nanoparticles. *Molecules* **2023**, *28*, 421. [CrossRef] [PubMed]

63. Nistor, G.; Mioc, A.; Mioc, M.; Balan-Porcarasu, M.; Ghiulai, R.; Racoviceanu, R.; Avram, Ș.; Prodea, A.; Semenescu, A.; Milan, A.; et al. Novel Semisynthetic Betulinic Acid−Triazole Hybrids with In Vitro Antiproliferative Potential. *Processes* **2022**, *11*, 101. [CrossRef]
64. Kazakova, O.; Șoica, C.; Babaev, M.; Petrova, A.; Khusnutdinova, E.; Poptsov, A.; Macașoi, I.; Drăghici, G.; Avram, Ș.; Vlaia, L. 3-Pyridinylidene Derivatives of Chemically Modified Lupane and Ursane Triterpenes as Promising Anticancer Agents by Targeting Apoptosis. *Int. J. Mol. Sci.* **2021**, *22*, 10695. [CrossRef] [PubMed]
65. Saha, S.; Ghosh, M.; Dutta, S.K. A Potent Tumoricidal Co-Drug 'Bet-CA'—an Ester Derivative of Betulinic Acid and Dichloroacetate Selectively and Synergistically Kills Cancer Cells. *Sci. Rep.* **2015**, *5*, 7762. [CrossRef] [PubMed]
66. Drag-Zalesinska, M.; Kulbacka, J.; Saczko, J.; Wysocka, T.; Zabel, M.; Surowiak, P.; Drag, M. Esters of Betulin and Betulinic Acid with Amino Acids Have Improved Water Solubility and Are Selectively Cytotoxic toward Cancer Cells. *Bioorg. Med. Chem. Lett.* **2009**, *19*, 4814–4817. [CrossRef] [PubMed]
67. Bobadilla, A.V.P.; Arévalo, J.; Sarró, E.; Byrne, H.M.; Maini, P.K.; Carraro, T.; Balocco, S.; Meseguer, A.; Alarcón, T. In Vitro Cell Migration Quantification Method for Scratch Assays. *J. R. Soc. Interface* **2019**, *16*, 20180709. [CrossRef]
68. Ghițu, A.; Pavel, I.Z.; Avram, S.; Kis, B.; Minda, D.; Dehelean, C.A.; Buda, V.; Folescu, R.; Danciu, C. An In Vitro-In Vivo Evaluation of the Antiproliferative and Antiangiogenic Effect of Flavone Apigenin against SK-MEL-24 Human Melanoma Cell Line. *Anal. Cell. Pathol.* **2021**, *2021*, 5552664. [CrossRef]
69. Polacheck, W.J.; Zervantonakis, I.K.; Kamm, R.D. Tumor Cell Migration in Complex Microenvironments. *Cell. Mol. Life Sci.* **2013**, *70*, 1335–1356. [CrossRef]
70. Bache, M.; Zschornak, M.P.; Passin, S.; Keßler, J.; Wichmann, H.; Kappler, M.; Paschke, R.; Kaluđerović, G.N.; Kommera, H.; Taubert, H.; et al. Increased Betulinic Acid Induced Cytotoxicity and Radiosensitivity in Glioma Cells under Hypoxic Conditions. *Radiat. Oncol.* **2011**, *6*, 111. [CrossRef]
71. Wang, H.; Wang, H.; Ge, L.; Zhao, Y.; Zhu, K.; Chen, Z.; Wu, Q.; Xin, Y.; Guo, J. Betulinic Acid Targets Drug-Resistant Human Gastric Cancer Cells by Inducing Autophagic Cell Death, Suppresses Cell Migration and Invasion, and Modulates the ERK/MEK Signaling Pathway. *Acta Biochim. Pol.* **2021**, *69*, 25–30. [CrossRef]
72. El-Desouky, S.K. A Cytotoxic Lupeol Fatty Acid Ester and Other Pentacyclic Triterpenes from Salvadora Persica Seeds. *Nat. Prod. Sci.* **2023**, *29*, 121–126. [CrossRef]
73. Nunez, C.V.; de Vasconcellos, M.C.; Alaniz, L. Editorial: Are Natural Products, Used as Antitumoral/Antiangiogenic Agents, Less Toxic than Synthetic Conventional Chemotherapy? *Front. Pharmacol.* **2022**, *13*, 1055516. [CrossRef]
74. Zhou, M.; Zhang, R.-H.; Wang, M.; Xu, G.-B.; Liao, S.-G. Prodrugs of Triterpenoids and Their Derivatives. *Eur. J. Med. Chem.* **2017**, *131*, 222–236. [CrossRef]
75. Moacă, E.A.; Pavel, I.Z.; Danciu, C.; Crăiniceanu, Z.; Minda, D.; Ardelean, F.; Antal, D.S.; Ghiulai, R.; Cioca, A.; Derban, M.; et al. Romanian Wormwood (*Artemisia Absinthium* L.): Physicochemical and Nutraceutical Screening. *Molecules* **2019**, *24*, 3087. [CrossRef] [PubMed]
76. Assay Procedure. Available online: https://www.abcam.com/en-tr/products/elisa-kits/human-bcl-2-elisa-kit-ab119506 (accessed on 30 January 2024).

Disclaimer/Publisher's Note: The statements, opinions and data contained in all publications are solely those of the individual author(s) and contributor(s) and not of MDPI and/or the editor(s). MDPI and/or the editor(s) disclaim responsibility for any injury to people or property resulting from any ideas, methods, instructions or products referred to in the content.